# Acclaim for the Previous Editions

'**A remarkably useful reference book**... a boon to all lay people who are virtual, hostages in the hands of doctors today.

*The Times of India*

**Very useful... provides the reader with knowledge about the how, the why, and the when of common drugs.** Designed as a family guide, it answers questions relating to the right use of drugs routinely prescribed by doctors. By incorporating the likely adverse effects and the necessary precautions, the authors have made the book very useful because the practitioners of today seldom have time to explain these points to their patients.

*The Tribune*

The authors have done a good job.

*Economic Times*

**Readable and informative**... aims to make the consumer more aware of what they consume at high costs... the book's purpose is to facilitate effective and non-hazardous drug usage...

*Health for the Millions*

**Amazing** that in this a small book, the authors have been able to condense more information than most medical practitioners seem to know.

*Prof Yash Pal, Former Chairman, UGC*

Contains valuable information... For ready reference, this volume is a welcome addition to the family shelf.

*Bhavan's Journal*

The authors need to be congratulated.

*National Herald*

A mine of information... the learned authors have done a yeoman service.

*Caravan*

Describes a number of common drugs prescribed for a host of afflictions from coughs and colds to stomach disorders, allergies, asthma, diabetes, blood pressure, anxiety, and insomnia amongst others. **It lists the generic and brand names, dosages, and known adverse effects... offering the reader necessary knowledge of modern medicine and facilitating non-hazardous drug usage.**'

*Femina*

# The Authors

**P C DANDIYA**

*MPharm, MSc, PhD (Toronto), FAMS*

Dr. P.C. Dandiya, is Emeritus Professor of Pharmacology at S.M.S. Medical College, Jaipur, and is the former President of the Pharmacy Council of India, Indian Pharmaceutical Congress, and the Indian Pharmacology Society. For his significant research contributions to Pharmacology he was awarded the S.Amir Chand Prize by the Indian Council of Medical Research and the Hari Om Ashram Award by the Medical Council of India. He is a fellow of the National Academy of Medical Sciences with 180 research papers and 14 books to his credit.

Dr. Dandiya has been a Visiting Professor to the Universities of London, Hawaii, Houston, Stanford, Toronto, and Copenhagen. Presently, he is also a de-facto visiting Professor at the Nanjing University in China. He was also the Pro-Vice Chancellor (Rector) of the Banaras Hindu University.

**J S BAPNA**

*MD, Phd, FAMS*

Dr. Jawahar S. Bapna is Adjunct Professor at Institute of Health Management Research, Jaipur. He has been the Director, Institute of Human Behaviour and Allied Sciences, Medical Superintendent of Guru Tegh Bahadur Hospital, New Delhi; Director-Professor and Head of the Department of Pharmacology, Maulana Azad Medical College, New Delhi and Jawaharlal Institute of Postgraduate Medical Education and Research, Pondicherry. He is a fellow of the International College of Neuro-psychopharmacology and has been the President of the Indian Pharmacological Society. He is a recipient of the Shri Amrit Mody Research Foundation Award and B Uvnas prize of the Indian Pharmacological Society. He has been an advisor to WHO, MSH and The Futures Group International, Danida. He has developed the Medicines Policy of Jharkhand, Uttranchal and Himachal Pradesh. He has contributed to the *Guide to Good Prescribing,* the best-selling book of WHO, published in 8 languages.

**GURUDAS KHILNANI**

*MD (Medicine), MD (Pharmacology), DHRM*

Dr. Gurudas Khilnani, is Professor and Head of the Department of Pharmacology, RNT Medical College, Udaipur. He is a founder fellow of the Indian Society of Cardiology. He had authored three books and has over 40 research publications to his credit. He is a resource person for International Course on 'Promoting Rational Drug Use in the Community' of WHO. He is a member of the Executive Committee of Indian Pharmacological Society, Rajasthan Medical Council and The Rajasthan Society for the Promotion of Rational Use of Drugs.

Revised
**10th Edition**
*Enlarged*

# THE COMPLETE FAMILY MEDICINE BOOK

Dr P C Dandiya
Dr J S Bapna
Dr G Khilnani

Orient Paperbacks
DELHI | MUMBAI | HYDERABAD

**Disclaimer**

**The information included in this book is general in nature and for reference and guidance only. It is not a substitute for medical advice and the readers are urged to consult their doctor before taking decisions which are medical in nature.**



**How to Order**

This book is also available on special quantity discounts from the publisher Orient Paperbacks, 5A/8 Ansari Road, Darya Ganj, New Delhi-110 002. Tel: (011) 2327 8877, Fax: (011) 2327 8879 email: mail@orientpaperbacks.com. On your business letterhead, kindly include information concerning the intended use of the books and the number of copies you wish to purchase.

www.orientpaperbacks.com

ISBN 13: 978-81-222-0482-7
ISBN 10: 81-222-0482-1

1st Published 1979
2nd Edition 1981
3rd Edition 1983
4th Edition 1987
5th Revised & Enlarged Edition 1991
6th Revised & Enlarged Edition 1995
7th Revised & Enlarged Edition 1997
8th Revised, Enlarged & Updated Edition 1999
9th Revised, Enlarged & Updated Edition 2005
10th Revised, Enlarged & Updated Edition 2010
Reprinted 2011

*The Complete Family Medicine Book*



Published by
**Orient Paperbacks**
(A division of Vision Books Pvt. Ltd.)
5A/8 Ansari Road, New Delhi-110 002

Printed in India at
Ravindra Printing Press, Delhi-110 006

# Preface

Since the first edition of this book was published in 1979, there have been remarkable changes and developments in the science of drugs: the general awareness about drugs has increased by leaps and bounds; new properties and knowledge about the mechanism of action of drugs have come to light; problems faced by the patient due to irrational combinations or unsuitability have become less frequent but drug-drug or drug-food interactions continue to cause avoidable side-effects; and drug laws (relating to prescription and distribution) have become stricter although their enforcement remains weak.

From the first edition of this book to the current tenth edition (about 30 years later), the readers have maintained a steady interaction with us through queries, doubts, suggestions and other feedback. In response, a concerted effort has been made to revise and expand information and to incorporate knowledge and developments in hitherto unexplored areas. 'Drug Abuse' and 'Sexually Transmitted Disease and AIDS', were added in the sixth edition in view of the alarmingly high increase of incidence in them and the urgent need for informed caution. A growing resurgence of interest in the ancient systems of Ayurveda and Unani Tibb prompted us to include a chapter on 'Commonly Used Ayurvedic and Unani Drugs'. With longevity on the increase, a new chapter on 'Drug Treatment in the Elderly' was added to the seventh edition. Queries about storage and administration of drugs were answered through an additional chapter on 'Medicines: Their Safe and Correct Usage.'

In thc ninth edition, three new chapters i.e. 'Drug Treatment in Osteoporosis', 'Treatment of Common Gynecological Ailments' and 'Antioxidants and Phytonutrients' were added while two chapters one on 'Digestive Enzymes' and on 'Ear Pain' were deleted. In the present edition, two chapters i.e. 'Exercise and You' and 'Routine Medical Exams' have been added in view of greater awareness in public on 'Live Healthier and Longer' concept of life. Besides, every chapter has been thoroughly revised, pruned and updated in view of the fast developments that have taken place in this period.

We would welcome suggestions from readers for future editions. You may send your feedback to the address given on the last page of the book.

# How to Use This Book

The book provides useful information about medicines employed in the treatment of various diseases and their symptoms. If you know the disease you will find out initial information about the medicines used for its treatment. To locate the chapter, consult the Contents or the Index of Diseases. This chapter will help you to become familiar with the concerned drugs, their doses and adverse effects, and also the precautions to be observed, both for treatment of the disease and to minimize the adverse effects. In general, the drugs or groups of drugs are arranged in the order of their importance.

A drug basically has two different names: 1) generic (chemical) name; and 2) proprietary or brand (trade) name, by which it is prescribed and sold. A drug usually has only one generic name but may be available under different trade names, each given by a different manufacturer. The Index of Medicines provides the generic and brand names of most commonly used drugs. *Whenever you buy a drug prescribed by your doctor, go through its contents, ingredients given in generic names on the container. Once you know the ingredients of the drug and its generic name, look up the Index to back the page numbers giving detailed information on the drug.*

In the text, the technical terms and generic names of the drugs are given in italics and brand names in small capital letters. In selecting one or two of the brand names out of the many available, we have, in general, taken the original manufacturer's or the most popular brands available in India.

Some drugs are sold by their generic names and in these cases no brand names are given. Usually, the name of a drug is followed by its detailed description, except at some places where all drugs used for a particular type of ailment are given in a table.

You may also consult Appendix 1 for understanding some common abbreviations used by doctors while writing a prescription, and Appendix 2 for some important normal values of the body's constituents or tests.

# Introduction

'Doctors needlessly endanger the lives of their patients by excessive and wrongful use of drugs. More and more people are falling prey to iatrogenesis (doctor-inflicted illness).'

—*R.H. Dastur, Veteran Physician*

In spite of the increasing dependence on modern drugs, the consumer or the patient remains starved for information. There is little time for a doctor-patient dialogue; doctors usually have little or no time to spend with each patient. Moreover, the patient often holds the doctor in such awe that he thinks twice before questioning his judgement. The resulting information gap often precipitates problems arising from errors in the frequency and duration of dosage, from the interaction of one drug with another, or of certain drugs with food, and many other such misadventures.

The resources available to refresh a doctor's knowledge of drugs, whether old or new, are not easily accessible. The most common 'educator' is a representative of the pharmaceutical company, who aided by chic appearance and a handful of samples, convinces the doctor of the wonders of his company's new pills. Subsequent to the visit of the pharma rep the first patient the doctor examines may be obliged to buy the new pills, no matter how worthless these be. Unlike other consumer goods, where the buyer is the chooser, in medicines, the patient buys them, but the choice is made by his doctor, and an erring doctor can be a big liability.

The wise old physician, Hippocrates, rightly said, 'For the sick the least is the best.' In contrast, the motto of modern medicine seems to be 'The most is the best.' It is common knowledge that in the present system of health care not only are too many drugs prescribed at one time, but also too often. Infact indiscriminate use of several life-saving and potent antibiotics has finally relegated them to the status of the 'not-so-effective' ones. We are therefore faced with the situation of needing newer and stronger antibiotics for infections which earlier responded to the so labelled 'not so effective' antibiotics. The newer generation of antibiotics are not only more toxic but also more expensive. These too, if used indiscriminately, may lose their effectiveness, and in time, even more potent agents maybe needed, perhaps even more toxic and expensive. How long this cycle will last is anybody's guess. With medicines, discretion is more important than adventurism. To use discretion one has to be knowledgeable. How many doctors instruct their patients not to take milk with *tetracycline,* the most important precaution with this class of drugs? (given with milk they may be as ineffective as chalk powder.)

The knowledge gap about drugs goes against the long-term interest of the individual, his family, and the community. In the enlightened world we live in it is essential that every individual knows the *how, why* and *when* of drugs that he and his family are likely to use some day. The purpose of this book is to facilitate effective and non-hazardous drug usage.

We would like to emphasize that this book is not intended to promote self-medication. In fact, the information available in it should act to discourage indiscriminate use of drugs resulting from lack of guidance on the one hand, and powerful commercial interests of pharmaceutical companies on the other. Knowledge, rather than ignorance, is more crucial to one's well-being, particularly, in the effective and safe use of drugs. Today the same drug is sold under a variety of trade names. A patient seldom discovers whether a doctor or doctors prescribing the medicine are prescribing the same drug or a different one. In all fairness he should know this.

Many potentially dangerous drugs, which are supposed to be given only on prescription are available freely at most chemist shops in India. In addition, a large number of drug combinations containing two, or more drugs in one preparation are sold in the market. Some are useful, while others are not only less useful, but highly toxic and more expensive. This adds to the cost of the treatment and the risk to health. The book attempts to inform the patient and the doctor on these.

This book has been designed as a family guide on medicines. It attempts to answer many questions in the mind of the patient and his family, and describes almost all the drugs used for common disorders, their correct use, and the need for medical advice. It will be of particular interest to housewives, chronic patients, and as they say, 'heads of families'. Doctors, pharmacist, and nurses may also find it very valuable. The book establishes that expensive drugs are not necessarily better drugs. With knowledge, understanding, and discretion, significant economy can also be affected in medical treatment.

*P.C. Dandiya*
*J.S. Bapna*
*G. Khilnani*

February 2010

# Contents

*Preface*
*How to Use This Book*
*Introduction*

1. **Drugs Used in Abdominal Pain** ... **13**
Anti-Spasmodic drugs • Other Drugs

2. **Drugs Used in Allergy** ... **16**
Specific Treatment • Symptomatic Treatment • Decongestants and Antihistaminics

3. **Drugs Used in Amoebiasis and Other Protozoal Infections** ... **20**
Intestinal Amoebiasis • Extra-Intestinal Amoebiasis • Giardiasis • Trichomoniasis

4. **Drugs Used in Anxiety** ... **24**
Anxiety Disorders • Phobia

**Drugs Used in Asthma**
(*See* Drugs Used in Bronchial Asthma)

5. **Drugs that Reduce Blood Lipid (Fat) Levels** ... **28**

6. **Drugs Enhancing Functional Capacity of the Brain** ... **32**
Stimulating Mental Activity • Stimulating Mental and Physical Activity • Cerebral Activators (Cognition Enhancers) • Alzheimer's Disease

7. **Drugs Used in Bronchial Asthma** ... **36**
Specific Treatment • Symptomatic Treatment • Chronic Asthma

**Drugs Used to Lower Cholesterol Level**
(*See* Drugs that Reduce Blood Lipid Levels)

8. **Drugs Used in Constipation** ... 42
Mild Purgatives • Strong Purgatives (Stimulant Purgatives) • Prokinetic Drugs

9. **Drugs Used in Cough** ... 48
Expectorants • Cough Sedatives and Suppressant

10. **Drugs Used in Diabetes** ... 54

11. **Drugs Used in Diarrhoea** ... 65
Anti-motility drugs • Infective Diarrhoea • Severe Diarrhoea • Irritable Bowel Syndrome • Ulcerative Colitis • Irritable Bowel Syndrome

12. **Drugs Used in Epileptic Disorders** ... 70
Grand mal (Tonic-Clonic) Seizures • Petit mal (Minor) Epilepsy • Proper Use of Drugs

13. **Drugs Used in Common Eye Diseases** ... 75
Eye Infections • Cataract • Dry Eyes • Glaucoma • Injuries • Role of Vitamin A

14. **Treatment of Common Gynaecological Ailments** ... 79
Vaginal Discharge • Dysmenorrhoea (Painful Menstruation) • Pelvic Pain • Premenstrual Syndrome • Menorrhagia (Excessive menstruation) • Scanty Menstruation • Menopause • Urinary Stress Incontinence

15. **Drugs Used in Disorders of the Heart** ... 84
Angina Pectoris • Unstable Angina • Myocardial Infarction

16. **Drugs Used in Heart Failure** ... 93
Increasing Contractility of the Heart • Controlling Sodium and Water Retention • Providing Long Term Benefits in CHF

17. **Drugs to Treat High Blood Pressure** ... 97
Treatment • Drugs • Factors Influencing Treatment of Hypertension

**Drugs Used in Insomnia**
(*See* Drugs Used for Overcoming Sleeplessness)

18. **Drugs Used in Disorders of the Joints** ... 109
Arthritis • Pain-relieving anti-inflammatory Drugs • Gout (*See also* Drugs Used in Osteoporosis)

19. **Drugs Used in Malaria** ... 114

20. **Drugs Used in Mental Depression** ... 118
(*See also* Drugs Used in Anxiety)

21. **Drugs Used in Major Mental Illnesses** ... 122
Serious Mental Disorders • Mania/Manic Depressive Illness

22. **Drugs Used in Migraine** ... 127
Acute Attack • Prevention of Future Attacks

23. **Drugs that Prevent Nausea and Vomiting** ... 132
Symptomatic Treatment • Nausea and Vomiting during Pregnancy • Motion Sickness

24. **Drugs Used in Osteoporosis** ... 136
(*See also* Drugs Used in Disorders of the Joints)

25. **Pain Relievers** ... 139
Non-narcotic and Narcotic Drugs

26. **Drugs Used in Parkinson's Disease** ... 149
Correcting Deficiency of Dopamine • Correcting Effects of Excess Acetycholine

27. **Drugs Used in Peptic Ulcers** ... 153
Antacids • $H_2$ Receptor Blockers • Anti-Cholinergic Drugs • Drugs Providing Protection to Mucosa • Eradication of H. Pylori Infection in Peptic Ulcer • Reflux Esophagitis

28. **Methods of Preventing Pregnancy** ... 160
Natural Methods • Spacing Methods • Oral Contraceptives • Emergency Contraceptives • Terminal Methods
(*See also* Drugs to be Avoided During Pregnancy and Breast-Feeding)

29. **Drugs Used for Overcoming Sleeplessness** ... 170

30. **Drugs Used in Sexual Inadequacies** ... 173
Erectile Dysfunction • Premature Ejaculation • Diminished Sexual Desire

31. **Sexually Transmitted Diseases and AIDS** ... 179
AIDS • Gonorrhoea • Syphilis

32. **Drugs for Treatment of Common Skin Disorders** ... 185
Scabies • Lice Infestation • Acne (Pimples) • Fungal Infections

33. **Drugs Used in Tuberculosis** ... 192
Preventive Therapy • Curative Therapy • First Line Drugs • Second Line Drugs

34. **Drugs Used in Worm Infestations** ... 198
Roundworm • Hookworm • Pinworm

35. **Antibiotics and Antifungal Drugs** ... 203
Anti-bacterial Drugs • New Antibiotics • Cephalosporin • Fluoroquinolones • Antifungal Drugs

36. **Antioxidants and Phytonutrients** ... 213

37. **Commonly Used Ayurvedic and Unani Drugs** ... 217
AIDS • Arthritis • Cancer • Diabetes • Heart Diseases • Hypertension • Respiratory Diseases • Liver Diseases • Skin Diseases • Tooth and Gum Paints • Anti-anxiety and anti-depressants • Memory-improving Drugs • Nerve Tonics • Miscellaneous

38. **Corticosteroids** ... 222
Arthritis • Rheumatic Heart Diseases • Allergic Diseases • Bronchial Asthma • Diseases of Eye • Skin Diseases • Shocks • Mineralocorticoid

39. **General Tonics** ... 227

40. **Slimming Drugs** ... 236
Drugs that Make You Feel Full • Drugs Acting on the Feeding Centre of the Brain

41. **Drug Abuse** ... 240

42. **Alcohol** ... 244
Chronic Alcoholism • Methyl Alcohol Poisoning

43. **Drugs and Your Child** ... 249
Immunization Schedule • Special Vaccines • Drugs Used in Diseases of Neonates & Children • Drugs to be Used with Caution

44. **Drug Treatment in the Elderly** ... 252

45. **Drugs to be Avoided During Pregnancy and Breast-Feeding** ... 255

46. **Smoking and Effects of Drugs** ... 260
Drug Interaction due to Smoking

47. **Medicines: Their Safe and Correct Usage** ... 263

48. **Exercise and You** ... 270

49. **Preventive Check-ups for a Healthy Body** ... 274

Appendix 1
*Abbreviations Commonly Used in Prescriptions* ... 277

Appendix 2
*Laboratory Tests* ... 278

Index of Diseases ... 280

Index of Medicines ... 281

1

# Drugs Used in Abdominal Pain

• • • • • •

Abdominal pain, one of the most frequently occurring symptoms, may originate from any organ in the abdomen, like the stomach, intestine, appendix, gall-bladder, pancreas, and kidneys. Therefore, any patient of abdominal pain of recent onset requires early and thorough evaluation for an accurate diagnosis. However, the commonest source of abdominal pain in the region of the stomach and intestines is the gastro-intestinal tract which consists of the stomach and intestines because it deals with outside material, that is, the food and drink we take. A little overeating may cause distension and indigestion. A spicy meal may lead to an increase in acid secretion and sour eructations. In these conditions some digestives or antacids are taken for relief. Very often flatulence, diarrhoea, dysentery, or an infection produces spasms of the walls of intestines, causing a griping type of pain called colic. This is a distressing situation, and suitable measures for immediate relief are necessary.

Various household remedies like massage, hot water fomentation, *churan, ajwain, jaljeera* and *pepper mint oil* but their success is usually limited. Therefore, the patient takes one of the preparations (mentioned in the table given later) which provides immediate relief. What is so special about these preparations that they provide such dramatic relief ? If you look at the table, you will find that all the preparations contain an anti-spasmodic (which prevents spasms of the smooth muscle of the intestine) which relieves colicky pain. However, if it is frequent or of a constant nature, the physician must be consulted. Under such circumstances continued and prolonged use of these drugs, instead of improving the condition, may produce serious adverse effects. Since an anti-spasmodic is the most common ingredient of all these preparations, we will elaborate a little on it.

### Anti-spasmodic Drugs

These are *atropine* or its synthetic substitutes (anti-cholinergic drugs) and are used for relieving the spasm of the muscles of the intestine. The action of almost all anti-cholinergic drugs is more or less the same. There are only slight differences in their potency or duration of action. The adverse effects caused and precautions to be observed with anti-cholinergic drugs have been discussed in the chapter on Drugs in Peptic Ulcers.

**Some Drugs and their Combinations for the Treatment of Intestinal Colic (Anticholinergic Drugs)**

| *Preparations (Brand Names)* | *Anti-spasmodic (Smooth Muscle Relaxant)* | *Analgesic (Pain Reliever)* | *Sedative (Causing Drowsiness)* | Others |
|---|---|---|---|---|
| ANTRENYL | *Oxyphenonium Br.* | — | — | — |
| BUSCOPAN (Tab/inj) | *Hyocine-N+ Butylbromide* | — | — | — |
| CATASPA | *Dicyclomine* | *Diclofenac* | — | — |
| CLOMIN | *Dicyclomine- HCl* | *Paracetamol* | — | — |
| CYCLOPAM (Tab/inj) | *Dicyclomine- HCl* | *Paracetamol* | — | — |
| COLIMEX | *Dicyclomine- HCl* | *Paracetamol* | — | — |
| DYSMEN | *Dicyclomine* | *Mefenamic acid* | — | — |
| MEFTAL-SPAS | *Dicyclomine- HCl* | *Mefenamic acid* | — | — |
| SPASMINDON | *Dicyclomine- HCl* | *Ethylmorphine* | — | — |
| SPASMO-PROXYVON | *Dicyclomine- HCl* | *Paracetamol Dextropropoxyphene* | — | — |
| NORMAXIN | *Clidinium Br. Dicyclomine- HCl* | — | *Chlordiazepoxide* | — |
| PIPEN Drops | *Pipenzolate* | — | — | *Activated Methylpoly-siloxane* |
| STELABID | *Isopropamide* | — | *Trifluoperazine* | — |
| NIM-SPAS CYCLOZOBID | *Dicyclomine* | *Nimesulide* | — | — |
| LIBRAX | *Clidinum* | — | *Chlordiazepoxide* | — |
| EPIDOSIN | *Valethomate* | — | — | — |

## Other Anti-spasmodics

*Dicyclomine* (COLIMEX COLINOL, CYCLOPAM 10 mg tab, 10 mg/ml-2ml inj. for IM ) is the most commonly used antispamodic agent found to be safer in usual doses of 10-20 mg thrice a day. It also prevents vomiting associated with colicky pain.

There are many preparations in which it is combined with *mefenamic acid* (MEFTAL SPAS for dysmenorrhea), *diclofenac* (DICLOSPAS for severe pain), *d-propoxyphene* (PARVON-SPAS for severe colicky pain), *nimesulide* (NIMSPAS) and *paracetamol* (COLIVAN-D). A combination of *clidinium* 2.5 mg with *paracetamol* (NORMOSPAS) is also available.These combinations are not superior and their use is irrational.

### **Drotavarine** (DROTIN, TROSPA 40 mg, 80 mg tab, 20 mg inj.)

It relieves colicky pain of gall-bladder, kidney and urinary passage and dysmenorrhoea (pain before and during menstruation). It relaxes smooth muscle directly and has no anticholinergic adverse effects. It is also used/prescribed with *mefenamic acid* (DROTIN PLUS) and *nimesulide* (NOBEL SPAS).

### **Fenoverine** (SPASMOPRIL)

This drug regulates the irregular movements in spasmodic conditions. It is used in post meal distension and pain. It is given in a dose of 100 mg, twice a day. It is useful in irritable bowel syndrome also.

**Tolterdine** (FLOCHEK, TOLTER 2 mg, 4 mg tab): It is useful to check urinary dribbling and incontinence in elderly due to a variety of causes in a usual dose of 2 mg twice a day. It should be avoided in enlarged prostate because it may precipitate retention of urine. It should also be avoided in glaucoma and ulceratine colitis.

**Mebeverine** (COLOSPA 135 mg)

It is like *fenoverine* but may cause constipation, dizziness and headache. It is prescribed for irritable bowel syndrome.

**Valethemate** (EPIDOSIN inj.)

It is commonly used in gynaecology to facilitate labour and is effective in relieving ureteric and bile duct colics.

Antispamodics for urinary bladder irritation and neurogenic bladder:

*Oxybutynin* (NOCTURIN, CYSTRAN 2.5 mg, TROPAN 5.0 mg) twice a day.

*Flavoxate* (URISPAS, URIKIND 200 mg) thrice a day

*Tolterodine* (DETRUSITOL, FLOCHEK 2 mg )

*Phenazopyridine* with *nitrofurantoin* (NEPHROGESIC)

*Phenazopyridine* (PYRIDIUM) 200 mg thrice a day.

**Combination Drugs**

A number of preparations provide a pain reliever with an antispasmodic drug. It is an example of shot-gun treatment and these combinations are not rational. At times peptic ulcer pain may resemble colicky pain (or an ulcer without symptoms) that may be aggravated by unnecessary use of pain relieving drug combinations. You should feel free to ask your doctor to prescribe you a safe drug.

# 2

# Drugs Used in Allergy

• • • • • •

The word 'allergic' is often used loosely and has become almost a part of our general conversation. In a way it has become synonymous with 'dislike'. Many ailments which cannot be immediately diagnosed are incorrectly attributed to allergy. Allergy is an unusual response of the body caused by substances like foods, pollens, house dust, feathers, fungus, insecticides, drugs, and chronic infection.

The common allergic diseases are allergic rhinitis and hay fever and the most common cause is pollen. Although we are all exposed to pollens, why do only a few of us suffer from allergy? Allergy is due to abnormal antibodies of the *IgE* type which are formed only in some susceptible individuals. Normally the antibodies are supposed to be protective. But the abnormal antibodies are fixed on special allergic cells called mast cells and on coming into contact with an allergen such as a pollen, release chemical agents such as histamine, serotonin, and slow-reacting substances. The release of these substances produce symptoms of allergy characterized by a running nose, itching, rash, and breathing difficulty.

## Treatment

The management of allergic reactions includes specific treatment aimed at removing the cause, blocking the effect of allergic reaction by immuno-therapy as well as symptomatic treatment. Some examples of allergen-avoidance are stopping use of such drugs, installation of air filters in air conditioners, keeping pets out of living room and removing dust collecting furniture and carpets.

## Specific Treatment

Specific treatment consists of removal of the offending agents. This is done by 'allergen testing'. Various extracts of possible offending agents are available and these are injected into the skin to detect the causative agent. However, in most cases it is difficult to identify the causative agent, but if it is found, desensitization of the individual can be carried out by injecting its doses. It has been found that through desensitization, the abnormal antibodies, that is, the *IgE* antibodies, are reduced or completely abolished and protective antibodies, that is, the IgG anibodies are developed.

## Symptomatic Treatment

The aim of symptomatic treatment is to check the release or antagonize the action of released chemical mediators of allergic reactions. The most important of these chemical mediators is believed to be histamine. For this reason antihistaminics are employed in almost all cases of allergy. Sometimes decongestants are combined with antihistaminics to enhance effects. Only in extremely severe cases are *corticosteroids* used (see chapter on 'Corticosteroids').

**Some Antihistaminics Drugs and their Sedative Properties**

| *Less Sedative* | *Moderately Sedatvive* | *Markedly Sedative* | *Newer Non-sedative* |
|---|---|---|---|
| Chlorpheniramine (ZEET) | Buclizine (LONGIFENE) | Dimenhydrinate (DRAMAMINE) | Fexofenadine (FEXO, ALLEGRA) |
| Clemastine (TOVEGYL) | Cinnarizine (STUGERON) | Diphenhydramine (BENADRYL) | Azelastine (AZEP nasal drops) |
| Cyclizine (MAREZINE) | Cyproheptadine (PERIACTIN) | Hydroxyzine (ATARAX) | Cetirizine (CETZINE) Levocetirizine (LEVOCET, TECZINE) |
| Dimethindine (FORISTAL) | Mebrophenhydramine (MEBRYL) Meclizine (DILIGAN) | Promethazine (PHENERGAN) | Ebastine (EBAST) Rupatadine (RUPAL,RALZAL, RUPIZ,RULIF) |
| Mebhydroline (INCIDAL) | Pheniramine (AVIL) | | Loratidine Desloratidine (DESLOR, LORFAST) |
| Methdilazine (DILOSYN) | | | Terfenadine* (TERFED) |

*withdrawn in many countries

### Uses of Antihistaminics

Besides their use in allergy, antihistaminics are useful for prevention and treatment of motion (travel) sickness and vomiting during pregnancy or following radiation. They are beneficial in the symptomatic treatment of Parkinsonism but ineffective in bronchial asthma. They are quite often used to treat common cold. In this condition anti-cholinergic effects of these drugs afford symptomatic relief by decreasing secretions of nose and respiratory passages.

***Adverse Effects:*** The most common adverse effects are drowsiness and sedation (except in nonsedative antihistaminics) which interfere with daytime activity, mental alertness, and reflex actions. Other side-effects include giddiness, ringing in the ears, weariness, fatigue, loss of appetite, nausea, vomiting, rapid pulse, fall in BP, constipation, abdominal pain, dryness of mouth, urinary hasitancy and blurring of vision. These adverse effects are more common in elderly people. Very high doses may induce fever.

***Precautions***

1. Avoid alcohol with these drugs as sedation of a dangerous level may occur.
2. Avoid driving and operating any kind of machine after taking these drugs as they cause drowsiness and accidents may occur.
3. If taken after a meal, the intensity of side-effects can be minimized.
4. Ointments containing these drugs should not be used for a prolonged period as allergic reactions have been found to be more common on local application of these drugs.

***Note:*** At times these anti-allergic drugs, when taken orally or more commonly, when applied on the skin, may cause allergic reaction. Is this not a paradox?

## Other Drugs for Symptomatic Treatment

### Hydroxyzine (ATARAX, PRUGO)

It is useful in sleeplessness due to itching (urticaria, dermatitis, eczema), anxiety and during post operative period. Its usual dose is 10-25 mg thrice a day.

### Ketotifen (ASTHAFEN, KETOVENT, KETOTIF)

This drug stabilizes the cell membranes of mast cells and thus prevents the release of histamine. Besides having antihistaminic properties, it is useful in preventing an attack of asthma. It does, however, cause drowsiness, a dry mouth, dizziness, nausea and weight gain.

### Cromolyn Sodium (IFIRAL, FINTAL)

Used as eye drops (2%) in allergic conjunctivitis and nasal spray (2%) in allergic rhinitis.

### Nedocromil

This drug is used 2 puffs, twice a day, in place of *cromolyn.*

Topical steroids like *flunisolide* (SYNTARIS) and *budesonide* (BUDECORT) are nasal spray.

## Non-Sedative Antihistaminics for Symptomatic Treatment

These new generation anti-allergic drugs do not reach the brain and do not produce sedation (*cetirizine* causes some sedation) which is common adverse effect of all the drugs available in this group. Therefore, these are used more often now in comparison to the older drugs described earlier. These drugs do not impair psychomotor activities such as driving and do not enhance effects of alcohol or *diazepam*. They are useful in allergic rhinitis, allergic conjunctivitis, urticaria, drug allergies and atopic eczema. They are not effective in motion sickness, vertigo and should not be used in pregnancy. These agents are less effective than older drugs in common cold.

## Decongestants Used in Symptomatic Treatment

These agents reduce the swelling of mucous membranes (shrinking effect) in allergic diseases by constricting small blood vessels. Some drugs are used by mouth such as *pseudoephedrine* (PSEUDAFED 60 mg tab) and *phenylpropanolamine.* The latter is rarely used alone. Many locally acting nasal decongestants are available. The best is saline (Salt- drops) available as *salin* nasal drops as it is devoid of adverse effects.

## Fixed Dose Combinations*

A number of decongestants are combined with antihistaminic drugs to increase their effects.

| Combinations | Brand Names |
|---|---|
| **Two drug combinations** | |
| *Cetirizine* 10 mg + *pseudoephedrine* 120 mg (long acting) | ALERCET- DC |
| *Cetirizine* 10 mg + *phenylephrine* 5 mg. | CETRIZET-DC, ZYNCET-D(10 mg) |
| *Fexofenadine* 120 mg + *pseudoephedrine* 180 mg. | ATIVA |
| *Loratidine* 5 mg + *pseudoephedrine* 120 mg | ROLETRA-D ,LORFAST-D |
| *Chlorpheniramine* 3 mg + *trithioparamethoxyphenylpropene* 12.5 mg | HEPASULFOL –AA. |
| *Desloratidine* 5 mg + *pseudoephedrine* 120 mg | NEOLORIDINE-D |
| *Levocetirizine* 5 mg + *pseudoephedrine* 120 mg | LAZINE-D, LEVOCET-D |
| *Cetirizine* 5 mg + *Ambroxol* 60 mg | CETZINE-A |
| **Three/ Four drug combinations*** | |
| *Cetirizine + phenlylpropanolamine + paracetamol* | Tab CZ COLD |
| *Chlorpheniramine + Guaicolate + ephedrine + paracetamol* | Tab SUDIN |
| *Pseudoephedrine + Chlorpheniramine + paracetamol* | RINOSTAT |
| *Chlorpheniramine + Dextromethorphan + Pseudoephedrine + Paracetamol* | Tab RESPREN |
| *Chlorpheniramine + Phenylpropanolamine + Paracetamol + Caffeine* | Tab RETHERMA- C |
| *Desloratidine + pseudoephedrine Ambroxol* | NUCOPE-AD |
| *Levocetirizine 5 mg + pseudoephedrine 30 mg + ambroxol 60 mg* | ALDINE-D |

* Third drug is usually paracetamol. One must avoid combinations because of unnecessary use of additional agent in allergic disorder

There are other decongestants which are used as nasal drops in allergic diseases such as allergic rhinitis or (seasonal or perennial). These nasal drops are:

1. *Xylometazoline* (OTRIVIN) 0.1% drops (Adults); 0.05% (Children)
2. *Oxymetazoline* (NASIVION) 0.05% (Adults); 0.025% (Children)
3. *Phenylephrine* (DRISTAN) 0.25% (Adults)
4. *Ephedrine* (ENDRINE) 0.75% (Adults)

***Adverse effects and Precautions:*** Some stinging sensation in the nose and mouth may occur and its regular use should be avoided because loss of smell and atrophic changes in the mucosal surface may occur. The decongestant of nasal drops may be absorbed leading to CNS excitation/ depression and rise in BP. Therefore, these drugs may be used occasionally and to clear blocked nose. After congestion can also occur with some drugs.

**A Word of Caution: Use of Phenylpropanolamine (PPA)**

Parents should not give OTC cough and cold remedies and decongestatnts to babies and toddlers. There is no sufficient evidence to show that such medications are actually safe. There is a risk of overdose toxicity also.A number of cases of strokes were reported from USA with the use of phenylpropanolamine as appetite suppressant. There is also a potential for psychiatric disturbances associated with use. In UK, Canada, Japan warnings have been issued and labels are changed. Its use should be discouraged.

# 3

# Drugs Used in Amoebiasis and other Protozoal Infections

Amoebiasis is a worldwide disease, particularly common in tropical countries and places where public hygiene and sanitation are poor. Amoebic infection is caused by an organism, *Entamoeba histolytica* (EH) which usually spreads through contaminated food and water. Since the causative organism of amoebiasis derives its nutrition from the normal bacterial flora of the large intestine, the latter is the chief site of infection. However, in some cases it may spread to other organs of the body of which the liver is the most susceptible. Based on the site of the infection, the disease has been divided into intestinal and extra-intestinal amoebiasis.

***Symptoms of Amoebic Infection:*** During the acute phase of intestinal amoebiasis the patient may have loose motions with or without mucus and blood, besides griping pain in the abdomen which may be severe at the time of evacuation. In chronic amoebiasis, a patient may complain of a dull pain in the lower abdomen, alternate constipation and diarrhoea, foul smell in the stools, formation of gases, and loss of appetite. Some people with amoebic infection may remain symptom-free or experience little discomfort but they may pass cysts in their stools (cyst passers) and are potential carriers of the disease which spread it to others.

***Extra-intestinal amoebiasis:*** It is usually associated with a previous history of intestinal amoebiasis. When the liver is involved, the patient may have pain in the right upper abdomen, fever, sweating, loss of weight, and anaemia.

***Importance of Diet:*** Success of the treatment of amoebiasis depends on drugs and also on proper diet and good hygiene. For quick recovery it is best to eat a diet rich in proteins and low in roughage and carbohydrates. Use of clean drinking water and avoidance of contamination are also equally important.

## Drugs for Intestinal Amoebiasis

The drugs used in treating amoebiasis can be divided into three categories according to their effectiveness.

**Metronidazole** (FLAGYL, METROGYL, UNIMEZOL)
This is a drug of choice in all forms of amoebiasis except in asymptomatic cyst carriers. Since most of it is absorbed in the intestines, another drug which acts in intestinal amoebiasis should be used along with it to avoid relapse and to eradicate the disease. It is given in a dose of 400-800 mg, 3 times daily, for 10 days.

***Adverse Effects:*** The incidence of adverse effects is low and include nausea, an unpleasant metallic taste in the mouth, a furry tongue, ulcers in the mouth, loss of appetite, distress, and pain in the abdomen. Less often it affects nerves and may, in rare cases, cause convulsions. Depression of the bone marrow may lead to a short lasting fall in white blood cell count. A relapse can occur if the full course is not taken.

***Precautions***

1. Avoid alcohol consumption with this drug as it causes a reaction in which severe vomiting and flushing occurs. Also avoid its use during initial months of pregnancy.
2. A patient suffering from epilepsy or any other nervous system disorder should avoid it.
3. It depresses the bone marrow. White blood cell count must be monitored by those taking the drug repeatedly.

**Tinidazole** (TINAGYL, TRIDAZOLE, TINIBA, TINI)
This is a related drug to *metronidazole* but has the advantage of a longer duration of action, thus reducing the frequency of intake. The duration of treatment is shorter. Its adverse effects and precautions are similar to *metronidazole* but the cure rate is higher. It has a few adverse effects only (metallic taste and nausea). It is given in a dose of 600 mg, twice daily for 5 days, or 2 g, once daily for 3 days.

**Secnidazole**
It is effective in a single dose and as a one-day treatment. The adult dose is 2 g (4 tablets of 500 mg each) taken once only.

**Ornidazole** (DAZOLIC, ORNIDA)
It is like *tinidazole* but less disturbance of taste is reported.

**Satranidazole** (SATROGYL)
It is a longer acting drug and can be taken as a single dose. It does not cause nausea, vomiting and metallic taste.

**Nitazoxanide** (NITCOL, ZOXANIDE 200 mg,500 mg)
It is effective against giardiasis, amoebiasis, trichomonas vaginal infections and other infections such as ulcer-causing H.pylori, ascariasis. It is well tolerated but may cause pain in abdomen, vomiting and headache.

**Diloxanide Furoate** (FURAMIDE)
It is an effective drug to kill active organisms in the intestinal lumen and is given along with *metronidazole* in intestinal disease. Its usefulness in acute amoebiasis with dysentery is doubtful. It is useful in the treatment of asymptomatic cyst passers.

### Dosage

In adults its dose is 500 mg, 3 times daily for 5-10 days and in children above 2 years, 20 mg/kg for 10 days.

***Adverse Effects:*** The drug is generally well-tolerated. It may cause flatulence, occasional nausea, and itching. It is a drug of choice for mild intestinal and asymptomatic amoeabiasis.

### **Diiodohydroxyquin** (DIODOQUIN) and **Lodochlorhydroxyquinoline** (ENTEROQUINOL)

Larger doses have caused SMON SYNDROME (subacute myelo-optico neuropathy), characterized by muscle pain and weakness, specially in the legs, diminished vision leading to blindness due to damage of the nerves of the eye. Although these symptoms regress following discontinuation of the drug, they are not always completely reversible. Such cases occurred mostly in Japan. Therefore, it should not be used.

### Other Drugs

*Tetracyclines* and *paromomycin* are also used in the treatment of amoeabiasis as they inhibit the intestinal flora essential for the multiplication of amoebae. *Paromomycin* is directly amebicidal. It is recommended that anti-amoebic drugs be given along with *tetracyclines* (see chapter on 'Antibiotics'). It is always best to have a course of *metronidazole* or *tinidazole,* to be followed by an intestinal amoebicidal drug.

## Drugs for Extra-intestinal amoebiasis

With the advent of *metronidazole* and *tinidazole* all drugs used in amoebic abscess of liver (commonest form of extra-intestinal amoebiasis) have become less important. Drugs like *emetine* and *dehydroemetine* are now rarely used.

### **Chloroquine** (LARIAGO, RESOCHIN)

It is a commonly used drug for malaria and has anti-amoebic effects on liver but no effects on intestinal amoebiasis. It is given for 21 days in hepatic amoebiasis (see chapter on 'Malaria').

**Treatment of Various types of Amoebic Infection**

| *Amoebic Infection* | *Dose* |
|---|---|
| Acute Amoebic dysentery | *Metronidazole* along with *diloxanide furoate* for 5 To 10 days |
| Chronic Amoebiasis and Cyst passers | *Diloxanide furoate* for 5 to 10 days or *Diiodoquin* for 2 weeks. |
| Hepatic Amoebiasis | *Metronidazole* with *diloxanide furoate* for 5 –10 days. Some patients may require chloroquine. Rarely *dehydroemetine* is used. It is a very toxic drug on the heart. |

## Drugs for Protozoal Infections

Protozoa are 'one-celled' infective organisms such as *Giardia lamblia, Trichomonas vaginalis* and *Entameba hystolytica.*

Giardia is a cosmopolitan protozoa and resides in the upper small intestines of human and animals. It is known as the "Grand old man of intestines". It causes abdominal pain, loose stools and bloating. Sometimes there is vomiting and impaired nutrient absorption. Infection can be treated by medicines shown in the table.

Trichomonas vaginalis is a common cause of "leucorrhea or 'white water discharge' in females. It can also infect urinary passage causing burning and prostatitis in males. Since infection is tranmitted during sexual contact, both the partners should be treated simultaneously.Vaginal infection results in irritation, smelling discharge, redness,burning during urination and pain during sexual act. It requires local medications to be inserted into vaginal canal (See chapter Sexually Transmitted Diseases & AIDS). Oral drugs are described below in the table.

**Dosage of Some Orally Given Drugs in Protozoal Infections**

| *Drug* | *Amoebiasis* | *Giardiasis* | *Trichomoniasis* |
|---|---|---|---|
| *Metronidazole* | 400-800 mg thrice a day (child-30-50mg/kg) | 2 g once a day for 3 days or 200 mg thrice a day (child10-15 mg/kg) | 2 g as a single dose or 250 mg thrice a day for 7 days (child 30-50 mg/kg) |
| *Tinidazole* | 600 mg twice a day for 3 5-10 days or 2 g once a day (child 10-15 mg/kg) | 150 mg twice a day for 7 days or 2 g single dose (child 30 mg/kg single dose) | 300 mg twice daily for 7 days or 2 g single dose (child 30 mg/kg single dose) |
| *Secnidazole* | 2 g single dose (child 30 mg/kg) | 2 g single dose (child 30 mg/kg) | 2 g single dose (child 30 mg/kg) |
| *Satranidazole* | 300 mg twice daily for 3-5 days (max 10 days) (only for adults) | 600 mg single dose | 600 mg single dose |
| *Ornidazole* | 500 mg twice a day for 5-7 days (child 10-125 mg/kg/day for 3 days) | 1.5 g once a day for 1-2 days (child 40 mg/kg) | 500 mg twice a day for 5 days |
| *Nitazoxanide* | 500 mg twice a day for 3-5 days | 500 mg twice a day for 3 days | 500 mg twice a day for 3-5 days |

# 4

# Drugs Used in Anxiety

First of all, let us understand what we really mean by 'anxiety'. In medical terminology, the meaning of this word is somewhat different from what it is used for in everyday life. *Anxiety* is not the same as *fear*. The situation of fear is of short duration: for example, 1) a fast driving car almost about to hit you; 2) a ferocious dog chasing you; 3) you are getting late for an important appointment; 4) you have to appear for an examination or interview. In all these situations the fear is short-lived. But in modern life, one faces several problems daily, of which some are persistent. These hazards or problems may be real or imaginary, for example, fear of losing a job. In either case the danger may last for weeks or month. The body chemistry is such that a compensatory mechanism immediately takes over the situation in a temporarily fearful state, but when the state becomes persistent or semi-permanent, the physiological compensatory mechanism fails and the chemically understood 'anxiety' state is established. This mental tension even leads to other physical problems, such as digestive disorders, headache or backache, continuous high blood pressure, and many other troubles. Sexual function is also suppressed by anxiety and impotence in men or frigidity in women may further aggravate the situation. About 2 to 3 per cent individuals from population have, at one time or other, suffered from anxiety. In some patients anxiety and depression coexists.

Some anxiety is healthy and indeed necessary. This does not call for any treatment which is given only when anxiety becomes a nuisance and even then, the aim of treatment is to keep it within reasonable bounds. A person relieved of all anxieties is to hold his job for long. Anti-anxiety drugs are usefully employed to lower the anxiety component (also termed as anxiety neurosis) and keep it within reasonable limits.

## Treatment

For a long time, sedatives, including alcohol, have been used for overcoming anxiety. Sleep-aids (sedatives) do decrease the anxiety and put you to sleep but the symptoms reappear as the effect of the drug wears off and then, the person repeats the same drug. This leads to habituation or addiction to these drugs. Indeed this is the main reason for developing addiction to alcohol and sleeping tablets. Availability of modern medicines have remarkably changed the treatment of anxiety related disorder such as anxiety, neurosis, panic attacks, phobic disorders and post traumatic stress disorder.

Anxiety reaction is usually associated with increased muscle tone and it can be overcome by modern drugs which cause muscle relaxation besides their ability to lower anxiety.

## Drugs

The currently used anti-anxiety drugs can be categorized as *benzodiazepines* and miscellaneous drugs as described :

**Diazepam** (CALMPOSE, VALIUM), **Chlordiazepoxide** (ANXIZIDE, EQUILIBRIUM, LIBRIUM) **Lorazepam** (ATIVAN, LARPOSE), **Alprazolam** (ZENAX, ALPRAX, ALPRAX-SR, ALPRAX-PLUS, RESTYL,TRIKA)

These are tranquillo-sedative drugs which fall into the category of *benzodiazepines* and have gained tremendous popularity. Since these drugs are known to counteract anxiety and tension, they have been indiscriminately used by both the patients and the physicians. In addition to their calming effect, these drugs cause muscle relaxation. The sleep produced by these agents is very refreshing. Of these, *diazepam* is the most popular. *Chlorediazepoxide* is longest acting and is useful in allaying day time anxiety. *Lorazepam* is far more effective when given by injection.

*Alprazolam* has fewer side-effects than others. At present it is very commonly used alone or along with *propranolol* and *sertraline* (Antidepressant).

***Dosage:*** The usual oral doses are *alprazolam* 0.5 mg-sustained release (SR) is better for round the clock effects; *chlordiazepoxide* 10-20 mg; *diazepam* 5-15 mg; *lorazepam* 2-4 mg; and *oxazepam* 10-30 mg.

***Adverse Effects:*** The adverse effects of these drugs are few. These include drowsiness, and a drunken or light-headed feeling, which are most likely to occur during the first two days of the treatment and usually disappear when the drug is continued. In some cases a reduction in doses may be necessary. Other adverse effects are ataxia or difficulty in walking, vertigo, increased appetite, weight gain, and a confused mental state, specially in patients suffering from impairment of blood supply to the brain. In these cases also, a reduction in the dose is helpful. Some women fail to ovulate while on regular treatment. In rare cases there may be hypotension (low blood pressure) and visual disturbances. Overdose may cause sluggish respiration, and coma.

***Precautions***

1. These drugs should not be taken continuously by patients suffering from liver or kidney disease.
2. Use of alcohol or anti-allergic drugs should be avoided while taking these drugs as the sedative effect is enhanced.
3. These agents may cause episodes of rage, excitement, hostility, and severe depersonalization reaction if administered to a patient suffering from schizophrenia.
4. These drugs should be used cautiously in infants and elderly.
5. Prolonged use of these drugs may cause addiction. They should not be withdrawn abruptly.

6. These drugs are not very effective in smokers and therefore, cigarette smoking should be avoided by the users.
7. Some concurrently used drugs reduce the effects of these drugs such as antacids (reduced absorption) and *rifampicin* (more inactivation of *benzodiazepines*). Conversely, contraceptive pills and d-propoxyphene (a commonly used pain reliever) increase the sedative effect and sometimes toxicity.

*Propranolol* (a drug used in heart disease) reduces symptoms of anxiety in a dose of 10 to 20 mg thrice a day. It is a valuable drug in stress induced anxiety such as examination fear, stage phobia and public appearance. It can be given along with *alprazolam* or *diazepam.*

**Fixed Dose Combinations Available to Treat Anxiety**

| | *Propranolol +* | *Alprazolam +* | *Sertraline* |
|---|---|---|---|
| AMBULAX | 20 mg | 0.25 mg | — |
| AMBULAX—M | 10 mg | 0.25 mg | — |
| AMBULAX-HD | 20 mg | 0.125 mg | — |
| ZEPRO | 20 mg | 0.25 mg | — |
| ZEPRO-M | 10 mg | 0.25 mg | — |
| ALPRAX-PLUS | — | 0.5 MG | 25 mg |
| ALPRAX-FORTE | — | 0.5 mg | 50 mg |
| ANXIT-PLUS | — | 0.5 mg | 25 mg |
| ANXIT-FORTE | — | 0.5 mg | 50 mg |

Some combinations have *melatonin* (3 mg-ALPRAX-Z) or *fluoxetine* an *antidepressant* (CORAL-F).

### Role of Antidepressants in generalized anxiety

Antidepressants are currently used as initial medicines because they do not cause problem of addiction or dependence. *Venlafaxine* (see treatment of depression) is used in a dose of 37.5 mg to 75 mg once a day. Other antidepressants such as *fluoxetine* and *paroxetine* are also useful.

### **Hydroxyzine** (ATARAX, VESPARAX)

This drug provides symptomatic relief in states of anxiety. Besides anti-anxiety action, it also has antiemetic (preventing vomiting) and anti-allergic properties. It has a significant sedative and hypnotic action that lasts for a short period. It is also useful in treatment of insomnia due to itching and urticaria (hives) and drug allergy. Its usual dose is 25 mg, 3 to 4 times daily. One may avoid concurrent use of CNS depressants with it.

### **Buspirone** (ANXIPAR, BUSCALM, BUSPIN)

This has all the properties possessed by the *benzodiazepines* but has least sedative action and does not produce cognitive impairment. No tolerance or dependence has been described. It does not have muscle relaxant effect. It is found to be useful in mild to moderate generalized anxiety. It has very slow action and full effect may take a few weeks. Initial dose of 5 mg, 3 times a day. Can be gradually increased even upto 60 mg/day.

***Adverse Effects:*** In high doses this drug can cause nausea, light headedness, headache and dizziness (avoid operating machines).

## Other Anxiety Disorders

**Phobia** is an unrealistic anxiety/fear in a particular situation. A brief description is given below.

**Agoraphobia** is the fear of open-spaces or marketplaces. It waxes and wanes and may disappear without treatment. Psychotherapy, familiarization and use of antidepressants (see chapter 'Drugs Used in Mental Depression') are helpful.

**Social phobia** includes Stage Phobia (public speaking, acting/performance), phobia in using public bathrooms and giving witness etc. Such people develop all the manifestations of anxiety and fear in above social situations. Many of them are shy and timid by nature since early in life. Psychotherapy, exposure treatment and some drugs (such as *sertraline*, *propranolol* or *clonazepam*) may help. A new drug *Gabapentin* (Cap NEURONTIN-300 mg) is found to allay social phobia. *Propranolol* (20-60 mg) is also useful to reduce anxiety and panic of social events like stage performance.

**Obsessive compulsive disorder** is a disorder in which person gets recurrent and unwanted ideas or impulses which are bizarre (obsessions). There is an associated compulsion to do some act repeatedly in response to obsessions e.g., repeated hand washing to avoid infection. This requires proper evaluation and treatment. The treatment includes behaviour therapy and use of antidepressants like *clomipramine* (CLOFRANIL 10, 25, 50, 75 mg) a time hounoured medicine used in depression, narcolepsy and obsessive neurosis in a dose of 10-50 mg daily; and *fluoxetine* (FLUDAC 20 mg) in a usual dose of 20-40 mg/day

**Panic attacks** are characterized by sudden appearance of anxiety and physical manifestations such as breathing difficulty, palpitation, tremor, choking, chest discomfort and fear of dying. Treatment includes psychotherapy and use of antianxiety and/or antidepressant drugs. Parenteral (intravenous/intramuscular) *diazepam* is given under supervision to avoid respiratory depression. Sublingual *lorazepam* 0.5-2 mg followed by *sertraline* 25-50 mg daily is the treatment given usually. *Clonazepam* (CLONORIL, REVOTRIL,CLONAFIT 0.25, 0.5, 1.0, 2.0 mg) is also commonly used because of less likelihood of rebound anxiety if stopped abruptly.

### Effective Medication: Principles and Guidelines

1. 'Less is more', the famous dictum of *Mies van der Rohe* about architecture, applies equally to these drugs. If used sparingly and in short courses, the problems of tolerance and loss of efficacy can be avoided, preventing the subsequent use of larger doses which may cause development of dependence on these drugs.
2. Doses should be matched to the patient's requirement for relief from symptoms and his ability to function without any mental impairment. For this reason, doses should never be standardized or routinized.
3. Traditional practice of divided doses of 3 or 4 times daily make no sense in this case. Most of these drugs stay in the blood for a long time. By giving a major portion of the daily dose of the drug sleep-inducing at bedtime, one may capitalize on its effect as well as assure some carry-over effect for the next day, which is precisely the sedation required during daytime activity. If necessary, the patient can take smaller doses during the daytime.

# 5

# Drugs that Reduce Blood Lipid (Fat) Levels

••••••

The blood circulating in the body consists of blood cells and a straw coloured liquid called plasma. Plasma is made up chiefly of proteins and water, and fats (lipids) are carried with these proteins. These are described according to their density. The low density and very low density lipoproteins which are called LDL and VLDL respectively, are considered to be harmful, whereas, high density lipoproteins which are called HDL, are useful as they remove LDL and VLDL from the blood. The fats which are carried by these lipoproteins are cholesterol and triglycerides. There are various reasons for a high level of fat in the blood. This is quite common in persons who are overweight or have familial genetic tendencies. In such persons, reducing body weight by controlling the diet and resorting to regular physical exercise is sufficient to lower the blood fat level. Certain disease conditions like diabetes, decreased function of the thyroid gland, and some metabolic disorders may be responsible for an increased blood fat levels. In these conditions proper control of the underlying disease will help in reducing blood fat.

**Recommended Lipid and Cholesterol Goals**

| *Lipids & Cholesterol forms* | *Desirable Blood levels (mg/100ml)* |
|---|---|
| Low Density Lipoprotein Cholesterol (LDL-C) | 80-160 |
| Very Low Density Lipoprotein Cholesterol (VLDL-C) | 10-50 |
| High Density Lipoprotein Cholesterol (HDL-C) | 30-70 |
| Compounds of Fatty acid with Glycerol (Triglycerides) | 60-170 |
| Sum total without proteins (Total cholesterol) | 150-220 |
| Total Cholesterol : HDL-C Ratio | 5 or less |

**How is Excessive Fat in the Blood Harmful?** Raised cholesterol is a major risk factor for heart disease. An excessively high quantity of cholesterol in the blood is likely to get deposited on the walls of the blood vessels and make them narrow. This narrowing of the lumen of the blood vessel is called atherosclerosis. The process of atherosclerosis may start at a young age but its manifestations are usually seen in older patients by which time it has advanced considerably. Atherosclerosis may lead to a defective blood supply to various vital organs of the body. In the brain, it may cause impairment of mental functions, paralysis, and unconsciousness. Another danger is the involvement of the heart. Narrowing of coronary arteries (those supplying blood to the heart muscle) may lead to a defective blood and oxygen supply to the cardiac muscle and cause disorders like angina or myocardial infarction which need treatment immediately.

## Preventive Measures

Various measures can be undertaken to minimize the occurrence of atherosclerosis. Life style changes are needed such as smoking should be stopped or reduced. The patient should exercise regularly and should not overeat. Saturated fats, such as butter, *ghee,* animal fat, hydrogenated oils, coconut oil, oxidized oils (left over after frying), should be avoided and replaced by unsaturated or polyunsaturated fats, like vegetable oils, corn oil, groundnut oil, mustard oil, cottonseed oil, and sunflower oil. Polyunsaturated fats reduce cholesterol by removing it from tissues. The calories from fats should be 30% or less and distribution of various fats should be equal (saturated fats = monounsaturated fats = polyunsaturated fats). Fish oils are rich in one type of polyunsaturated fatty acid called as Omega-3 fatty acid. There are reports of reduction of triglycerides and antiatherogenic effects of fish oils. Fresh fruits and green vegetables have high levels of antioxidants which are useful. The dictum is 'Never a day without fruit.' Sugar intake should be reduced. Total caloric intake should be lowered so that there is a gradual decrease in weight. It has been observed that the above-mentioned measures help in reducing plasma fat in most cases. However, for patients in whom these measures are ineffective in lowering the plasma fat, drugs may be employed. It must be remembered that once a heart attack has occurred, the reduction of plasma lipids will decrease the chances of future attacks.

***Blood cholesterol: How much reduction is beneficial?*** Conventional normal value may be too high for Indian cases because various studies have shown that we are genetically more prone to heart disease (and are likely to have more complications at young age!) and tolerate cholesterol levels poorly. Hence lower values are recommended. Obviously aggressive reduction of blood cholesterol reduces chances of atherosclerosis. The table below gives the treatment goals to be achieved by drugs or diet according to the number of risk factors as per NCEP-ATP III guidelines.

| *Risk factor* | *10 year risk%* | *Goal of reduction of LDL-C* | *Drug treatment at this level of LDL-C* |
|---|---|---|---|
| Very high(CHD)* | >20% | <70 mg% | >100 mg% |
| High(>2 risk factors) | >20% | <100 mg% | >130 mg% |
| Intermediate | 10-20% | <130 mg% | >160 mg% |
| Low(0 1 risk factor) | <10% | <160 mg% | >190 mg% |

CHD* = Coronary heart disease

The goal of treatment is to reduce LDL-C to <100 mg% if patient has CHD(Optimal <70 mg%). For subjects without heart disease the treatment goals are shown in the table.

***Should High Triglycerides (TG) be treated?*** Studies have shown that TG if elevated >150 mg% also carries a definite risk (14% in males and 37% in females) and therefore should be treated by dietary regulation (if between 150-199 mg%) or drugs (if over 200 mg%). A value above 500 mg% is always treated with diet, avoidance of alcohol and use of hypolipidemic drugs.

## Drugs which Reduce Elevated Blood Lipids

***Statins:*** This is an important class of drugs which reduce formation of cholesterol by blocking enzyme (HMG COA- Reductase). Different statins differ in their potency and maximum reduction in lipid levels. In general LDL–cholesterol is reduced by 30-35% by comparable doses. HDL-cholesterol (good effect) increases by 5-15% and triglycerides reduce by 10-30%. If cholestyramine is used together, LDL- cholesterol may further reduce to 60-70% of pretreatment levels. The statins are preferably taken at night because of the fact that cholesterol forming enzyme has maximal activity at this time. *Rosuvastatin* and *atorvastatin* can be taken any time because they are longer acting. Mild adverse effects are nausea, headache, bowel upset and sleep disturbance. Muscle pain may occur rarely (in 1 out of 1000 patients). Actual myopathy may occur if *Gemfibrozil* or other drugs (*Erythromycin, Ketoconazole or Cyclosporine*) are also taken. Liver enzymes may also increase in blood. Various drugs available are:

**Drugs that Reduce Elevated Blood Upids**

| *Drug* | *Usual dose/day* | *Peculiarity/Effects* |
|---|---|---|
| *Lovastatin* (ROVACOR tab 10 mg, 20 mg) | 10-40 mg | First clinically useful drug |
| *Simvastatin* (SIMCARD tab 10 mg, 20 mg) | 5-20 mg | Twice potent to *Lovastatin* |
| *Pravastatin* (PRAVATOR tab 10 mg, 20 mg) | 10-40 mg | Decreases fibrinogen level and there by reduction in clot formation |
| *Atorvastatin* (ATORVA tab 10 mg, 20 mg) | 10-40 mg | Antioxidant effect |
| *Rosuvastatin* (FORTUIS tab 10 mg, 20 mg) | 10-40 mg | Longer action |
| *Fluvastatin* | 20-40 mg | — |

### Combinations

Since a patient with heart disease also suffers from vascular disease and high lipids a few combinations containing *Atorvastatin* are available to treat them simultaneously. POLYCAP: *Simvastatin* 20 mg + *Atenolol* 50 mg + *Hydrochlorothiazide* 12.5 mg + *Aspirin* 10 mg (enteric coated) and is promoted for the treatment of coexisting heart disease and high fat levels to reduce multiple risk factors and cardiovascular risks, prevention of strokes.

### The Fibrates (Fibric Acid Derivatives)

This is another important class of drugs. Their use results in a fall in triglycerides by 20-25%, cholesterol (LDL- C) by 10-15% and, an increase in HDL-C by 10-15% and these effects are due to activation of fat metabolizing enzyme (lipo-protein lipase) and less formation of triglycerides by liver. These drugs are effective when triglycerides and cholesterol are raised.

**Some Fibrates and their Characteristics**

| *Drug* | *Dose/day* | *Peculiarity/Adverse effects* |
|---|---|---|
| *Gemfibrozil* (GEMPAR NORMALIP) 300 mg cap. | 300-600 mg twice a day before meals | Bowel upset, loose motions, myopathy with statins, no increase in gall stone formation |
| *Bezafibrate* (BEZALIP 200 mg, 400 mg) tab. | 200 mg twice a day with meals | May decrease fibrinogen & blood glucose also-bowel upset and skin rash |
| *Fenofibrate* (FENOLIP, LIPIGARD 200 mg) cap | 200 mg once a day with meals | Greater reduction in LDL-C, longer action, uric acid reduced by 30%-GIT upset, liver and muscle damage in rare cases. |

NB: *Clofibrate* is no longer used.

### Resins: Cholestyramine, Colestipol and Colesevelam

These resins bind with bile acids in the small bowel and thus allow unabsorbed bile salts and cholesterol to pass into stools. Liver tries to make more bile salts from its cholesterol and therefore levels of LDL- C decrease. *Cholestyramine* is given in a dose of 4 g three times a day. The granules should be made into a paste before taking. Dry powder cannot be swallowed. These drugs are unpalatable and can cause a lot of bowel upset (gases, heart burn, constipation, nausea). Loss of fat soluble vitamins can cause deficiency symptoms of Vitamin A,D,E and K. A number of drugs *(warfarin, statins, digoxin)* are poorly absorbed if taken together. Therefore, resins are useful as adjuncts only. Colesevelam is better tolerated than others.

### Ezetimide (Ezetip, Lipezet 10 mg tab)

This drug prevents absorption of cholesterol from small bowel. It reduces LDL- cholesterol levels and further reduces LDL- C by 25% and triglycerides by 14%. It is well tolerated but occasional abdominal pain, diarrhoea, joint pains, headache, dizziness may be there. Its usual dose is 10 mg once a day regardless of meals. It is usually combined with statins.

### Nicotinic acid (Nialip 500 mg tab)

It is Vitamin $B_3$ *(Niacin* or *nicotinamide)* derivative and reduces tryglycerides and VLDL-C (20-50%) rapidly and followed by LDL-C (15-25%) subsequently. It is the most effective drug to raise good cholesterol (HDL- C) by 15-30 %. It acts on liver and prevents formation of triglycerides. Starting dose is 100 mg thrice a day with meals and gradually increased to 2 gm to 6 gm per day.

***Adverse Effects:*** It is a poorly tolerated drug. It causes dyspepsia, flushing, itching and sensation of heat (skin blood vessels widen). It also causes diarrhoea, darkening of skin, worsening of diabetes, joint pains in gout and irregular heart beats. Flushing can be reduced by concurrent use of *aspirin* (NIASPRIN). It is never given in pregnancy. It increases fall in BP due to drugs used for the treatment of high blood pressure.

### Other Drugs

*Guggulipid* (GUGULIP 25 mg tab) is a plant derivative (gum guggul) which lowers lipids modestly. It may cause loose motions.

Recently *Resveratrol* (RESVITA) obtained from red grape seeds has been marketed. This contains omega-3 fatty acids .

*Polycosanol* (POLYCOBAL) also reduces LDL- C and total cholesterol. It is obtained from sugarcane.

### Role of Vitamins in Atherosclerosis Prevention

*Homocysteine* is a sulfur- containing amino acid whose levels are increased in a number of cases with heart disease and strokes. Raised levels accelerate the process of atherosclerosis and this can be slowed by the use of folic acid (5 mg/day), *methyl cobalamin* ( an active form of Vitamin $B_{12}$), and *pyridoxine* (Vitamin $B_6$). Other Vitamins A,C, and E have antioxidant properties and thus remove the free radicals from tissues (free radical are injurious and allow atherosclerosis to progress). Therefore, 'healthy heart nutrients' supplementation may be needed (along with lipid lowering drugs) to tackle the complex process of atherosclerosis.

# 6

# Drugs Enhancing Functional Capacity of the Brain

The brain is the most vital organ of the human body. It has billions of neurons interconnected with one another and has varied functions. The brain is the center of all mental activities and controls physical activities to a very large extent. The intelligence of an individual is considered to be dependent on the quality of his brain functions. Since time immemorial the human being has been attempting to enhance the functional capacity of the brain. It is the desire of many to increase their physical activity through the brain. Parents are generally very concerned about the memory power of their offspring and one of the great desire to do something arises when a child is mentally retarded. In such cases the former are prepared to try any remedy prescribed by a doctor, *Vaidya, hakim* or even a sage who is supposed to be full of wisdom.

All sorts of drugs have been tried to increase the functional capacity of the brain. A number of plant products, minerals, and even animal organs have been ascribed for this purpose. In *Ayurveda, Brahmi* preparations have been employed for this purpose and a number of *Ayurvedic* and *Unani* manufacturers of formulations have come out with several so-called brain tonics, some of which have been shown to bring temporary benefits, and others none when experimentally tested.

The drugs currently in use can be divided into two groups: 1) those stimulating the central nervous system; 2) those which increase cerebral activity. Those stimulating the central nervous system can be further subdivided into two types: a) stimulants of mental activity; b) stimulants of mental as well as physical activity.

## Drugs that Stimulate Mental Activity

### Caffeine

This is found in tea, coffee, and cocoa. It stimulate the central nervous system, causing elevation of mood and increased alertness. It lessens the feeling of tiredness and fatigue. With limited doses, the ability to concentrate increases and the work output is enhanced. It causes constriction of cerebral blood vessels, which may be helpful in the relief of headache and migraine. It also causes irritation in the stomach and increases the production of acid.

The *caffeine* content of an average cup of tea is 30 to 45 mg, coffee- 80 to 100 mg, and a cola-drink bottle, 30 mg. *Caffeine* is available in various tonics, medicines for headache and migraine, pain relievers and antihistaminics used in the treatment of the common cold.

***Dosage:*** The minimum dose of *caffeine* necessary to cause stimulation ranges between 100 mg and 300 mg. However, if your daily intake of tea or coffee is very high, you may need a higher dose for the stimulant effect. Smokers also need more *caffeine* for the same effect than non-smokers. Several 'pain-killer' tablets in the market contain very low doses of *caffeine* (less than 30 mg) which serve no useful purpose.

***Adverse Effects:*** The adverse effects of *caffeine* vary from person to person, but in general, a dose of 1,000 mg or more may cause restlessness, irritability, excitement, insomnia, trembling, palpitation, fast breathing and increased urination. Still higher doses may cause ringing in the ears, flashes of light in front of the eyes, and mental confusion.

***Precautions***

1. A strong cup of tea or coffee should not ordinarily be taken late in the evening or at night, since in some persons it causes disturbance of sleep or insomnia. In Western countries, tea and coffee without *caffeine* is available and has become extremely popular for night consumption.
2. If you are suffering from hyperacidity or a peptic ulcer, restrict your intake of tea or coffee. You may add more milk or take these drinks with meals.
3. Many people can tolerate *caffeine* and develop a psychological dependence on it, but this is not of any serious consequence.

## Drugs that Stimulate Both Mental and Physical Activity

### Amphetamine (DEXEDRINE)

This brings about an increase in mental as well as physical activity. It makes a person 'high', and for this reason has been extensively abused by young persons and has been given nicknames like 'Pep Pills' and 'Speed'. Students take it at the time of examinations to keep awake for long hours. However, it may cause a state of confusion rather than allowing for longer study hours, and thus, may do more harm than good, when used by students.

*Amphetamine* has been used to treat patients of narcolepsy (who keep falling asleep during the day for short periods), hyperkinetic syndrome (overactive children), and bedwetting. *Amphetamine* has been extensively misused in competitive sports to improve performance. Participants in national and international sports can now be subjected to urine examination for the presence of this drug and proven use of the drug disqualifies them from competitions.

***Adverse Effects:*** The adverse effects of *amphetamine* include restlessness, dizziness, trembling, hyperactivity, tenseness, irritability, weakness, insomnia, fever, euphoria, confusion, increased libido (sexual desire), anxiety, deliriousness, and hallucinations. It may even cause suicidal or homicidal tendencies in mentally ill patients. Fatigue and depression follow stimulation. Other adverse effects are palpitation, precipitation of anginal pain, dryness of the mouth, nausea, vomiting, diarrhoea, and abdominal cramps.

**Modafinil** (PROVAKE-100 mg, 200 mg):
It promotes wakefulness in sleep disorders such as narcolepsy, obstructive sleep apnoea (breath holding spells in obese at night) and work-shift sleep disorder. Its usual dose is 100 to 200 mg once a day preferably in morning.

## Cerebral Activators (Cognition Enhancers)

While the use of CNS stimulants has declined due to their non-specific nature of actions, a new class of drugs called 'Cerebral Activators' has been introduced. It is claimed that these drugs improve the brain functions particularly in dementia- a condition of brain characterized by loss of intellect and memory. These may have a role in the treatment of Alzheimer's disease also. However, their use is limited and the claims regarding their efficacy are not always fully substantiated.

**Piracetam** (NORMABRAIN, NEUROCETAM, NOOTROPIL)
This drug is supposed to directly improve the efficiency of the higher functions of the brain such as learning, memory, thought, and consciousness both in normal and deficient situations. It does not have a sedative or psychostimulant effect. These changes are brought about by increase in nerve to nerve message activity and energy supply to nerve or those parts of brain which are involved in learning and memory. It variably improves brain function in senile dementia and mental retardation in children. The drug should be taken with caution in kidney or liver disease, and during pregnancy.

***Dosage:*** The recommended dose for adults is 800 mg, three times a day. For children, the usual dosage is 50 mg/kg of body weight in 3 divided doses.

**Dihydroergotoxine** (CERELOID, HYDERGINE 1 mg tab, 0.3 mg Inj)
It produces a short lasting memory improvement in dementia and stroke patients. It may cause stuffiness of nose and fall in BP.

**Pyritinol** (ENCEPHABOL)
This improves disturbed cerebral metabolism and activates glucose metabolism. It also improves cerebral micro-circulation. It has been tried in cerebro-vascular accidents, disturbed cerebral development in children and adolescents, in post-anaesthetic recovery, and alcohol withdrawal state. Its efficacy is uncertain.

***Dosage:*** The prescribed dose is 200 mg. three times daily for 6 to 8 weeks.

***Adverse Effects:*** It may cause disturbances, increased excitability, loss of appetite, headache, tiredness, nausea, vomiting, and diarrhoea.

**Ginkocer** (GINKOCER, BILOVAS)
This is a dried extract of *Ginkgo biloba.* Besides bringing about some action like *Piracetam* and *Pyritinol*, the drug causes inhibition of the platelet-activating factor. It has been tried in the treatment of multi-infarct dementia (repeated minor strokes lead to dementia) because it improves blood supply in small brain vessels in the stroke area.

### Other Drugs

Other drugs of this group are, *Nimodipine* (NIMODIP, VASOTOP) which is useful after subarchnoid haemorrhage, *Nicergoline (SERMION), Glutamic acid (GLUTANEURAL-500 mg)* and *Piribedil* (TRIVASTAL-50 mg). Trivastal is advocated for the treatment of tinnitus (painful ringing sensation in elderly) and giddiness also. It has antiparkinson activity.

## Drugs for Alzheimer's disease

Alzheimer's disease is a condition in which there is a breakdown or loss of the higher functions of brain due to loss of communication among brain cells. Clear communication among brain cells is vital for the brain to function properly. Poor networking and loss of cells leads to poor cognitive skills (thinking, reason, self care). The treatment requires social and family support and drugs. The drugs are not curative.

### Rivastigmine (EXELON, RIVADEM)

This drug increases levels of a chemical (Acetylcholine) which is needed for nerve to nerve message transfer in the brain. It has shown improvement of brain function in Alzheimer's disease. Cognition, apathy, delusions and hallucinations (see chapter) improve with its use. Its usual doses is 1.5 to 3 mg twice a day.

### Donepezil (ARICEP, DONECEPT, DOPEZIL)

It also improves cognitive functions by increasing acetylcholine levels in remaining nerves in the brains of Alzheimer's patient. It has a longer duration of action, so it is given once (5 to 10 mg) daily at night.

**Memantine** (AXURA, ADMENTA tab. 5 mg, 10 mg) is a new drug which can be used alone or along with *rivastigmine.* It may occasionally cause dizziness.

Other drugs tried are *Tacrine, Galantamine* and *antioxidant vitamins* (Vit. E, C). Interestingly *Ibuprofen* a pain reliever has been shown to slow the course of disease. A new class of pain relievers (Cox- 2 inhibitors) are also being evaluated to treat this otherwise incurable disease.

# 7

# Drugs Used in Bronchial Asthma

Bronchial asthma is characterised by chronic inflammation of the bronchial tubes resulting in narrowing of airways due to allergens, dust and fumes, infection and stress. There are more secretions and swelling of inner lining of airways (bronchi) and occasional blockage due to thick mucus (sputum). Patients longs for a mouthful of breath. Every moment of the day!

**What Happens During an Attack of Asthma?** The best description of asthma is given in a story of a patient who came to a doctor and gasped. 'Doctor, if you can take my air out, I swear, I will never breathe in again.' During an asthmatic attack there is difficulty in breathing, more especially in breathing air out. The chest is distended in a desperate effort to drive out the air through the obstructed airway. The obstruction of the airway causes a wheeze (a whistling sound) which becomes faint as the severity increases due to poor movement of air. Besides difficulty in breathing, coughing, and a sense of constriction in the chest, apprehension and anxiety may be experienced which disrupts the normal activity. If the attack is prolonged, lasting for several hours and does not respond to the usual treatment, it is called status asthmaticus or acute severe asthma. In this the patient may get fatigued and may die of respiratory arrest. Vigorous emergency treatment is essential to save the life.

**Causes of Asthma:** Asthma is caused by obstruction of the airway, chiefly due to bronchoconstriction, that is, constriction of the passages of air in the lungs, and to a lesser extent by secretions and swelling of the respiratory passages. There can be various causes for bronchoconstriction but three factors which possibly interact with each other are worth considering, as their removal may help in curing asthma. These are: 1) allergic reactions, 2) infection of the respiratory tract, and 3) psychological factors. However, it must be emphasized that in most cases the underlying cause is unknown and the only alternative is to provide symptomatic treatment with bronchodilator drugs.

**Allergic Reactions:** Reaction to inhaled or ingested substances to which a person is allergic appears to be the commonest cause of asthma. This is called allergic asthma. It can be either seasonal or non-seasonal. Seasonal asthma is the more common of the two and is due to inhaled pollens, moulds, and eating of certain vegetables and fruits. A mite found in house dust appears to be a main bug responsible for 'house dust allergy'. Non-seasonal asthma may be due to allergy to feathers, animal-dander, foods (Tartrazine is a yellow food additive which cause allergy), and drugs like *penicillin, aspirin,* and *indomethacin. In some susceptible persons use of propranolol may precipitate asthma.*

**Infection of the Respiratory Tract:** Respiratory infection is a common cause of asthma in young children, the very old, and in most of the severe cases. These patients initially suffer from a common cold which progress into bronchial asthma.

**Psychological Factors:** Emotional stress and strain play an important role in asthma. Asthmatics are usually irritable and stubborn. The disease can also be a factor in aggravating their suffering and emotional behaviour. They have a peculiar psychological make-up or 'asthmatic personality'. A dry cough at night, exercise, crying or a hearty laugh have also precipitated acute attack in some cases.

## Treatment

With the advancement in the methodology of treatment, the life expectancy of asthmatics have been considerably increased than in the past. The management of bronchial asthma includes specific treatment aimed at removal of the cause and symptomatic treatment.

### Specific Treatment

If the cause of the asthma can be discovered, every effort should be made towards its removal to provide complete and permanent relief. If the patient develops symptoms of allergy, such as skin rashes, itching and pruritus and running nose the possible allergen (substance causing allergy) should be identified. Its removal is the most effective way of controlling allergic asthma. If this is not possible, desensitization by using an extract of specific allergen should be attempted. In many cases of allergic asthma, the specific allergen is not identifiable and anti-allergic drugs are tried. A few patients of seasonal asthma are benefited by temporarily moving to another town before the onset of a particular season, but this is not always feasible.

If infection is the cause, the person should protect himself from stress and strain due to extremes of weather. Frequent attacks of common cold may lead to asthma. Intensive treatment with a specific antibiotic must be instituted immediately. The most common offending organisms are *Pneumococci* and *Haemophilus influenzae.* In these infections, broad-spectrum antibiotics like *Amoxycillin, Cefuroxime* or *Ampicillin* are usually effective (see chapter on 'Antibiotics').

### Symptomatic Treatment

Two types of medications are used 1) for treatment during acute attack; known as *relievers or quick relief medications* and 2) for preventing the recurrence of the attack known as controllers.

## Quick Relief Medications

### Adrenergic Beta-Receptor Stimulants: Salbutamol (ASTHALIN, BRONKOTAB, VENTORLIN), Terbutaline (BRICANYL), Adrenaline

Stimulation of the adrenergic beta-receptors of the lungs causes relaxation of the bronchioles and opens up the respiratory airway. *Salbutamol* and *terbutaline* are most effective.

### Salbutamol (ALBUTEROL)

It is the most commonly used drug to produce dilatation of narrowed airways in asthma. For acute attack it is given by inhalation (patient inhales the drug by a deep inspiration with nose pinched: adequate training is needed for best effects). Two types of inhalers are available:

**Asthma Devices**

These are used to increase delivery of drug directly into airways and to reduce the systemic adverse effects.

**Dry Powder Inhalers (DPIs)** are compact devices available in various user-friendly shapes and are easy to use and refill with a capsule. A capsule containing powdered *salbutamol* is broken and rotated in a device (ROTAHALER) during deep inspiration and the drug reaches into lungs.

**Metered Dose Inhalers (MDIs)** are propellant which makes a mist during use. Metered doses (100 µg to 200 µg per puff) of *salbutamol* can be pushed from the canister in which *salbutamol* liquid is placed with propellants. The mist (aerosol) is inhaled so that drug reaches into lung.

Both these devices require proper use and 'hand-mouth coordination'.

**Spacers** are patient friendly devices and are available for children and adults. These increase the delivery of drug and reduce wastage.

Other varieties of devices available are Acculahers, multihalers, valve-holding chamber MDIs.

It is recommended that *'Leaflet of patient information' dispensed along with a particular brand should be carefully read.* Patients are instructed to gargle after the use of inhaled steroids to avoid hoarseness and throat irritation.

***Adverse Effects:*** Tremor, palpitation, restlessness, nervousness, throat irritation and swelling over ankles (foot) may occur. Inhaled *salbutamol* causes less adverse effects than tablets.

**Some Preparations of Salbutamol**

| *Brand Name* | *Dose* |
|---|---|
| ASTHALIN | *Salbutamol* (Tab. 2 µg, 4 µg) Usual dose 2 to 4 µg three to four times a day. |
| VENTORLIN Syrup | contains 2 µg *salbutamol*/ 5 ml |
| ASTHALIN MDI | 100 µg/ puff inhaler, ROTACAPS 200 µg/puff |
| ASTHALIN Respiratory solution | 5 mg/ ml to be used with nebulizer. |
| AEROCORT inhaler | contains 50 µg/ puff *Beclomethasone* + 100 µg/ puff *salbutamol* |
| AEROCORT ROTACAPS | contains 100 µg/ puff *Beclomethasone* + 200 µg/ puff *salbutamol* |
| BUDESOL RESPULES | contains 2.5 *salbutamol* and 0.5 µg *budenoside* |
| BRONCHO PLUS | contains *salbutamol* 2 µg with *theophylline* 200 µg |
| THEOASTHALIN | As above, *Theoasthalin-SR-Salbutamol* 4 µg with *thephylline* 300 µg long acting formulation |
| DUOLIN | 0.5 µg *ipratropium* and 2.5 µg *salbutamol* |
| ETO-SABETOL | contains *salbutamol* 2 µg, *theophylline* (etophylline) 200 µg and *Bromhexine* 8 µg |

*Levo-salbutamol* (LEVOLIN 1mg, 2mg and respiratory solution 0.31 mg in 2.5 ml) is related to *salbutamol* in its effects.

*Terbutaline* (BRICANYL) is another drug effective in acute attack and has similar properties to *salbutamol.* Its doses and preparations are:

**Some Terbutaline Preparations**

| *Brand Name* | *Dose* |
|---|---|
| BRICANYL TABLET | 2.5 to 5 mg; dose 2.5 to 5 mg thrice a day |
| BRICANYL INHALER | (Misthaler) 250 µg/ puff 1 to 2 puff three times a day |
| BRICANYL SYP. | 1.5 mg/ 5 ml for children |
| BRICANYL SOLUTION | 10 mg/ ml for the use in nebulizer |
| BRICANYL INJECTION | 0.5 mg/ ml to be used by intramuscular route |
| THEO BRIC | Terbutaline 2.5 mg + theophylline 100 mg |
| THEOBRIC SR | Terbutaline 5 mg (SR) + theophylline 300 mg (SR) |

If these drugs are used for very long time, there is reduction in the effect due to the fact that airways loose responsiveness to them. Therefore, preventive treatment must be used simultaneously.

**Adrenaline and Isoprenaline:** These are effective medicines but cause disturbance of heart rhythm rarely used now days.

### Direct-Acting Drugs: Theophylline, Aminophylline, Deriphylline, Doxophylline

*Theophylline* and its preparation, *aminophylline,* cause dilatation of bronchioles by direct action. *Aminophylline* which contains *theophylline* and *ethylenediamine* as a dissolving agent is very frequently used for providing immediate relief during an acute attack of bronchial asthma. In this condition, *aminophylline* is given in a well-diluted solution by the intravenous route. *Theophylline* is also given by the oral route along with *ephedrine* and other drugs, for prevention of recurrence of asthmatic attacks. *Theophylline* is more effective when given at night to prevent occurrence of night time attacks.

### Dosage

The average oral dose of *theophylline* is 100-200 mg given three to four times a day. This is generally not tolerated by most patients. *Deriphylline* causes less gastric irritation and is better absorbed. To provide immediate relief, *aminophylline*, containing 250 mg of *theophylline,* is diluted in 20 ml of 5% glucose and injected intravenously, very slowly, over a period of 5-10 minutes.

Some commonly used *theophylline* preparations are DOXOBID which contains *doxophylline* 400 mg; PHYLOBID which contain 200 and 400 mg; TR PHYLLIN cap which contains 125mg 250 mg; and DERIPHYLLIN RETARD which contains 150mg, 300 mg and 450 mg.

***Adverse Effects:*** *Theophylline* is irregularly absorbed and an effective dose given by mouth causes irritation in the gastro-intestinal tract. So it should never be taken on empty stomach. The most common adverse effects are nausea, anorexia, and vomiting and nervousness. A very quick intravenous injection of undiluted *theophylline* may cause a sudden fall in blood pressure, and irregular beating of heart.

### Corticosteroids: Role in Bronchial Asthma

These are invaluable in critically ill cases. They are used either as topical inhaled steroids or by oral or by IV route. Intravenous *hydrocortisone* 100 to 200 mg given every six hourly for 1 to 2 days, is used in the management of acute severe bronchial asthma *(status asthmaticus)*. Although given intravenously, steroids are not quick acting so inhaled treatment is continued. In some cases oral *Prednisolone* is given to prevent recurrent attacks of asthma.

Inhaled steroids are also useful in long term treatment in many cases. Here inhaler is used to deliver drug into lungs. Some drugs used are:

| *Drugs/Brand Names* | *Dosage* |
|---|---|
| Beclomethasone dipropionate (BECLATE) | 100 to 200 μg MDI |
| Budesonide (PULMICORT) | 100 μg, 200 μg, 400 μg/ MDI |
| Fluticasone propionate (FLOHALE) inhaler | 25 μg, 50 μg, 125 μg/ puff |
| Flunisolide (SYNTARIS nasal spray) | used as nasal spray in allergic rhinitis |
| Ciclasonide(OSONIDE) | 80 μg, 160 μg MDI |

A major problem with steroid inhalers is throat irritation, hoarseness of voice and fungal growth over throat. This can be drastically reduced by doing gargles with fresh water after inhaler use every time. Very minute amounts of drug reaches into blood so systemic effects (see chapter on 'Corticosteroids') are negligible. It is to be understood that inhaled steroids are not used in the treatment of acute attack but have preventive role only.

### Drugs Used for Prevention and Long term Treatment of Chronic Asthma-Controllers

**Bambuterol** (BAMBUDIL, BETADAY)

It is given orally in as dose of 10 to 20 mg once a day. It is a longer acting bronchodilator.

**Salmeterol** (SALMETER, SEROBID)

It is used by inhalation (MDI) in a dose of 25 μg twice a day. It is also available in combination with *fluticasone* (SEROFLO MULTIHALERS, ROTACAPS, ESIFLO, SERETIDE ACCHALER contains 50 mg salmeterol + 100 to 500 mg *Fluticasone*). SEROFLO has 3 strengths (100, 250 and 500 ug of *fluticasone* and thus dose can be tailored according to need).

**Formoterol** (FORATEC)

It is also given by inhalation route 12 to 24 μg twice a day. DUOVA Rotacaps contain *Formoterol* 9μg (forte-18 μg) with formoterol 12 μg

**Ipratropium Hydrobromide** (IPRAVENT 20 μg/ puff)

It is used as 20 to 40 μg inhalation two to four time a day. It is more effective in chronic bronchitis with asthma like problems. It can cause dryness of mouth and palpitation. Nebulised *ipratropium* along with *salbutamol* are given in refractory asthma.

*Tiotropium* acts like *ipratropium* and is used in a dose of 18 μg daily by inhalation. (TIOVA,TIATE 18 μg).

TIOMATE contains *Formoterol* 12 μg with 18 μg of *tiotropium*.

**Montelukast** (MONTAIR, MONTELAST 4 mg tab), **Zafirlukast** (ZUVAIR 10 mg tab)
**Montelukast** 10 mg + **Levocetirizine** 5 mg (REKAST-L)

These prevent airway inflammation and are effective orally. They are useful in patients who can not take glucocorticoids. Adverse effects are mild as headache and skin allergy. MONTAIR Plus contains 10 mg *bambuterol* with 10 mg *montelukast*.

**Sodium cromoglycate** (CROMOLYN, CHROMOTOP)

It stabilizes mast cells (cells responsible for formation of chemicals which cause asthma) and prevents release of constrictor chemicals. It is given by inhalation.

*Fintal* 1 mg MDI is used in 2 puffs four times a day. It is well tolerated by most patients but sometimes irritating cough and brochospasm may occur. It has preventive value only.

*Ketotifen* (ASTHAFEN, KETASMA) acts like *cromolyn* but can be given orally in a dose of 1 mg twice a day. Adverse effects are sedation, weight gain, nausea and dizziness.

*Omalizumab* (XOLAIR) is a new preparation raised against IgE, the root cause of spasm in asthma. It will soon be available in India.

### Combination Drugs

Anti-asthma drugs have a big market as the patient has to take them for a prolonged period of time. Pharmaceutical companies, specially the multinationals are cashing in on this by bringing out new drug combinations and increasing prices. There are a number of drug combinations available in India for asthma. If one drug of a group is unable to provide satisfactory relief, another drug from a different group can be tried or two drugs can be given together, depending on the response of the patient. For Bronchodilator cough syrups see chapter 'Drugs Used in Cough'.

# 8

# Drugs Used in Constipation

Most people are extremely particular about two rituals every morning: defecation and a bath. One of the most important concerns relating to cleansing of the bowels daily is the belief that all ailments from ague to plague are caused by constipation and if the bowel is not cleansed at least once a day, purgatives are necessary.

**What Really Constitutes Constipation?** Constipation is a condition in which the bowels are evacuated after a longer interval or with difficulty and the person is not satisfied. What the right interval should be, is difficult to generalise since it varies from person to person. Some evacuate their bowels once, others twice a day, while there are still others who do so only once in 2 or 3 days and yet have sound health.

**Causes of constipation:** Some may have constipation on account of a change of environment or emotional tension, but the normal rhythm returns after a few days, and should not be a source of worry. The most important causes of constipation are a disregard of the call of nature to pass a motion and an improper diet. When the rectum is full, it sends signals to the central nervous system for their movement and if this is repeatedly ignored, it gradually leads to failure of the rectum to signal the urge. Other causes of constipation may be a disease or abnormality of the gastro-intestinal tract, adverse effects of drugs, drying of the stools (faecal impaction), obstruction of the intestines, and severe illness in which the food and intake is too little. In case of prolonged constipation in infants or intermittent constipation with diarrhoea, the physician should be consulted to rule out surgical problems. If there is a painful disorder of rectum and anus such as fissure in anus, the person tends to avoid defecation due to pain. This must be treated properly.

**What Can be Done About Constipation?** If you are suffering from constipation, and have been taking purgatives, try to stop these gradually. Your system will probably return to normal if you take enough soups, vegetables, and fruits. However, if you are the worrying type you may take mild laxatives only as a temporary measure without making it a habit. Remember, disregarding the call for a motion is the worst you can do to your constipation. Do not wait unnecessarily. Your diet should be made up of high roughage foods containing a lot of wholegrain cereals; leafy vegetables like spinach, raw carrots, cucumbers, salads, prunes, figs, papaya, water melon, and other fresh fruits. Your intestines will soon gain the normal tone. If all these measures fail, you are a candidate for mild purgatives or laxatives. Never take strong purgative. They are needed only under exceptional circumstances and should be used under the care of a doctor. In elderly bed ridden individuals, longer lasting constipation leads to fecal impaction and leaking of fecal material. This is wrongly interpreted as diarrhoea (Paradoxical diarrhoea) and unnecessarily antidiarrheal are used. They actually worsen the constipation! The correct treatment is to evacuate rectum by gloved finger and do a cleansing enema.

## Mild Purgatives

Mild purgatives or laxatives are those which promote defecation, causing minimum adverse effects. Drugs included in this group are:

### Bulk Producing Drugs

**Isabgol** (SAT ISABGOL, NATURE CARE, FIBOGYL, IGOL, ISOGEL, NATUROLAX, CREMAFFIN), **Agar-agar** (AGAROL), **Methyl Cellulose** (FIBROPIL), **Psyllium** (ISOVAC), **Calcium Polycarbophil** (FIBOTAB)

These have high proportion of non-absorbable material called as 'fiber'. These drugs absorb water to increase the bulk in the intestines and make the stools soft. The onset of their action is slow, about 12 to 24 hours. They are the safest purgatives for the treatment of chronic constipation. Of the three, *isabgol* is most commonly used in India. An advantage of these agents is that there is reduced absorption of dietary cholesterol so LDL-cholesterol levels decrease.

### Dosage

*Isabgol* is given in a dose of 3.5 to 5.6 g. *Psyllium* is given with water or milk in a dose of 3 to 5 g daily. *Calcium Polycarbophil* is given in a dose of one to two tablets once or twice in a day. Unlike other drugs in this group *polycarbophil* does not produce gases. *Agar-agar* is given in a dose of 4 to 16 g, and *methyl cellulose* 1 to 6 g in divided doses.

***Adverse Effects and Precautions:*** Those agents which are derived from vegetable sources are devoid of toxic effects. Occasionally flatulence may occur, but this can be relieved by increasing the fluid intake. the chronic use of *isabgol* may decrease plasma cholesterol by interfering with the absorption of bile acids but it does not cause any harm and may, in fact, do good to an obese patient. Always take plenty of fluids along with these drugs to obtain maximum benefit and to avoid the possibility of intestinal obstruction which has been reported to occur in rare cases.

### Stool Softeners

**Dioctyl Sodium Sulfosuccinate or Docusate** (CELLUBRIL, DOSLAX, LAXICON), **Sodium Picosulfate** (COLOX, CREMALAX)

This is an effective stool softener for the treatment of constipation in some cases. It is a detergent which softens the stools by allowing more water into it.

## Dosage

The daily dose of *Dioctyl Sodium Sulfosuccinate* varies from 50 to 500 mg, depending on the severity of the condition. The action starts after 24 to 48 hours. COLOX syrup should be taken in a dose of 5 mg/tsf and CREMALAX in 10 mg at night.

***Adverse Effects and Precautions:*** Adverse effects of this drug are quite rare. It has been reported to interact with mineral oils to increase their absorption. It can cause pain in abdomen, bitter taste in the mouth and liver toxicity. It should not be taken concurrently with mineral oils.

## **Liquid Paraffin** (CREMAFFIN, AGAROL)

This is a traditional remedy for constipation. It is an inert oil which lubricates the intestines and forms a film or coating around the stools to make their passage smooth and comfortable. It softens the stools by preventing the absorption of water into the intestines. It allows the stools to pass through the intestines with a minimum of friction. It is often recommended for patients with heart attack, hernia, and for pregnant women, as well as after surgery on the rectum or abdomen, and in cases in which straining to evacuate may be harmful. CREMAFFIN contains 11.25 ml milk of magnesia and 3.35 ml/15 ml suspension of paraffin. Liquid paraffin is given in a dose of 15 to 45 ml as such or as an emulsion. Its action starts after 12 to 24 hours.

***Adverse Effects:*** It is unpleasant to swallow due to oily in nature. If taken regularly, it may cause deficiency of fat soluble vitamins such as A, D and K. It may, at times, leak through the gastro-intestinal tract and cause not only an annoying but embarrassing situation. On accidental inhalation liquid paraffin has also been reported to cause lipoid pneumonia in elderly and weak persons. Although it promotes and facilitates the passage of stools, it delays healing, and therefore, its use is not preferred after surgery for piles. Simultaneous use of *docusate* increases its absorption so effect is lost.

## Osmotic Purgatives

Sodium and magnesium salts are used as osmotic purgatives. The main action is to increase the volume of fluid in the large bowel so that it gets distended and evacuations occurs.

## **Magnesium Hydroxide** (MILK OF MAGNESIA 8% suspension)

This is a mild purgative which can be used even in pregnant women and children. It absorbs water from the intestines to form the bulk and make the stools soft. Besides purgative action, it counteracts acidity in the stomach. Its usual dose is 15-30 ml. Its action starts after 2-6 hours.

***Adverse Effects:*** It is a mild purgative and does not have any adverse effect except to produce flatulence in some people.

***Precautions***

1. Take plenty of fluids along with this purgative.
2. Patients with chronic kidney disease who may have difficulty excreting magnesium, should be wary of MILK OF MAGNESIA.

## **Magnesium Sulfate** (MAGSULF or EPSOM SALT)

Magnesium Sulfate is a useful purgative for preparation of bowels before surgery, X-ray examination, colonoscopy and some times to remove dead tapeworms after drugs & poisoning.

This is an osmotic purgative which causes total evacuation of the bowel in 1 to 3 hours. Therefore it is given early in the morning in a dose of 5 to 15 g.

**Lactulose** (DUPHALAC, LIVO-LUK, LOOZ)

It is undigestable sugar and retains water. It is useful in constipation and is given in doses of 4 to 10 g twice a day and acts within 6 to 18 hours. It is broken down in large bowel by resident bacteria into sugar which have osmotic effect. An important use of lactulose is in liver failure. Here it reduces formation and absorption of ammonia which is responsible for causing coma (20 g twice a day). 10g sachet of *Lactitol* (ENCELAX) can be used in place of *lactulose. Sorbitol* (BIOFFIN) can be taken in a dose of 15 to 60 ml 1 to 3 times a day.

*PolyEthyleneGlycol* (PEG) solution (PEGLEC) is used to wash large bowel before surgery and colonoscopy.

**ENEMA**

*Tap water enema* 500 ml – quick acting

*Phosphate enema* (PRACTOCLYSS) 120 ml is available as an easy to use plastic dispenser.

Mineral oil 100 to 250 ml given by rectum to soften and lubricate fecal masses.

Glycerin enema (SULABH, NEOTOMIC)

## Strong Purgatives (Stimulant Purgatives)

They stimulate the musculature of the large bowel and also increase fluid secretion in the bowel. There is passage of semisolid/ liquid stools in 6 to 8 hours. Often cramping abdomen pain may also occur. Irritant substances such as senna (sennosides), *phenolphthalein, bisacodyl* (*Dulcolox* tab and suppositories) and castor oil are included in this class. Because of excess of fluid and ions loss (potassium and sodium) bowel movements ultimately may be reduced (colonic atony). The uterus at full term gets stimulated and therefore they are never used in pregnancy. These are mostly used after deworming treatment, before X-ray examination of bowels and before abdominal surgery.

**Some Strong Purgatives**

| *Drugs/Brand Names* | *Dosage* |
|---|---|
| *Phenolphtalein* (AGARAOL, CREMAFFIN-C, emulsion) | 60-130 mg at bedtime |
| *Bisacodyl* (DULCOLAX, JULAX tab 5, 10 mg; suppository 5 mg) 5mg and 10 mg-acts within 1 hour | *Adult* 10 mg at night; (acts within 8 hours) *child* 5 mg at night; (acts within 8 hours) Suppository (acts in an hour) inserted anally. |
| Senna (SOFSENNA, GLAXENNA 12 mg tab., EVACUOL granuels 18 mg, SENNOSIDE A & B in 5 gm sachet) | 1-2 tab. at bedtime |

***Adverse Effects:*** The irritation of the intestines may cause griping or cramping pains in the abdomen. Sometimes there may be erosion of the inflamed mucosa passage of mucous in the stools and colonic atony (inactivity of large bowel). Other adverse effects include an excessive loss of fluids and electrolytes. *Phenolphthalein* turns stool pink in colour (harmless but patient needs this information). Allergic skin rashes may occur with *phenolphthalein, senna* and *bisacodyl.* Colonic mucosa may develop dark pigmentation on regular use of *senna.*

***Precautions***

1. These agents should not be taken regularly for treatment of chronic constipation.
2. If there is any previous history of abdominal pain, avoid the use of these drugs.
3. These should never be used by pregnant women as premature uterine contractions may cause abortion.
4. These are secreted in the milk and should not be used by feeding mothers.

We suggest that purgatives should be avoided as far as possible especially the strong ones. Most cases of constipation get cured without the aid of drugs. If a purgative must be taken, then simple, cheap, and effective *isabgol* is the best option. Cashing the agony of a constipated person, pharmaceutical companies are trying their level best to alleviate this malady by flooding the market with expensive preparations containing various combinations of purgatives. In our opinion, no combination is superior to an individual purgative.

***Note:*** Castor oil has been used for long number of years but its use has gradually declined as more user friendly drugs are now available. In many western countries, specially in Europe, *Senna* tea is very popular. It does not contain any tea and does not taste like tea. However, people feel warm by drinking a hot decoction of *senna* leaves which also helps move their bowels the next morning.

## Prokinetic Drugs

A new class of drugs are now available which increase the bowel movements primarily by their effects on receptors present in musculature. They are devoid of osmotic effects. These drugs are slow acting and are therefore useful in chronic functional constipation due to reduced bowel activity seen in diabetes, irritable bowel syndrome and atonic constipation. Drugs available are:

**Mosapride** (MOSID, NORMAGUT)

It acts like *cisapride* but no adverse interactions are reported. It is given in a dose of 5 mg thrice a day.

**Itopride** (TONATE, ITOKINE-T ITONORM, ITOTOR-OD)

It is used in a dose of 50 mg thrice a day.

**Tegaserod** (TEGIBS 2 mg, 6 mg tab., TIBS)

It is used to treat constipation in irritable bowel syndrome in a dose of 2 mg to 6 mg twice a day before meals. Adverse effects are pain in abdomen, diarrhoea, headache and dizziness. This agent is withdrawn in USA.

***Note:*** *Cisapride* has also been withdrawn due to its cardiac adverse effects but it is available in India. We discourage its use.

**Purgative abuse**

Some people are obsessed with bowel evacuation and start taking purgatives regularly. This is harmful. Long term use results in deficiency of nutritive vitamins and proteins, imbalance of fluid and electrolytes, and swelling of intestinal mucous membrane. It is better to seek medical advice and use purgatives judiciously.

**Don't use strong purgatives if you have**

- Acute abdominal pain and constipation — unless diagnosis is ascertained
- If constipation is due to intestinal obstruction
- Pregnancy
- Underfunction of thyroid.

# 9

# Drugs Used in Cough

A cough is a sudden expiratory thrust of air from the lungs. It is essentially a protective reflex. Coughing is useful when it effectively removes secretion or extraneous material from the respiratory tract, that is, when it is productive. It is useless when it is unproductive. It has been said that more people have died from an inability to cough rather than from the act of coughing. Does this mean that coughing is always useful and should never be prevented? No. The unproductive or useless cough is often very troublesome and needs to be stopped.

**Causes of Cough:** The causes of coughs are many and need not be restricted to the respiratory system. A cough may be a manifestation of a disease of the heart or lungs. Cough is a usual manifestation of respiratory allergy, bronchial asthma, obstruction of airway passages by foreign bodies *(supari, pan masala)*. How then do we discover the actual cause? Consideration of such factors as duration of the cough, its tendency to occur at particular times, the nature of the sputum brought up, and other complaints of the patient, all help in establishing its source. A short cough is usual in upper airways infections such as the common cold, infection of throat and sound box while prolonged coughing is characteristic of chronic bronchitis and bronchiectasis. A cough with bloody sputum should suggests investigation for tuberculosis or cancer. In children whooping cough occurs in bouts and is followed by deep inhalation (whoop). A similar situation is croup but here there is inspiratory difficulty. Coughing and expectoration of sputum are often most troublesome in the early morning and at bedtime, especially in chronic bronchitis. Three common causes of cough at night are post-nasal drip, bronchial asthma and reflux esophagitis(heart burn). These causes are often ignored because these are unrelated to lungs.

## Treatment

Removal of the underlying cause is essential when the cough is indicative of a more serious disease. For example, the use of anti-microbial agents in infective conditions of the upper airways and chest, use of acid suppressants in the evening and treatment of heart failure by diuretics or proper surgical treatment in appropriate cases. *Enalapril, lisinopril* and *ramipril* are some of the commonly used blood pressure lowering drugs which may cause dry cough. These should be stopped instead of giving cough suppressants if cough occurs with their use. In this chapter we will restrict ourselves to drugs meant to provide symptomatic relief for a cough.

**Commonly Used Mucolytic Drugs**

| Brand Names | Mucolytic agent | Other ingredients |
|---|---|---|
| AMBRODIL | Ambroxol | — |
| AMBROLITE | Ambroxol | Salbutamol |
| AMCOLD | Ambroxol | Cetirizine |
| BISOLVON | Bromhexine | — |
| BRICOREX EXPECT | Guaiaphenesin | Terbutaline |
| BROZEDEX | Bromhexine/Guaiaphenesin | Terbutaline |
| MUCOLITE | Ambroxol | — |
| RELENT | Ambroxol | Cetirizine |
| SEDOSOLVIN | Bromhexine | Dextromethorphen/ Chlorpheniramine |

*Alex-sugar free cough formula is available for diabetic patients.

Paediatric drops have higher content of active ingredients as compared to syrups therefore doses are not similar.

**Some Commonly Available Cough and Cold Preparations for Children**

| Brand Names | Antihistaminic | Decongestant | Fever/ Pain reliever | Other |
|---|---|---|---|---|
| ALEX PAED. DROPS | Chlorpheniramine | Phenylpropanolamine | — | — |
| ARINAC SUSPENSION | — | Pseudoephedrine | Ibuprofen | — |
| CINARYL DROPS | Phenylpyraline | Phenylephrine | Paracetamol | — |
| FEBREX PLUS DROPS | Chlorpheniramine | Phenylpropanolamine | Paracetamol | — |
| PEDIA-3 SYRUP | Chlorpheniramine | Pseudoephedrine | Paracetamol | Dextrome-thorphen |
| SINAREST PAEDDROPS | Chlorpheniramine | Pseudoephedrine | Paracetamol | — |
| SUDIN KID SYRUP | Diphenhydramine | Phenylpropanolamine | — | Bromhexine |
| Guaiaphenesin | | | | |

As everyone knows, a mild tickling at the back of one's throat induces a bout of cough. This is exactly what happens when the pharynx and larynx (parts of the throat) get irritated by infection or irritants, such as dust, fumes, or smoke. Therefore, our aim should be to reduce the irritation and this can be achieved by adopting such simple measures as giving up smoking, sucking cough lozenges or candy sugar, inhaling water vapours — either plain or medicated, and staying in a warm humid environment till the irritation is relieved.

For coughs originating from parts still lower down in the respiratory tract, numerous medications are available. Broadly these are of two types.

## Expectorants

These help in the production of more watery secretion in the respiratory passages and stimulate coughing by a reflex action from the stomach. Some examples of expectorants are *menthol, guaiacols, ammonium chloride, sodium citrate, potassium iodide, vasaka, balsam* of *tolu,* and volatile oils. Their action is usually very weak. The best expectorant is warm water!

**Some Commonly Prescribed Cough Suppressants**

| *Brand Names* | *Cough Suppressant* | + | *Antihistaminic* | + | *Decongestant* | + | *Other* |
|---|---|---|---|---|---|---|---|
| ALEX CAPSULES | *Dextromethorphon* | | *Chlorpheniramine* | | *Phenylpropanolamine* | | *Paracetamol* |
| ALEX COUGH LOZENGE | *Dextromethorphon* | | — | | — | | — |
| ASCORIL-D SYRUP | *Dextromethorphon* | | *Tripolidine* | | *Phenylpropnolamine* | | — |
| BENYLIN COUGH SYRUP | *Dextromethorphon* | | — | | *Pseudoephedrine* | | — |
| CHERICOF SOFGEL | *Dextromethorphon* | | *Chlorpheniramine* | | *Phenyl Propanolamine* | | — |
| CHERANA COUGH LOZENGE | *Noscapine* | | *Chlorpheniramine* | | — | | — |
| COREX SYRUP | *Codeine* | | *Chlorpheniramine* | | *Menthol* | | — |
| COREX DX SYRUP | *Dextromethorphan* | | *Chlorpheniramine* | | *Menthol* | | — |
| DELETUS-D SYRUP | *Dextromethorphan* | | *Tripolidine* | | *Phenylpropanolamine* | | — |
| DETIGON LINCTUS | *Chlophedianol* | | — | | *Menthol* | | *Ammonium Chloride* |
| EPHEDREX SYRUP | *Dextromethorphan* | | *Diphenhydramine* | | *Phenylpropanolamine* | | — |
| GRILINCTUS | *Dextromethorphan* | | *Chlorpheniramine-* | | *Guaiphenesin* | | — |
| MITS LINCTUS | *Codeine* | | *Chlorpheniramine* | | — | | — |
| CODEINAE CO SYRUP | | | | | | | |
| PHENSEDYL | *Codeine* | | *Chlorpheniramine* | | — | | — |
| PRENOXID | *Prenoxdiazine* | | — | | — | | — |
| SUDIN-D SYRUP | *Dextromethorphan* | | *Diphenhydramine* | | *Phenylpropanolamine* | | — |
| SUPRESSA | *Dextromethorphan* | | — | | — | | — |
| TUXYLIX | *Pholcodine* | | *Promethazine* | | *Phenylpropanolamine* | | — |
| TUXYNE | *Dextromethorphan* | | *Loratidine* | | *Pseudoephedine* | | *Caffeine, Aspirin* |
| ZEDEX | *Dextromethorphon* | | — | | *Menthol* | | *Bromhexine, Ammonium Chloride* |

A number of preparations contain drugs which produce liquefied and thin sputum (mucolytics). These drugs are *acetylcysteine* (MUCOMELT-A), *bromhexine, ambroxol, carbocysteine.* There are also available as a single ingredient preparations (see table). In other preparations antihistaminics are combined with expectorants. The idea is to suppress cough of allergic origin and help expectoration of sputum. In some of them a pain reliever is also added and such combinations are useful in common cold, coryza and influenza. These, however, cannot be considered to be ideal preparations.

### *Adverse Effects*

1. Ammonium salts may cause gastric irritation or abdominal pain and are nauseants.
2. Mucolytics *(bromhexine, ambroxol)* may cause running of nose and excessive formation of tears. They are irritant to stomach also.
3. Skin rash may occur in allergic individuals.

**Commonly Used Bronchodilator Expectorants**

| *Brand Names* | *Bronchodilators* | *Others* |
|---|---|---|
| ASTHALIN LIQUID | *Salbutamol* | *Guaiaphenesin* |
| BRICAREX LIQUID | *Terbutaline* | *Guaiaphenesin* |
| BRONCOREX LIQUID | *Terbutaline* | *Bromhexine, Guaiaphenesin* |
| MUCOSOL LIQUID | *Terbutaline* | *Bromhexine* |
| TUSQ-X LIQUID | *Terbutaline* | *Bromhexine, Guaiaphenesin* |
| VENTORLIN LIQUID | *Salbutamol* | *Guaiaphenesin* |

## Cough Sedatives Which Act on Cough Centres in Brain (Antitussives)

When the cough is dry, hacking, without production of sputum and is annoying (disturbs sleep) and hazardous (in patients of hernia, piles, heart disease and recent eye surgery) it is required to

**Selecting an Appropriate Cough Preparation**

Single ingredient preparations are hard to get as most are combinations with antihistaminics and decongestants. The choice of a suitable preparation is critical. As always, it is necessary to have a clear idea of what is intended to be achieved before starting its use.

1. For simple suppression of a dry hacking (useless) cough, linctus or syrup of *codeine, dextromethorphan* or *pholcodine* may be useful.
2. To increase bronchial secretion slightly and to liquefy the existing phlegm, plain or medicated vapour inhalation and expectorants may be used.
3. For a cough originating in the pharyngeal region, lozenges are effective. Warm saline-gargles sooth the inflamed throat. Some lozenges have benzocaine (a local anesthetic). This inhibits cough reflex.
4. If a bronchospasm is the cause of cough, bronchodilators can be used.
5. Steam inhalation directly or through vaporizer helps to cough out secretions easily.

Equally important are simple precautionary measures such as avoidance of alternate exposure to hot and cold (especially in infants who, after a warm bath, are exposed to the chill of a cold room), resisting the temptation to suck ice, or of having a cold drink immediately after an exhausting game on a hot summer evening, avoiding a smoggy or dusty atmosphere and giving up smoking. So next time when you have a cough, ponder a while on its cause and how you could have avoided it.

**Some Commonly used Cough Expectorants**

| *Brand Names* | *Expectorant ingredients* + | *Antihistaminic* + | *Other* |
|---|---|---|---|
| AVIL EXPECTORANT | *Ammonium chloride, menthol* | *Pheniramine maleate* | — |
| BENADRYL COUGH FORMULA | *Ammonium chloride, menthol* | *Diphenhydramine* | *Alcohol* |
| BRONOLAX* | *Ammonium chloride* | *Diphenhydramine* | *Ephedrine, Codeine* |
| CLISTIN DMR* | *Ammonium chloride, Sodium citrate* | *Chlorpheniramine* | *Dextromethaphen* |
| COFURA EXPECTORANT | *Ammonium chloride, Menthol, Sodium citrate* | *Diphenhydramine* | — |
| COSOME EXPECTORANT | *Bromhexine* | *Chlorpheniramine* | *Phenylpropanolamine* |
| DASLIN EXPECTORANT | *Ammonium Chloride, Sodium citrate, Menthol* | *Diphenhydramine* | *Alcohol* |
| DILOSYN EXPECTORANT | *Ammonium Chloride, Sodium citrate, Menthol* | *Methdilazine* | — |
| GRILINCTUS* | *Ammonium chloride* | *Chlorpheniramine* | *Dextromethorphan Guaiaphenesin* |
| PIRITON | *Ammonium chloride, Sodium citrate* | *Chlorpheniramine* | — |
| POLARAMINE EXPECTORANT | — | *Dexchlorpheniramine* | *Pseudoephedrine, Guaiaphenesin* |

*These drugs have combinations of expectorants and sedatives.

be controlled or suppressed by drugs. Most of these drugs act in the brain, on an area which is responsible for sending messages of coughing.

**Codeine** (CODINE LINCTUS/TAB, COREX, EXIPLON)
It has been in use for dry cough but constipation is the main adverse effect. It should not be used in bronchial asthma. It is given in a dose of 2 to 3 times daily.

**Dextromethorphan** (ALEX, DELETUS-D, CLISTIM-DMR, LASTUSS-LA)
It is a common ingredient in lozenges (COF-Q LOZENGE, ALEX) and syrups. Antihistaminics and decongestants are also combined. It does not cause constipation but should not be used in newborns and during pregnancy. Dizziness, drowsiness and difficulty of walking are adverse effects (usual dose 10 to 20mg two to three times a day). *Pholcodeine, oxeladin, chlorphedianol* are found in some preparations.

**Noscapine** (COSCOPIN LINCTUS, NOSCAPAX tab)
It does not have sedative effect and no addiction is reported. It is equal in efficacy to codeine in a dose of 15 to 30 mg three times a day. In some preparations antihistaminic or decongestant drugs are combined. It can cause nausea, vomiting and headache and is never given in asthmatics.

*Pholcodine* is given in a dose of 10 to 15 mg three times a day, *Noscapine* 15 mg three times a day and *Pipazethate* 40 mg three times a day.

***Note:*** These preparations should not be used for children as there are cases of drowsiness and coma occurring due to inadvertent use.

*Cough sedatives which act peripherally on throat and air passages: Benzonatate* is given in a dose of 100 to 200 mg three times a day, and *Levodropropizine* (RAPITUS) 30 to 60 mg three times a day.

*Pharyngeal Demulcents*

- Act by soothing,coating inflammed surface and by increasing salivary flow. Irritation is reduced so cough decreases!
- Linctuses/Syrups/Lozenges — medicated with menthol
- Lemon drops
- Aromatic Tincture Benzoin with steam inhalation — increases watery mucus and protects mucosa

# 10

# Drugs Used in Diabetes

••••••

Diabetes is the term generally used for the condition *diabetes mellitus (DM)* in which there is absolute or relative lack of insulin in the body. Insulin, a hormone synthesized and secreted by the pancreas, is responsible for lowering the circulating levels of the blood sugar (glucose). In diabetes, the blood sugar which should normally be in the range of 70 to 110 mg per 100 ml of blood, increases and may appear in the urine.

In year 2000, the total burden of diabetes in the world was 171 millions which is projected to rise to 366 millions by 2030. For India, the corresponding figures are 31.7 millions and 79.4 millions respectively*. The diabetes starts early at a younger age than the western population and patients may or maynot be overweight. There is a considerable socio-economic burder of diabetes**. It has been estimated that over 2% of India's population suffers from this disease Diabetes has a hereditary component and often runs in families. If both the mother and father are diabetic, there are more than 90% chances that their children will also be diabetics. If one parent is diabetic, there are 40% chances of diabetes in children.

***Symptoms of Diabetes:*** A diabetic person has three important symptoms which usually indicate the presence of the disease. There is an increased appetite, thirst and excessive formation of urine. However, the diagnosis is confirmed by urine or blood sugar check or when a patient suffers from some of the complications of diabetes such as delayed healing of wounds, premature vascular disease, a neuritic pain, or diminution of vision. It is vital to know that you are diabetic before you discover it as a result of some complication. An early diagnosis may not only retard serious complications but may also prevent the shortening of life expectancy. Quite often patients are without symptoms and a high blood sugar may be a coincidental finding during routine annual check- ups. Nevertheless, even it there are no obvious symptoms it must be confirmed and treated.

---

* http://www.who.int/diabetes/facts/worldfigures/en/

** Ramchandran, *A. Socioeconomic Burden of Diabetes Journal of Assoc. Physicians of India,* 2007; Vol 55(Supplement) pp.9-12.

**Confirmatory Test**

| Blood sugar (mg%) | Normal | Impaired glucose tolerance | Diabetes |
|---|---|---|---|
| Fasting | <100 | 100-125 | >126* |
| 2 hr post glucose** | <140 | 140-199 | >200 |

*Fasting blood glucose, if >126 mg% is diagnostic if confirmed on subsequent day.
** 75g glucose dissolved in 300 mg of water is taken after an overnight fasting by the persons who are on at least 150 –200 gm of carbohydrates daily for 3 days before the test
The factors which may influence the Glucose Tolerance Test (GTT) are emotional or physical stress, fever, endocrinal disorders, heart or liver disease, infective illness, and drugs like *thiazide* diuretics, *corticosteroids*, and contraceptives.

If fasting blood glucose is more than 126% and/or casual (random) reading is 200 mg% or more, in the presence of symptoms, there is no need to do glucose tolerance test. However, if fasting blood glucose is less than 126 mg% and symptoms are suggestive, an Oral Glucose Tolerance Test (OGTT) is performed. For this, the patient is given a carbohydrate diet (containing more than 150g of carbohydrates) for three days before the test. His activity is kept at a normal level, as prolonged bedrest may show false positive results. The patient is asked to go for the test on an empty stomach; his fasting blood and urine samples are collected and then he is given 75g glucose (100g glucose in pregnant women). Glucose is taken in 250ml of water in five minutes. His blood and urine sample are collected at hourly intervals for two hours for an estimation of the glucose concentration.

***Types of Diabetes Mellitus:*** Based on the functional state of the pancreas and the age of onset, diabetes has been divided into two categories: 1) Insulin dependent diabetes mellitus (IDDM) or *type-1*, and 2) Non-insulin dependent diabetes mellitus (NIDDM) or *type-2*.

IDDM starts in childhood, adolescence, or young adult life. Patients in these categories have an abrupt onset of symptoms, proneness to ketoacidotic coma, and require exogenous insulin for normal well-being. The exact cause of IDDM is not known. It is thought to be allergic (auto-immune) or infective (viral infection by picorna group) in origin. In contrast, NIDDM starts at an older age, usually above 40 years, and increase slowly with a few symptoms. Patients of NIDDM are not dependent on exogenous insulin for normal well-being. It usually besets those people whose pancreas still has some capacity to synthesize and secrete insulin. Therefore, it is relatively

**Monitoring and Control**

The control of diabetes means the following:

*Fasting blood glucose:* 90-130 mg%.

*2 hr blood glucose:* 150 mg% or less

Glycosylated haemoglobin <8 mg%

Pay now and benefit later is a dictum all diabetics should know. It has been proved that tight control of elevated blood glucose may prevent or delay microvascular (small vessels) complications. It prevents organ damage (kidney, heart, nervous system and eye).

A blood test ,HbA1c (Glycosylated haemoglobin) gives state of control over 8-12 weeks and fructose levels in blood give idea of control over preceding 1-2 weeks. Monitoring is done by home glucose measurement in urine *(Glucotest, diastix, strips)* or blood *(Glucometer* ACCUCHEK). Recently, a low cost glucometer (ONE-TOUCH HORIZON) is made available which is affordable for regular home blood glucose monitoring. For early detection of complications other blood tests (lipids, creatinine) urine albumin levels, eye examination and electrocardiogram are done annually.

easy to manage NIDDM as compared to IDDM, in which the only alternative is to replace the insulin. There are four pillars to manage diabetes- 1) ***Diet*** 2) ***Insulin*** 3) ***Exercise*** and 4) ***Tablets*** *[**DIET**-* to remember]

## Treatment

Role of Diet and Exercise: The basic treatment of diabetes still constitutes the control of diet. However, it is difficult to change the dietary habits and most diabetics find it almost impossible to adhere to a strictly regulated diet (a diabetic has more weakness for sweets than a non-diabetic). Fortunately, according to the latest concept in treatment, drastic restrictions in diet are not necessary. The nutritional requirements of a diabetic person are the same as that of a non-diabetic. At one time it was believed that the carbohydrate intake should be cut down drastically, but now it is not considered to be that important. In diabetes, the metabolism of fats and proteins is directed in such a way that these are broken down into glucose. These effects have been correctly described as 'in diabetes, the fats and proteins burn in the flame of carbohydrates'. A drastic cut in carbohydrates further enhances the breakdown of fats and proteins, leading to serious consequences. For this reason it is recommended that 40% of the patient's diet should be made up of carbohydrates in the form of cereals, vegetables, and fruits. *Direct sugar, such as sweets, syrups, candies, and pastries are best avoided.* Fat should be restricted to 60 to 80 g per day; it is known to increase the risk factors of atherosclerosis in diabetics. Unsaturated fats like *til,* groundnut, *kardi* or sunflower oil are preferable to saturated fats like butter, *ghee,* animal fat, coconut oil, and hydrogenated vegetable oils.

The principal aim of dietary management is to have smaller and frequent meals to avoid a sudden increase in blood sugar which occurs after meals. The total caloric intake should be about 20 calories per kilogram of body weight. To this 200 to 300 calories per day should be added if the patient is a thin, young male and the same amount should be deducted if the patients is an old, obese female. However, the tendency of many patients to regard the prescription of a high carbohydrate diet as license to venture into the area of sweets and pastries should be curbed.

In type-2 diabetes, the patient is usually overweight, and reducing the caloric intake and regular exercise to restore the normal body weight help in controlling the disease if it is mild.

## Drugs

Oral anti-diabetes and insulin preparation the drugs used in Diabetes Mellitus.

### Oral Anti-Diabetic Drugs

These are effective in type-2 diabetes in which at least a part of the pancreas is functioning. Oral anti-diabetic drugs, given orally, are more commonly employed than insulin which is always required to be given by injection. They decrease blood sugar either by enhancing insulin secretion from the pancreas or by increasing its effects on body tissues. They show the best results in obese people who have recently become diabetic. They are divided into four groups and are given in the table on next page along with their common trade names, average daily doses, and the duration of action.

## Sulfonylureas

These are effective in the mild type of type-2 diabetes in which daily insulin requirement is less than 40 units. *Sulfonylureas* can be given along with insulin or even replaced by the later or vice versa, depending upon the extent of rise of blood sugar. *Tolbutamide* and *Chlorpropamide* are seldom used now a days. *Glibenclamide* (also named as GLIBURIDE in USA) is the most commonly used drug in one or two doses (before breakfast and dinner). *Glipizide* is faster acting drug. *Gliclazide* may delay occurrence of retinopathy due to reduction of free radicals and antiplatelet effects. Glimepiride has strong effects on tissues to utilize glucose.

**Oral Anti-Diabetic Drugs**

| *Drugs* | *Brand Names* | *Dose/day* | *No. of Doses/day* |
|---|---|---|---|
| I. Sulfonylureas | | | |
| *Tolbutamide* | RASTINON, ORINASE | 0.5 to 1.0 g | 2 to 4 |
| *Chlorpropamide* | DIABINESE, CHLORFORMIN | 0.25 to 0.5 g | 1 |
| *Glibenclamide (glyburide)* | DAONIL, BETANASE | 2.5 to 10 mg | 1 to 2 |
| *Gliclazide* | DIAMICRON, AZUCON | 40 to 240 mg | 1 to 2 |
| *Glipizide* | GLYNASE, GLUCOLIP | 5 to 20 mg | 1 to 2 |
| *Glimepiride* | AMARYL, GLIMER | 1 to 4 mg | 1 |
| II. Biguanides | | | |
| *Phenformin* | DBI-TD, DBI | Rarely used | — |
| *Metformin* | GLYCIPHAGE, GLYCOMET | 0.5 to 2.0 g | 2 to 4 |
| III. Glitazones | | | |
| *Rosiglitazone* | ROSICON, ENSELIN | 2 to 8 mg | 1 to 2 |
| *Pioglitazone* | PIOGLIT, PIOZONE | 15 to 45 mg | 1 |
| IV. Meglitinides-regulate post meal blood sugar | | | |
| *Repaglinide* | EUREPA | 1.5 to 6 mg | 3 to 4 |
| *Nateglinide* | GLINATE | 180 to 480 mg | 3 to 4 |
| V. Inhibitors of glucose absorption | | | |
| *Acarbose* | GLUCOBAY, K-CARE | 50 to 100 mg with each meals | 2 to 3 |
| *Miglitol* | MIGTOR, DIAMIG | 25 to 50 mg with each meals | 2 to 3 |
| *Voglibose* | VOLIBO | 0.2 to 0.3 mg with | 2 |

***Adverse Effects:*** The adverse effects of these drugs are few and generally mild. The most common adverse effects encountered are gastric uneasiness, diarrhoea and allergic skin rash. In rare cases, these drugs may cause depression of bone marrow. *Chlorpropamide* has been reported to affect the liver and may cause jaundice and intolerance to alcohol is reported with *chlorpropamide* and *glibenclamide.* If the dose is too high, these may cause an excessive lowering of blood sugar. This is specially true of *glibenclamide.*

### *Precautions*

1. The drug should be taken with meals to minimise gastric distress.
2. These drugs should be used cautiously by patients of heart, kidney, or liver disease.
3. Alcohol should be restricted when taking these drugs. Their interaction may cause a feeling of unpleasantness and flushing of the face (alcohol intolerance).

4. Certain drugs like *co-timoxazole, warfarin* and *alcohol* enhance the action of *sulfonylureas,* and care should be taken if these are used concurrently. Sometimes it may be advisable to reduce the dose of *sulfonylureas* if any one of these drugs are being taken.
5. These drugs should not be taken during pregnancy.
6. They should be given with caution to the old or debilitated and to those who eat poorly and irregularly.

**Note:** Many large scale trials have been done to find the impact of drug induced control of diabetes on its complications. The UKPDS and DCCT studies finally reported that oral medicines do not increase the cardiovascular complications as was thought earlier. Intensive control by diet and drugs can prevent or delay the complications in DM-2.

### Biguanides

**Phenformin,** (DBI-TD, DBI), **Metformin** (GLYCIPHAGE, WALAPHAGE)

These drugs decrease the intestinal absorption of carbohydrates, promote their oxidation in the tissues and also reduce conversion of fats and proteins into glucose in the liver. They usually reduce elevated blood glucose levels only and do not produce hypoglycemia (fall in blood glucose levels below normal).

***Adverse Effects:*** *Phenformin* causes abdominal discomfort, nausea, vomiting, and diarrhoea in 15% to 25% of cases, but with its sustained release preparation, the frequency of these adverse effects is much less. The most serious adverse effect of this drug is lactic acidosis (accumulation of lactic acid in the body) which not only causes muscular pain in the legs and difficulty in breathing, but can also prove to be fatal. The drug may also cause allergy in the form of skin rashes and itching; in rare cases it may cause allergic shock. *Phenformin* is rarely used in India. *Metformin* is a better tolerated and most commonly used drug. It is taken independently or combined with other drug(s). It is less likely to cause lactic acidosis. It is also effective in young females with polycystic ovarian disease with infertility.

#### *Precautions*

1. In case of severe abdominal discomfort is severe, the drug should be taken along with or after meals.
2. If there are any symptoms of lactic acid accumulation such as pain in the muscle, the drug should be stopped immediately. Also stop the drug if allergic reactions occur.
3. *Metformin* decreases the absorption of vitamin $B_{12}$ in high doses.
4. It should be used cautiously by those suffering from a heart, kidney, or liver disease.
5. It causes harmful effects to the unborn child and should not be taken during pregnancy.
6. It should be used with caution by the old or debilitated and by those who eat very poorly or irregularly.

### Thiazolidinediones (Glitazones)

**Pioglitazone,** (PIOZONE, PIOGLIT), **ROSIGLITAZONE** (ROSICON, ROSINORM)

**Pioglitazone:** It enhances entry of glucose in muscles and fats and reduces formation of glucose from fats and proteins in liver. These effects are due to enhanced effects of insulin on tissues and are brought about by changes in functions of gene that regulates fat metabolism. An added advantage is that bad lipids (triglycerides) are reduced and good lipid (HDL) levels are increased. It is not useful in juvenile (type-1) DM. For type-2 DM it can be used alone or in combination with *metformin* or *glimepiride.*

***Adverse Effects:*** The drug may increase body weight. It may cause headache, muscle pain and anaemia. Hypoglycemia usually does not occur when *pioglitazone* is used alone. One requires monitoring of liver function. Women taking oral contraceptives may have unwanted pregnancy due to adverse interaction. Therefore, other methods of preventing pregnancy should be adopted. Congestive heart disease may worsen and swelling over feet is also reported. *Pioglitazone* should be avoided in such cases.

**Rosiglitazone:** It has same effects except changes in lipid levels do not occur. There are less adverse drug interactions of *rosiglitazone* as compared to *pioglitazone*. Excessive fall in blood glucose may occur more frequently with *pioglitazone* than *rosiglitazone* when *levofloxacin* is used concurrently.

### Meglitinides

**Repaglinide** (EUREPA, RAPILIN), **Nateglinide** (GLINATE, NATELIDE)

These drugs release insulin in response to meals and therefore regulate post-meal hyperglycemia (rise in blood glucose after meals) in adults. These should be avoided in liver disease. *Repaglinide* is ingested 10 to 30 minutes before meals. Side effects are mild headache, dyspepsia, joint pain, weight gain. It can be given with other drugs.

**Acarbose** (DIABOSE, GLUCOBAY,K-CARB Tab,50 mg)

It inhibits the enzyme which is present in the intestines. This enzyme is needed to convert carbohydrate into glucose. Therefore when taken with meals, it reduces the rise of blood glucose as it is not formed and absorbed from intestines. It may cause gaseousness and loose stools. Acarbose should always be taken *with meals. Miglitol* and *voglibose* are similar acting drugs but cause less distension and gases.

### Combined Drug Therapy

Since antidiabetic drugs lower blood glucose by independent and differing mechanisms, these drugs are sometimes combined for better effect if one drug given alone fails to control the diabetic state. Thus in secondary *sulfonylurea* failures, *biguanides* can be added. The following combinations are readily available:

**Some Oral Anti-Diabetic Drugs**

| *Combination Drugs* | *Brand Names* |
|---|---|
| *Glimepiride* 1mg + *Metformin* 500 mgSR | GLYCIPHAGE-G, GLYCOMET-GP K-GLIM-M, AMARYL-M |
| *Glimepiride* + *Metformin* + *Pioglitazone* 15 to 30 mg | TRIBET, GLYCIPHAGE-GP |
| *Pioglitazone* + *Metformin* | GLUCONORM-P, PIOGLIT-MF, WALAPHAGE-PZ |
| *Glibenclamide* 5 mg + *Metformin* | GLUCORED, DUOTROL-SR, DAONIL M |
| *Glibenclamide* + *Metformin* + *Pioglitazone* | TRIGLYCOMET |
| *Glipizide* + *Metformin* | DIBIZIDE-M,GLYNASE-MF, GLIPIMET |
| *Gliclazide* 80 mg + *Metformin* | DIANORM-M, GLYCHEK-M Forte, GLYCINORM-M, WALFORMIN. |

Note the subtle differences in the names of these medications. Therefore be sure what actually are you taking.

The drugs given below have also been marketed for better control of a diabetic's blood sugar: *Guargum* (CARBOTARD, DIAT-AIM) and *Glucomannan* (DIETMANN) which contain a high molecular weight hydrocolloidal material which forms a gel in the gastro-intestinal tract and slows carbohydrate absorption. It reduces sudden rise in blood glucose after food intake. One sachet of *glucomannan* (1g) is taken before main meal. The dose of *guargum* is increased gradually by starting with a 2.5g dose once or twice a day and when tolerated It is increased to 1 sachet (5g) taken two or three times a day. *Chromium picolinate* increases insulin action on tissue as it acts as a co-factor for insulin action. It is used in doses of 200 $\mu$g to 500 $\mu$g /per day.

### Newer drugs

**Incretins:** These are interesting drugs as they induce insulin release following oral glucose and meals.

**Exenatide:** It is obtained from the saliva of venomous lizards and at present drug controller of India has permitted its use by subcutaneous injections in 'difficult to control' cases.

*Sitagliptin* (100 mg, once a day, orally) is not yet available in India. *Pramlintide* is undergoing trials.

## Insulin

In the history of medical research, there has perhaps been no episode more dramatic than the discovery of insulin. Dr. Fredric G. Banting, a young physician, started his work on 10 dogs. Mr Best and Mr Noble, two undergraduate students, were asked to assist him for 4 weeks each. Mr Best assisted Dr Banting throughout the entire work.

On July 27, 1922, they removed the pancreas from a dog, chopped it into small pieces in a chilled mortar frozen in saline, and prepared an extract. When 5 ml of this extract was injected into a normal dog, it caused the blood sugar to fall from 200 mg to 110 mg per 100 ml. They

### What is the Role of Insulin in Our Body?

All cells in our body need energy in order to function normally. This energy is derived from the food we eat which is made up of carbohydrates, proteins, and fats. After digestion, the carbohydrate, which mainly comes from cereals and starch such as wheat, rice, fruit, etc. is converted into glucose, or simple sugar. This glucose is the main source of energy for all the body cells. Excess glucose is stored in the liver and muscles as a compound called glycogen.

The glucose must enter cells for generation of energy. It can enter the cells only if the insulin, which is a hormone, is available in adequate amount. When the insulin is either inadequate, absent, or abnormal, it is difficult for the glucose to enter the cells and provide energy.

In addition to helping glucose enter the cells and providing them with energy, insulin is also involved in the storage of glycogen in the liver and muscles. Thus, it is involved in storage of reserve energy. In between meals when the cells need energy, glycogen is converted back into glucose and burnt for energy needs.

Normally, pancreas releases insulin proportional to the amount of food we eat. The beta cells monitor blood glucose levels regularly and release the amount of insulin necessary to use the glucose in the blood. In diabetes, the pancreas either does not produce insulin or produces too little of it. Thus, the blood glucose cannot be used effectively by the cells and excess glucose cannot be stored in the liver. It goes as a waste in urine.

repeated the study on another dog from which the pancreas had been removed and found that the blood sugar fell more dramatically from 300 mg to 170 mg per 100 ml. It was from this extract that insulin was later isolated as the chemically active principle.

On January 11, 1922, a patient of diabetes was first treated with the pancreatic extract and Mr Banting and his professor, Dr Macleod, received the Nobel Prize in Medicine and Physiology. Banting shared his part of prize with Mr Best, his student.

## Insulin Preparations

Insulin is ordinarily obtained from beef or pork. Pork *insulin* is nearer to human insulin as compared to beef. In recent years human insulin has been prepared by a semi-synthetic process and is available for use in several countries including India. The advent of *recombinant DNA* technology for the manufacture of insulin greatly reduces the cost. It can be safely used by persons allergic to insulin of animal origin. At present most of the insulin preparations in use are highly purified porcine or human varieties.

*Insulin* and its preparations are used in cases of type-1 and the severe type of type-2 diabetes and for those patients of diabetes in whom controlled diet or oral anti-diabetic drugs have failed to maintain satisfactory blood glucose levels. *Insulin* is also given when it is not advisable to give oral anti-diabetic drugs, such as in pregnancy and to patients of heart, liver, or kidney disease Furthermore, if disease is of a severe nature, causing breakdown of fats and proteins and resulting in coma, it is advisable to use soluble insulin which is then a life-saver. It is also used in conditions of stress like surgery and infection.

Preparations of insulin and their varying periods of onset and duration of action are given in the following table:

**Different Insulins and Their Action Time**

| *Group* | *Insulin Preparations/ Appearance* | *Time of peak action/hrs.* | *Duration of action/hrs.* | *Can be mixed with* |
|---|---|---|---|---|
| Fast Acting | *Crystalline (regular) soluble and clear* | 2 to 4 | 6 to 8 | Lente |
| | *Semi Lente-Cloudy* | 3 to 6 | 12 to 14 | — |
| | *Human regular* | 2 | 6 to 8 | — |
| Intermediate Acting | *Lente-Cloudy* | 8 to 10 | 20 to 24 | Regular/ semi-Lente |
| | *NPH(isophane) Cloudy* | 8 to 10 | 20 to 24 | |
| | *Human NPH* | 6 to 7 | 10 to 20 | — |
| Long Acting | *Ultra Lente-Cloudy Protamine Zine-Cloudy* | 14 to 20 | 24 to 36 | Regular |

Lente = Semi Lente 30% + Ultra Lente 70%

**Storage:** *Insulin* should never be stored in the freezer compartment of the fridge or allowed to freeze, should this happen, the *insulin* should be discarded. Similarly, after use do not keep it near gas stove in kitchen near TV cabinet or on the top of refrigerator.

## Choice of Insulin

The choice of an *insulin* depends upon the condition of the patient. In emergencies such as diabetic coma, *crystalline insulin* (only soluble insulin) is preferred because of its quick onset of action. It is repeated at 6-hour intervals given intravenously usually, until the situation is under control. *Crystalline insulin* is also employed in combination with intermediate-acting insulin preparations for quick action. However, a dose of intermediate-acting *insulins* taken before breakfast is effective in controlling most cases of diabetes, other than some cases of juvenile diabetes in which there is a marked rise in blood sugar during the night and in which, an additional evening dose may be needed. The use of long-acting preparations, with the hope of a single injection for controlling diabetes, has been disappointing and is not advocated. Premixed mixture of crystalline and lente insulin *(Biphasic insulin)* are convenient for tighter control of fasting and post meal blood glucose elevation. A large number of such preparations are available in the market. A convenient device is insulin pen (NAVOLET) which has premixed insulin mixture and can be put into packet by executives or others who are on the move. At present it is expensive.

## Newer Insulins

Newer *insulins* are now available. They are 3 to 5 times more expensive. They have the advantage that *insulin* allergy, fat loss at the site of injection, and sometimes, fat accumulation, occur less frequently. The possibility of the formation of anti-*insulin* antibodies is also less. At present these are increasingly used.

**Newer Insulins (Available in India as 40 units/ml)**

| Pork Insulins | Characteristics | Human Insulins | Characteristics |
|---|---|---|---|
| 1. ACTRAPID, RAPIDICA | Neutral, Short action | ACTRAPID HM | Short acting |
| 2. ILETIN-L | Insulin, Zinc suspension | HUMAN INSULATARD | Purified NPH insulin |
| | | HUMAN MONOTARD | Purified insulin Zinc suspension |
| 3. ILETIN- NPH | Insulin NPH | HUMAN MIXTARD | Premixed 30:70 & 50:50 |
| 4. LENTARD, ZIMULIN | Premixed 30:70 mixture | HUMAN RAPIMIX | Premixed 30:70 |
| 5. MIXTARD | Premixed 30:70 mixture | HUMAN ZINULIN | Premixed 30:70 |
| 6. RAPIMIX | Premixed 30:70 mixture | HUMINSULIN 30:70 & 50:50 | Premixed 30:70 & 50:50 regular + NPH |
| | | HUMINSULIN-L & HUMINSULIN-N | Human Ultra lente (long acting PZI) |
| | | INSUMAN 25/75 | Premixed 25% short 75% intermediate |
| | | INSUMAN 50:50 | Premixed 50% short 50% intermediate |

### Insulin Pen-devices

Several types of insulins are also available as pen like devices NOVOPEN-3, INSULATARD NOVOLET, NOVOMIX-30 FLEXPEN, LANTUS OPTIPEN. It must be remembered that these pen devices usually have 100 units/ml instead of 40 units/ml of insulin. Also it must be noted that U-40 syringes may not be used for U-80 and U-100 vials as available in western countries.

**Newer Insulin analogues**

| Type | Onset | Peak | Duration |
|---|---|---|---|
| Insulin-Lispro(HUMOLOG) | 5 to 15 min | 60 to 90 min | 3 to 4 hours |
| Insulin-Aspart(NOVOMIX) | 5 to 15 min | 60 to 90 min | 3 to 4 hours |
| Insulin Glulisine | 5 to 15 min | 60 to 90 min | 3 to 4 hours |
| Insulin glargine(LANTUS) | 90 min | Flat levels | 18 hours |

**Nasal Insulin Inhalers:** In order to avoid injections inhaled insulin is developed. This will soon be available for use in India.

## Artificial Pancreas and Pancreatic transplantation

Battery operated devices with glucose sensors are now available for difficult to treat children with type-1 DM. They are costly. Pancreatic transplantation (Islet cells are injected into portal vein which goes to liver) is still a dream.

***Dosage:*** The dose varies with the severity of the condition and the response of the patient. Repeated estimation of blood sugar during the treatment is helpful in adjusting the dose. In general, the treatment is started with an intermediate-acting preparation and a dose of 10 to 15 units is given; 2/3 dose is given before breakfast and 1/3 dose before dinner. This is increased by 5 units per day with a constant monitoring of glucose levels of blood and urine till satisfactory control is achieved.

All the preparations of *insulin* are ineffective orally and have to be injected under the skin. Recently, computer-assisted, battery-driven implantable devices (insulin pumps) have become available, which inject *insulin* appropriate to the requirements. Usually highly purified *insulins* are used in these devices. It will be a major breakthrough in this field if someone discovers a drug as effective as *insulin* that can be given orally.

***Adverse Effects:*** The most common adverse effect is hypoglycaemia. Hypoglycaemia may be caused by the delay or omission of meals and unexpected exertion. The symptoms of hypoglycaemia include intense hunger, sweating, palpitation of the heart, tremors, weakness, and irritability. These symptoms can be recognized early and can be relieved by sugar, glucose or sweets in 10 to 20 minutes. If you are taking acarbose with insulin injection then use glucose only and not household sugar. It is to be noted that long standing diabetics may not notice all of these symptoms of low blood sugar.

*Insulin* may cause allergic reaction at the site of the injection, characterized by stinging and itching sensations associated with reddening and swelling of the skin. Generalized allergic reactions are rare. Human *insulin* does not cause allergic reactions. Repeated injections of insulin at the same site may cause depression or elevation at the injection site (Lipodystrophy). Rarely patient may not respond to insulin (due to insulin resistance). These problems are uncommon with human insulins.

**Alcohol Consumption: Never 'One for the Road....'**

The question of whether a diabetic can take alcohol is often asked. There can be no hard and fast rule but if you are on *insulin*, alcohol can cause enhanced and more prolonged decrease in blood glucose by enhancing insulin action.

This means that if you are a gentleman and suffer from diabetes, behave like a 'gentleman'. If invited over for cocktails, do go, take a drink or two and come back home for your frugal supper. Don't stay beyond the second round.

If you do, you will also stay for the last one 'for the road', synonymous, for diabetics with 'for the hospital'. The decision has to be yours and not your host's. Flushing and palpitation may occur in those who have genetic tendency and are taking *chlorpropamide* and *glibenclamide* and yet consume alcohol.

***Precautions***

1. If you are taking *insulin* by self-injection, use disposable insulin syringes only.
2. If you are likely to miss a meal or going to exert physically, reduce the dose of *insulin.*
3. If any symptoms of hypoglycaemia appear, take sugar or glucose.
4. If any allergic reaction occurs, consult the doctor immediately.
5. Rotate the site of insulin injection i.e., start from one thigh, then rotate to abdominal wall then forearm then upper arm after one side rotate to the next side.

**Artificial Sweeteners**

In order to satiate our taste for sweets artificial sweeteners are now available in the market.

*Saccharin* (SWEETEX drops and pellets) is an old one and is 300-500 times as sweet as sugar. It gives a bitter after-taste and is associated with bladder cancer. Its use is discouraged.

*Cyclamate* is also associated with cancer therefore should not be used.

*Aspartame* (EQUAL-18 mg) It is 180-200 times as sweet as sugar but it cannot be used for baking and cooking. Its calorie value is negligible.

*Sucralose* (SUGAR-FREE pellets, one pellet is equal to 1 tsp of sugar, SUCRALITE granules) is 600 times as sweet as sugar and can be used with cooking.

*Acesulfame* (SWEET-ONE) can also be used during baking and cooking.

*Neotame* (NUTRASWEET) is 8000 times as sweet as sugar.

Fructose is a natural sugar and it does not need insulin for utilization. Therefore it only mildly raises blood glucose levels.

Sugar containing alcohols (Polyols) such as *sorbitol* and *xylitol* are commonly used in sugar-free icecreams, and as vegetable and fruit sweeteners. In excess these may also raise blood glucose levels.

**Can diabetes be prevented?**

Work is being done to achieve this. Attempts to delay the occurrence of frank diabetes in those who are likely to develop type-1 diabetes by the use of immune suppressants have shown a limited success. Prevention of occurrence of type-2 diabetes by regular exercise and *metformin* shows that such treatment may actually reduce the risk of developing. Studies are being carried out in India in pregnant mothers to find out the glucose abnormalities and their value in finding out the probability of diabetes in neonates.

# 11

# Drugs Used in Diarrhoea

Diarrhoea is one of the great killers of children in India. It is characterized by frequent passage of liquid or semisolid stools and may be accompanied by abdominal (griping) pain. When diarrhoea is associated with abdominal pain and passage of blood and mucous due to infection or inflammation of the intestines, it is called dysentery. In these conditions there is an excessive loss of fluids and salts from the body. Diarrhoea associated with vomiting, may lead to serious consequences like dehydration shock and death. Infants, children, and elderly debilitated persons are more susceptible to dehydration, and for this reason diarrhoea is a more serious problem in them than in young adults.

**Causes of Diarrhoea:** Diarrhoea may be non-specific as is caused by fear, anxiety or apprehension, and indigestion. People on the move are often afflicted with traveller's diarrhoea due to the change in environment. Specific diarrhoea is caused by infection in the intestines, a systemic disease, or by drugs. Three mechanisms operate in causing diarrhoea: 1) Increased formation of fluid; 2) Increased activity of gut (bowels) and 3) Bacterial overgrowth.

**What Is to Be Done for Diarrhoea?** The first step is to discover the cause of diarrhoea. Infection in the intestines is a common cause by contaminated food or water. It may also be due to viruses (in children), bacterial toxins or bacterial infection. In last cases treatment with anti-bacterial drugs is necessary.

In India diarrhoea is very common during the wedding season when one feast follows another. In such cases, diarrhoea comes under control by itself or may require symptomatic treatment. Certain food like ice-creams, cheese, chocolates (all have lactose, sugar) and soft drinks (fructose sugar) can cause diarrhoea. This type of diarrhoea occurs in those who have lactose iIntolerance.

Diarrhoea may be secondary to some diseases like cholera, typhoid, allergic disorders, or a complication of diabetes. It can be controlled by treating the underlying disease. Chronic (longer lasting) diarrhoea is due to malabsorption syndrome, wheat allergy or tuberculosis.

Some drugs like broad-spectrum *antibiotics (ampicillin* and *tetracyclines)* and *purgative* may cause diarrhoea. In these cases reduction of doses or withdrawal of the drug is suggested. A potentially serious condition is pseudomembranous enterocolitis which occurs on use of powerful antibiotics.

## Treatment and Drugs

In most cases diarrhoea is due to a short lasting disturbance but is associated with loss of fluid and salts. Thus the greatest problem caused by diarrhoea is dehydration (excessive loss of fluids and salts like sodium, potassium, calcium, and magnesium). To replace these fluids and salts, a rehydration powder WHO-ORS formula dissolved in water, should be given at frequent intervals.

### Drugs

Diarrhoea leads to dehydration which accounts for more than two-third of the deaths due to diarrhoea. This dehydration can be prevented by ensuring that the fluid lost in diarrhoea is replaced by increasing the intake of fluids available at home and an oral rehydration solution. Home- available fluids (HAF) include *chhach, lassi, neembu pani,* light tea, *daal ka pani, chawal ka maand*, and salt-sugar solution. In the case of a child, more of these home-available fluids should be given as the requirement is higher.

Besides oral rehydration salts (ORS) which contain a mixture of sodium chloride, sodium bicarbonate or citrate, potassium chloride and glucose can be given for greater efficacy in the form of solutions in water. In children the ORS is able to reduce the significant number of deaths due to diarrhoea (by at least 90%). Ever since the ORS has been made available, this has made the job of treating such patients easy and with great success at low cost. ORS recommended by the UNICEF/WHO is available at all chemists' shops under various trade names. This is also available at all government hospitals and dispensaries free of cost. Similar preparations with different composition are also available, but it is advisable to insist on WHO formula when buying ORS.

## Anti-motility drugs in diarrhoea

Since intestine movements are increased, a number of drugs are used to oppose such excessive activity of gut. But overall utility is limited and these are often misused.

**Preparing and Using ORS-WHO Formula**

1. Take 5 glasses full of boiled, cooled and clean drinking water. Mix one packet of ORS. Stir till solids are dissolved.
2. Use entire solution in 24 hours. Prepare fresh solution daily.
3. Give ORS after every loose stools.
4. Children below 2 years should be given 50 to 100 ml (¼ glass).
5. Children between 2 to 10 years should be given 100 to 200 ml (½ glass).
6. Children above 10 years should be given as much as they are able to drink.
7. Continue giving ORS in small sips even when vomiting occurs.
8. If breast-feeding, continue.

**Preparing ORS at home:** Take 3 finger pinch (½ teaspoonful) of common salt and two finger scoops (5 teaspoonful) of sugar in one litre of boiled and cooled water. Add lemon or orange juice to your taste.

**Diphenoxylate** (LOMOTIL)

*Diphenoxylate* is a drug related to the painkiller *pethidine.* It is available in combination with *atropine,* an anti-spasmodic drug which relieves gripping or colicky pain. The combination is marketed under the name of LOMOTIL containing *atropine* 0.025 mg and *diphenoxylate* 2.5 mg.

***Adverse Effects:*** If taken in larger doses over a period of time, it may cause addiction. In children, LOMOTIL has been reported to produce adverse effects due to the retention of toxic substances in the intestines as a consequence of decreased mobility. The toxicity in children includes dryness of the mouth, blurring of vision, urinary retention, distension of abdomen due to toxin stay (toxic paralytic ileus) marked respiratory depression, coma, and even death. Some of these symptoms can appear even with near therapeutic doses. *For this reason, its use has been banned in children below the age of six years.*

**Loperamide** (LOPAMIDE, RIDOL, IMMODIUM, 2 mg)

It has a poor penetration through the blood-brain barrier and therefore does not cause addiction and sedation in therapeutic doses. It is more potent than *diphenoxylate.* The average daily adult dose is 4 to 8 mg and should not exceed 16 mg. It is not recommended in children less than 2 years of age.

***Adverse Effects:*** Abdominal cramp and skin rashes is the main side-effect of this drug. Some precautions should be observed as for LOMOTIL. These are never given if diarrhoea is due to ulcerative colitis, diverticulitis or irritable bowel syndrome

**Racecadotril** (REDOTRIL,RACELOC,ROMELAST cap 100mg)

This is newer drug which reduces fluid secretion and its loss in stools. It is useful in viral and watery diarrhoea in diabetics in a dose of 100 mg three times a day. It may cause nausea, thirst, giddiness and headache. It is safer than *diphenoxylate* and *codeine. Codeine* was the time tested drug but because of its addiction potential and availability of newer and safer agents it is rarely used for its antimotility effects.

**Isabgol** (SAT ISABGOL)

It is generally used in the treatment of constipation, but is also effective in mild diarrhoea (see 'Drugs Used in Costipation').

## Drugs Used in Infective Diarrhoea

The drugs in this group are used for overcoming diarrhoea due to infection. These include *furazolidone, sulfonamides,* and *antibiotics.*

**Furazolidone** (FUROXONE)

This drug has been found to be effective in controlling diarrhoea due to a large variety of micro-organisms. An important feature of this drug is that micro-organisms do not develop resistance to it. It is a valuable agent in the treatment of gastro-enteritis and infections which are resistant to *sulfadiazine, tetracycline* or *chloramphenicol.* It is also available in combination with *metronidazole* — an antiamoebic drug. The usual adult oral dose is 100 mg, four times a day. Children require 5 to 10 mg/kg body weight in 3 to 4 divided doses (FUROXONE 25 mg/ml).

***Adverse Effects:*** Adverse effects of this drug are minimal. It may cause nausea, vomiting, headache, and in rare cases, allergic reaction in the form of skin rashes.

***Precautions***

1. The drug should not be taken on an empty stomach.
2. If the nausea and vomiting are experienced, the doses should be reduced or the drug should be withdrawn.
3. The drug should be stopped if symptoms of allergic reaction occur.

**Neomycin, Colistin Sulfate** (WALAMYCIN)

*Neomycin* is an antibiotic found to be of special value in the treatment of diarrhoea in infants because of its local action. It is usually given in combination with other non-specific anti-diarrhoea drugs.

**Ampicillin** (AMPICILLIN, CAMPICILLIN)

Nowadays *ampicillin* is a drug of choice in the treatment of bacillary dysentery (see 'Antibiotics and Antifungal Drugs')

**Norfloxacin** (NORFLOX, UROFLOX)

It is a *fluoroquinolone* which is effective against microbes causing diarrhoea and urinary infection. Usual dose is 400 mg twice a day. Manufacturers forbid its use in children. Unfortunately a large number of preparations contain pediatric syrups/ dispersable tablets which have been used. This drug can cause cartilage damage. Adverse effects are nausea, vomiting, headache, dizziness, dry mouth, loss of sleep and convulsions. Its use should be restricted.

## Drugs Used in Severe Diarrhoea

In severe types of dirrhoeas and in diarrhoea associated with vomiting, immediate attention is necessary. Besides the use of powerful drugs for treating the diarrhoea, the fluid and electrolyte balance should be corrected to avoid dehydration. Dehydration is characterized by hot and dry skin over the abdomen, dry tongue and lips, sunken eyeballs, and shock. In such cases, fluids should be infused through an intravenous drip and anti-spasmodics and antibiotics, if needed should be given.

### Role of Probiotics in antibiotic associated diarrhoea

Use of broadspectrum antibiotics (*tetracycline, ampicillin, cephalosporins*) may cause diarrhoea by killing useful resident bacteria of large bowel and growth of diarrhoea causing microbes.

Some resident organisms are needed to maintain intestinal luminal envirnment hostile to infections. *Lactobacillus acidophilus, Saccharomyces boulardi* (yeast) and *bifidobacreium* are probiotics which are used alone or along with vitamins and antibiotics to avoid antibiotic induced *diarrhoea* in adults and children. In addition, some of these are used alone in symptomatic treatment of diarrhoea. BECELAC contains *loperamide, B-complex* and *Lactobacilli;* SPORLAC, BABYLAC contain *Lactobacilli* (60 to 120 lacs of spores); ABSOLUT contains *Lactbacilli* with multivitamins; ZEDOTT-Plus contains *Racecadotril* with *lactobacilli;* ECONORM STIBs contains *sacchromycetes boulardi* (250 to 500 mg) in sachets; MOX-P, MOXIKIND-LB,

BLUMOX-P contain *amoxicillin* with *lactobacilli;* and LACTODO-LB contains *efadroyl* with *lactobacilli.*

These combinations increase the cost and offer little advantage. The effect of probiotis alone in childhood diarrhoea is only modest. In some studies benefit of *bifidobacteriun* is shown in childhood diarrhoea.

## Drugs* Used for Ulcerative Colitis

A number of drugs are available for the treatment and shown in table below:

| *Drug* | *Brand Names & dose* | *Precautions* |
|---|---|---|
| *Sulfasalazine* | SALAZOPYRIN 500 mg tab; 1 to 2 tab. 3 times a day | May cause sulfonamide like allergic reactions |
| *Mesalazine* | MESACOL 400 mg tab; 3 to 6 tablet/day, suppository 500 mg | Can cause pain in abdomen, skin rashes, and decrease in bone marrow activity; never given in case of kidney or liver diseases |
| *5- Amino salicylate* | ENEMA; 1 to 2 gm daily | As above |
| *Prednisolone* | WYSOLONE 5, 10 mg tab; 40 mg/day | See *corticosteroids* |
| *Hydrocortisone* | ENTOFOAM 10% enema | |
| *Balsalazine* | COLOREX, INTAZIDE 750 mg tab; 2.25 G to 6.75 G/day | Watch for allergic reactions |

* *Olsalazine* is not available in India presently. Severe ulcerative colitis may require surgery and spealized therapy.

## Drugs Used in Irritable Bowel Syndrome

Irritable bowel syndrome (IBS) is a common functional disorder of intestines. A patient with IBS has complaints such as abdominal pain, constipation or diarrhoea. Investigation reveal normal structures. Many patients are treated unnecessarily with antiamoebic and antibacterial drugs.

Treatment depends on the nature of complaints. Many patients improve with eating more fibres (*Isabgol* husk may be added). In others, fibre rich diet increases gaseousness and bloating.

Two types of drugs are useful in this disorder:

1. Those who have loose stools can benefit from *diphenoxylate* or *loperamide*. Antidepressants and *diazepam* also helps.
2. Those who have constipation require drugs like *cisapride*, *mosapride* and *tegaserod* (see chapter 'Drugs That Prevent Nausea and Vomiting'). *Tegaserod* (TEGIBS 2 mg, 6 mg cap) is a new drug available in India. It is used in IBS when constipation is the main complaint (spastic colon).

# 12

# Drugs Used in Epileptic Disorders

Y ou may have witnessed, at some time, a typical roadside scene where a person has suddenly fallen down and people have gathered around him, saying that he has had an attack of *mirgi*. Well, *mirgi* is nothing but a Hindi name for epilepsy. Epilepsy is characterized by fits with loss or disturbance of consciousness, leading to an inability to maintain posture. There may be other symptoms like increased muscle tone, followed by decreased muscle tone, frothing at the mouth, and the eyeballs moving upwards followed by convulsive movements of the arms or legs. An attack of epilepsy may occur at any time and it is usually difficult to predict its onset. However, some patients do get a warning signal or aura in the form of flashes of light or sounds. This is the description of grand-mal and major epilepsy (also called as generalised tonic-clonic seizures). Other forms are absence seizures (minor epilepsy or petit mal epilepsy), atonic seizures (akinetic unconsciousness with muscle relaxation resulting in fall); myclonic epilepsy (shock like intermittent muscular contractions) and infantile spasms (seen in infants).

Atonic epilepsy is a variant of petit-mal in children. There is a history of falls and transient lapses in class. The performance becomes poor. Therefore parents and teachers should note a recent poor performance of a good student and act accordingly! Infantile spasms also begin in infancy and mental retardation may be associated with it. It requires rigorous treatment for control.

***Causes of Epilepsy:*** The exact cause of epilepsy is not known in primary epilepsy. It has been suggested that some localized areas of the brain become hyperexcitable either due to changes in its vascular supply or other unknown reasons. Various factors such as changes in the blood gases, decrease in blood sugar and calcium, stress and strain, may precipitate an attack of epilepsy too. Seizures may be due to brain infection, metabolic disturbances, toxic effect of drugs, withdrawal after longer use of alcohol and tranquilizers, eclampsia or brain tumors. Head-injury is another common cause of epilepsy.

## Drugs Used in Grand mal (Tonic-Clonic) Seizures

It has been estimated that about 70-80% of epileptic patients can benefit from drugs currently available.

**Diphenylhydantoin or Phenytoin** (DILANTIN SODIUM, EPTOIN) **Mephenytoin** (MESANTOIN), **Fosphenytoin**

These drugs categorized as *hydantoins,* are to be preferred in the treatment of grand mal epilepsy. They are also useful in psychomotor epilepsy to some extent. The advantage of these agents is that there is very little or no sedation. These are used either alone or in combination with other drugs. They are also available in combination with *phenobarbitone* (DILANTIN-P).

*Fosphenytoin* is a newer injectable drug for intravenous administration which is considered to be safer than *phenytoin.*

***Dosage:*** *Diphenylhydantoin* is given in an initial oral dose of 0.3 to 0.6 g per day, while *mephenyton* is given in an oral dose of 0.3 to 0.8 g per day. The drug is continued for several years and some patients require it for life long.

***Adverse Effects:*** The adverse effects of these drugs depend upon the duration of exposure and the doses administered. In the normal course of treatment the adverse effects are not severe and can be made bearable by adjustments of doses. These drugs may cause gastric irritation which can be avoided if they are taken after meals. About 20% patients receiving these drugs experience swelling of gums. This can be minimized by good oral hygiene. A few cases may develop allergy which may be in the form of mild skin rashes, or severe depression of the bone marrow. Prolonged use may raise the blood sugar levels, and may cause osteoporosis owing to the disturbance in the metabolism of Vitamin-D which regulates the calcium of the body. Even in adequate doses unwanted growth of hair on face, coarsening of facial features and acne can be embarrassing, especially in the cases of females. *Phenytoin* may also produce anaemia due to reduced absorption of folic acid.

***Precautions***

1. Abrupt discontinuation of the therapy may bring on severe epileptic attacks.
2. The dose should be reduced gradually over one to two weeks under supervision.
3. Periodic blood examination should be done in patients receiving these drugs.
4. Patients receiving these drugs for a prolonged period should be given vitamin-D and calcium supplentation to avoid thinning of the bones.

**Carbamazepine** (TEGRETOL , MAZETOL, CARBATOL , MAZETOL-SR 200 mg)

This drug belongs to the category of *iminostilbenes* and is used in the treatment of psychomotor and grand-mal epilepsy. Now a days it is considered to be a first choice for grand-mal epilepsy. It provides partial or complete relief to at least 65% of the patients. *Carbamazepine* has also been found to be useful in the treatment of neuralgia (a condition in which there is severe neural pain in some area of the face) uncontrollable hiccoughs, manic depressive illness and acute mania. It is preferred in young girls because it does not have cosmetic adverse effects of *phenytoin.*

***Dosage:*** The average daily oral dose of *carbamazepine* is 0.4 to 1.2 gm in three divided doses. Sustained release tablets can be taken twice a day.

***Adverse effects:*** Its adverse effects may be mild, causing nausea, anorexia or loss of appetite, drowsiness, and sedation. The drug may also cause pigmentation or discolouration of skin in about 3% cases and rarely depression of the bone marrow. Dose related neurotoxicity-ataxia, double vision, unsteadiness and occasionally seizures, may occur. Water retention with low blood sodium concentration may occur in elderly.

***Precautions***

1. The drug should not be taken on an empty stomach.
2. Periodic examination of the blood is recommended.

**Phenobarbital** (LUMINAL)

This drug, which is a barbiturate, has been in use in the treatment of grand mal epilepsy since 1912, and is still employed since it is inexpensive and has low toxicity. This is employed either alone or in combination with *diphenylhydantoin.*

***Dosage:*** The usual daily oral dosage of *phenobarbital* is 0.1 to 0.3 g given in divided parts.

***Adverse Effects:*** The adverse effects of this drug is mild in nature. The most common effect is drowsiness which can be minimized by giving the drug in divided doses at suitable intervals. Moreover, the patients soon develop tolerance to this adverse effect. These drugs may cause impairment in learning and memory and mild allergic reactions which are in the form of skin rashes in 1 to 2% cases. Severe types of allergy are extremely rare. Like *phenytoin,* long term use of *phenobarbital* may cause vitamin D and folic acid deficiency.

***Precautions***

1. Do not stop these drugs abruptly as this may precipitate a severe epileptic attack.
2. Keep away from children.
3. Consumption of alcohol and other depressant-drugs may cause marked sedation and should be avoided.

**Primidone** (MYSOLINE)

*Primidone* is a useful agent in the treatment of grand mal and psychomotor epilepsy. It is generally given in combination with *diphenylhydantoin* in order to achieve better results in the treatment of grand mal epilepsy and myoclonic seizures.The average daily oral dose of *primidone* is 0.5 to 2 g.

***Adverse Effects:*** The most common complaint is lethargy, drowsiness, and dizziness. Sometimes the drug may cause visual disturbances. Allergic reactions in the form of skin rashes are very rare. Violent psychotic reaction is possible in patients with an unstable personality.

### Newer drugs Used in Grandmal/Psychomotor Epilepsy

**Oxcarbazine** (OXECARB. OXETOL 150,300 mg)

It is considered to be safer and with a fewer adverse effects of *carbamazepine.*

**Lamotrigine** (LAMITOR, EPITIC, LAMIDUS 25 mg, 50 mg)

A broad spectrum anti-epileptic effective in refractory cases. Its adverse effects are dizziness, unsteadiness, double vision and skin rash.

**Gabapentin** (NEURONTIN-300 mg, 400 mg)
It is an add-on drug for the treatment of resistant partial seizures. It can be used as first line drug for diabetic neuropathic pain and post theraupetic neuralgia. It is also useful in manic depressive illness and prevention of migraine. Its unwanted effects are mild sedation and unsteadiness.

**Topiramate** (EPITOP, TOPIVAL, TOPIRAIN 25, 50 mg, TOPAMATE-25, 50, 100 mg tab)
It is used as an add-on drug for the treatment of refractory grand mal and partial seizures. Adverse effects are poor concentration, unsteadiness, sedation, weight loss and occasional formation of kidney stones. Psychiatric symptoms may also appear. It is also useful in migraine prevention.

**Levetiracetum** (TORLEVA, LEVROX 250, 500 mg)
It may be used as an adjunct in difficult cases as well as in the treatment of partial seizures withs secondry generalized fits.

*Tiagabine* and *Vigabatrin* are some of the other drugs.

## Drugs Used in Petit Mal (Minor) Epilepsy

**Ethosuximide** (ZARONTIN)
This drug is commonly used in the treatment of petit mal (absence seizures) epilepsy. *Ethosuximide* has gained more popularity because of its less toxic nature. It is not effective against grand mal fits.

***Dosage:*** The average daily oral dose of *ethosuximide* is 0.5 to 1.5 g.

***Adverse Effects:*** In quite a few patients this causes nausea, vomiting, and abdominal distress. Some patients may experience drowsiness, dizziness, or headache, but these usually decrease on continued use. In some cases of unstable personalities, these agents may cause aggressiveness, agitation, anxiety, restlessness, or euphoria (a false sense of well-being). A few cases of depression of the bone marrow due to an allergic reaction have also been reported.

***Precautions***

1. It should not be taken on an empty stomach.
2. On prolonged use, a periodic blood examination is advisable.

**Sodium Valproate** (ENCORATE, EPILEX, VALPARIN, VALPROL)
This is a new drug and its chemical structure is quite different to the other drugs described for epileptic disorders. It is a valproic acid derivative and is useful in the treatment of grand mal, petit mal, and other type of seizures. It is supposed to benefit the patient by increasing the concentration of GABA, a neurotransmitter in the brain. It is considered to be superior to *ethosuximide* in absence seizures. *Divalproex* (DEPAKOTE, DIVALPRO, ENCORATE CGRONO, EPILEX CHRONO-125,250 and 500 mg) is a special form of valproic acid used in various epilepsies and in bipolar mental disorder and migraine.

***Dosage:*** Initially given in doses of 600 mg per day, it should be gradually raised to 2,000 mg or more per day. *Divalproex* is used in a dose of 0.5 to 1.5 g/ day (two divided doses).

***Adverse Effects:*** This drug may cause loss of appetite, nausea, drowsiness, and vomiting. Therefore, it should be taken after meals. Other effects are curling and loss of hair (alopecia), fall in platelet count. The most dreaded but rare problem is severe liver damage in children below 3 years.

***Precautions***

1. The drug should not be taken on an empty stomach.
2. It should not be taken if there is a pre-existing liver disease.
3. It is excreted in the form of ketone bodies in the urine, so it will give false positive test for these substances. (Caution in diabetes).
4. It is never used during pregnancy because it may cause defects of backbone and spinal cord in babies.

*Clonazepam* (CLONORIL 0.5 mg, 1 mg) is used in absence seizures, resistant grand mal seizures. *Clobazam* (FRISIUM 5 mg, 10 mg) is effective in refractory epilepsy. *Lorazepam* (LARPOSE, ATIVAN) is given intravenous slowly to control rapid repetatitive or persistent epilepsy fits (status epilepticus).

## Proper Use of Drugs

Anti-epileptic drugs control seizures and are required for longer duration. They must be taken regularly and in optimal doses. All the drugs have tendency to change the disposition of a number of other drugs needed for concurrent disease. Therefore, ask your doctor about change in dosages in case you are suffering with diseases such as diabetes, high blood pressure or painful disorder while on anti epileptic drugs. Drugs should never be stopped suddenly because precipitation of severe convulsions may threaten life. Duration of treatment is prolonged for several years. Some doctors advocate for gradual withdrawal of medications if patients is without seizures for last 5 years. If the control is not adequate the doctor may advise a blood level estimation of the drug. So far as possible pregnancy should be avoided during treatment but if a woman conceives the drugs should not be stopped. A doctor may substitute safer drugs under supervision to avoid birth defects. Folic acid should also be taken by women from 4th month onwards to reduce chances of neural tube defects and bleeding in newborn.

A family member should carefully learn to help patient during convulsions. The person in seizure must be rolled on one side, a watch kept on breathing and a pillow is placed under his head. The family physician must be informed, and the patient must never be left alone. A diary of fits should be maintained by the sick with addresses or contact numbers of treating doctor/ relatives and should be kept in the wallet.

# 13

# Drugs Used in Common Eye Diseases*

* * * * * *

Blindness is a major health problem the world over. It is estimated that out of 37 million blind people worldwide, 12 million are from India, of which 75% are cases of avoidable blindness. The factors causing visual disability, are discussed briefly in this chapter.

## Eye infections

### Bacterial infections

Infection of eye membrane (conjunctivitis) and eyelids (blepharitis) occurs both in children and adults. It may occur in a newborn baby (neonate) too. It is usually caused due to poor hygiene. There may be discharge from the eye. The eyelids may adhere to one another and it may be difficult to open the eye. Sometimes a boil may appear on the eyelash with pus in it (stye). In this case eyelash should be removed by a specialist followed with proper medication. Fomentation of the eyes with boiled water and a pinch of boric acid powder also provide some relief. **Infection of cornea** may be a severe condition, which if left untreated may cause complete blindness, hence it requires aggressive treatment.

**Treatment:** Antimicrobial eye drops or ointments like — *Chloramphenicol* 0.4% (MYCIN), *Gatifloxacin* 0.3% (GATE, GATIFAX), *Moxifloxacin* 0.5% (VIGAMOX, OCCUMOX), *Tobramycin* 0.3% (OBRA, NEBRACIN), etc. should be used.

### Trachoma

Once a major cause of blindness, Trachoma is a slowly developing, contagious infection of eye caused by *Chlamydia trachomatis.* The patient feels irritation in the eye with redness. If cornea is involved, it may lead to blindness.

**Treatment:** *Sulfacetamide* (ALBUCID, LOCULA, OPTISOL), *Azithromycin* 1% ( ZAHA), *Tetracyclin* eye ointment.

---

* Chapter contributed by Dr Pradeep Mathur, Professor of Ophthalmology, S.M.S. Medical College, Jaipur.

### Fungal infections

Injuries due to wooden stick, thorn or vegetable matter can cause fungal infection. This leads to a corneal ulcer, which is difficult to treat and needs a specialist's intervention.

**Treatment**: *Natamycin* eyedrops 5 % (NATAMET), *Itraconazole* 1% eyedrops (ITRAL), *Fluconazole* eyedrops 0.3% (ZOCON).

### Viral infections

Epidemic keratoconjunctivitis is usually seen after rainy season and is caused by *Adenovirus*. It has no specific treatment and is self limiting. *Herpes,* a common viral infection, can also cause corneal ulceration.

**Treatment:** *Acylovir* 1% eye ointment (ACIVIR).

### Allergic conjunctivitis

It could be seasonal keratoconjunctivitis seen usually in summer season. Patient has complaints of eye discomfort and redness. It is treated with combination of anti-allergics and low dose of steroids. Another form of allergy is due to use of medication, for which the use of the drug should be stopped.

**Treatment:** *Sodium cromoglycate* 2% (ALLERCROM), decongestants (ANDRE, MEZOL, PHENIL), *Olapatidine* 0.1 % (WINOLAP, OLOPAT), soft steroids like *Fluoromethlone* (FML, FLOMON), *Lotoprednol* (LOTEL, LOTEPRED).

## Cataract

Cataract is loss of transparency of the natural lens. The most common cause of cataract is ageing. It may also be congenital or due to injury to the eye, serious infection of eye and diabetes mellitus. The chief symptom of cataract is a gradual decrease of vision. An entirely opaque lens is 'ripe' while the one that retains some transparency is 'immature'.

Treatment of 'immature' cataract during the period of dimming of vision comprises of wearing accurately prescribed spectacles. The ultimate treatment of cataract is removal of this opaque lens surgically and implanting an artificial lens after proper calculation of its power. One should not wait for the maturity of cataract. At present the latest treatment is phacoemulsification in which the incision is small and a foldable lens is implanted. However, spectacles may be required for near vision after cataract surgery (may not be needed if intraocular lens is multifocal).

## Dry Eye

It is a common cause of eye discomfort affecting a majority of people. It specially affects those working on the computers, due to decrease in their eye blink rate, and those wearing contact lens. The patient complaints of redness and grittiness of eyes along with fatigue. There occurs deficiency of tear film in such people, who should be treated with tear supplements. The patients are advised to blink more frequently. Some commonly available tear supplements are *Carboxymethyl cellulose* (TEAR NATURAL, SOFT DROPS), *Hydroxypropyl cellulose* (MOISOL).

## Glaucoma

Glaucoma is a condition in which the pressure inside the eyeball is raised causing damage to the optic nerve. The major risk factors for the development of glaucomatous optic nerve damage include the high level of intra-ocular pressure, increasing age, black race and a family history of glaucoma. Broadly it can be classified into various types, of which POAG (primary open angle glaucoma) detected late because there are no obvious symptoms. It is an acquired condition, with onset typically after age 50. It affects both eyes but often asymmetrically. In early and even moderate stages, the patient is usually asymptomatic. Abnormalities of the visual field occur. In more advanced stages, the patient may become aware of an enlarging scotoma (defect in visual field) particularly when it encroaches on fixation. If left untreated, vision may be lost. Other form of glaucoma known as Angle closure glaucoma presents with severe pain, redness and marked diminution of vision can be devastating. Blindness can result in 2 to 3 days from onset. Glaucoma can be treated with long term medication or surgically.

**Treatment:** Commonly used drugs for chronic open angle glaucoma are *Timolol maleate* 0.5% eyedrops (TIMOLET, TIMO-5, GLUTIM), *Betoxalol* 0.5% e/d (OPTIPRESS, BETAPRESS), *Levubunolol* 0.1% e/d (BETAGAN), *Brimonidin* 0.2% e/d (ALPHAGAN, BRIMOCOM), *Latanoprost* 0.005% e/d (XALATAN, LATOCOM) used once a day. *Pilocarpine* 2% e/d for acute glaucoma (narrow angle type) 3 to 4 times a day provides quick relief and reduction of eye pressure. Surgical iridectomy (removing piece of iris) or laser iridotomy (cutting a hole in iris) provides permanent treatment in some cases.

## Injuries

Injury to eye can be due to roadside accident, chemical or mechanical injuries, burns or foreign bodies.

**Roadside accident:** The eyes are well protected by the bony structures surrounding them. A large blunt object can only damage the eyelids. A black eye (black area below or on side of the eye), which commonly occurs during roadside accidents, is due to blood beneath the thin skin of the eyelids and is usually associated with swelling. The vision may be unaffected. Cold compresses for 10 minutes every hour for a day will reduce the swelling. If the injury is severe or vision is affected, the doctor should be consulted.

**Burns:** A chemical substance burns the eye and requires thorough washing with water. No time should be wasted in finding a neutralizing agent for the chemical substances. The most effective method is to plunge the entire face into a container of water and then open the eye under water. Heat burn requires treatment similar to chemical burn. Bandaging or closing the lid will prevent the movement of eyeballs and reduce pain. No lotion should be used for washing the eyes.

**Foreign body:** Dirt or dust in the eye may cause sensation of a foreign body being in the eye. It may come out by washing the eyes. If not, it should be removed by a physician.

## Vitamin-A Deficiency

Vitamin-A deficiency most commonly affects the eyes, the clinical condition being xerophthalmia and keratomalacia. Xerophthalmia denotes the entire spectrum of ocular abnormalities arising from vitamin A deficiency. These include night blindness, retinopathy, conjunctival and corneal xerosis (dryness), corneal ulceration and softening. The eye instead of looking clear appears muddy and wrinkled. It becomes dry, hazy (like ground grass) and unwettable. There may be greyish, triangular, foamy, rough and raised patches on the eye (Bitot's spots). These are present in both eyes. It may progress to ulcer in the eyes. Severe deficiency of vitamin A in children may cause keratomalacia (softening of a part or the entire eyeball). The process is rapid one. It is a grave medical emergency and if not treated promptly, may lead to necrosis and perforation of the eye ball resulting in blindness. It is often associated with protein energy malnutrition.

**Sources of Vitamin A**

| Source | μg |
|---|---|
| *Rich Sources* | |
| Cod liver oil | 10,000 to 100,000 |
| Shark liver oil | 9,000 to 16,000 |
| Liver of other animals | 6,000 to 10,000 |
| *Good Sources* | |
| Butter | 720 to 12,000 |
| *Ghee* | 600 to 700 |
| Egg | 300 to 400 |
| Carrot | 325 to 650 |
| Green leafy vegetable | 325 to 2,000 |
| Mango (Ripe) | 375 to 750 |
| *Fair Sources* | |
| Milk | 50 to 60 |

* 1g = 1,000,000 micrograms (μg)

**Treatment:** The vitamin A deficiency can be prevented by adequate nutrition contained in the food mentioned above. A shortcut has been suggested by National Institute of Nutrition, Hyderabad, which consist of the administration of 200,000 IU (66,000 $\mu$g) of vitamin A every six month to pre school children who are unlikely to have adequate nutrition. Excess of vitamin A produce toxic effects. Commonly available preparation such as injection AQUASOL-A contains 50,000 IU of vitamin A.

# 14

# Treatment of Common Gynaecological Ailments*

• • • • • •

A man can do almost everything a woman does with one big exception i.e., he cannot conceive and give birth to a child. He lacks the apparatus for this multiplication which a woman possesses. Because of this additional equipment a woman may suffer, due to the impairment of this complicated equipment, which takes place off and on. In India the number of specialist doctors i.e. the gynaecologists and obstetricians are few in proportion to the female population, and for this reason a large number of women suffer discomfort, pain and illness. This may not always be of short duration unless treated in time. All female ailments may not need drug treatment, some can be alleviated by other procedures. In this chapter we will try to cover both of them.

## Vaginal Discharge

Abnormal vaginal discharge is a common complaint at all age groups. The discharge may be due to excessive (physiological) formation of secretions or due to a variety of infections. When it is not due to infection, the discharge does not have any foul smell and does not cause irritation and itching. This is called as Leucorrhoea and is seen around ovulation, during sexual excitement and before menstruation. This type of discharge can be due to hormonal changes also.

A foul smelling discharge causes much irritation and is due to infections. Non-specific vaginitis occurs commonly in debilitated women, pill users, pregnancy and diabetics. Specific infections occur due to candida (fungus), trichomonas (one celled parasite) or bacteria. Poor hygiene predisposes to such infections.

If a discharge has blood, some serious cause should be considered. It can be tumor (cancer) or polyp (a mass) inside the genital tract. If there is a painful ulcer on vulva, it can be due to virus *(Herpes)*. Sometimes a foreign (extraneous) body such as Copper-T and tampoons may cause infection and need removal. Thinning of layers of vagina may occur at menopause so an estrogen cream may help.

---

* Chapter contributed by Dr Rakesh Khuteta, Professor of Gynaecology, S.M.S. Medical College, Jaipur.

### Treatment

General health should be improved with maintenance of personal hygiene. Anxiety should be allayed. A number of drugs are available (See chapter on antibiotics). Some commonly used drugs are given below :

| *Ailment* | *Drugs* |
|---|---|
| For Non-specific Vaginitis | *Povidone Iodine* (BETADINE) vaginal pessary, one moistened pessary twice a day for 10 to 14 days. |
| For Bacterial Vaginits & Chlamydia | *Ceftriaxone* 250 to 500mg *IMorDoxycycline* (MICRODOX) 100 to 200mg/day for 7 days or *Azithromycin* 250mg twice a day for 3 days |
| For Trichomonas | Tab *Metronidazole* 200-400mg three times a day (Treat Spouse also) |
| For Candida | Vaginal creams such as *Miconazole*-2% (GYNODAKTARIN) *Clotrimazole*-2% (CANDID GEL) or CANDID pessary 200mg for 3 nights or *Ketoconazole*-2% (KETOVATE CREAM) or Oral capsule *Fluconazole* 150 mg once a week |

*Lactobacilli* (MYCONIP, vaginal tab), is used to restore vaginal acidity and thus bacterial growth is reduced. It is useful in leucorrhoea and recurrent vaginits. A number of fixed dose combinations or kits are available for treatment of mixed vaginal infections *Tinidazole* 1g (2 tablets) + *Fluconazole* 150mg (one cap.) in a single dose (AZOSTAT, NUFORCE) and *Azithromycin* – 1g + *Fluconazole* 150mg + *Secnidazole* 2g (AZITHRAL-XP).

### Dysmenorrhoea (Paindful Menstruation)

It means painful menstruation. Pain may be cramping in the lower abdomen and its severity to cause disturbance in day to day activity. It occurs in 5-10% females. It is called primary when there is no obvious cause. It occurs in teenagers and is usually relieved after pregnancy. (However, this therapeutic marriage may not be recommended). It is relieved by pain relievers and antispasmodics (see chapter 'Pain Relievers').

Endometriosis (placement of endometrial lining in other pelvic organs such as tubes, cervix or colon) is a common cause of secondary amenorrhoea and requires proper treatment with oral contraceptives or with *Danazol* (LADOGOL, DANOZEN 100mg). *Danazol* has anabolic and progesterone like effects and it suppresses ovarian function so less estrogen is formed. Its usual dose is 200-400mg/day. If no relief is obtained, surgical removal of such tissues is recommended.

### Pelvic Pain

It is a common symptom of a large number of underlying causes. It can be acute or chronic. The underlying mechanism is irritation of membrane overlying abdominal organs (peritoneum) by infection or blood. It is due to gynaecological and non-gynaecological causes.

*Acute Causes:* Pelvic inflammatory disease (PID), ruptured ectopic (tubal) pregnancy, ruptured (bursting) cyst of ovary or abortion.

*Chronic Causes (longer standing):* Pelvic inflammatory disease (Tuberculosis), endometriosis, IUCD users chronic cervicitis or tumors.

In addition to the above causes related to female genital tract, many diseases of large bowel, kidney and spine (back bone) present with lower abdominal and back pain, appendicitis, stone in ureter or urinary bladder, lumbar-disc prolapse, and amoebiasis are some of the causes.

After ascertaining diagnosis by PV (Per Vaginal) examination, ultrasound, urine examination and biopsy (if required), a gynaecologist usually prescribes pain relievers and antispasmodics as described in chapter on Pain Relievers Anxiolytic drugs help if psychosomatic trouble is detected. A number of antibiotics are available in combination with *metronidazole, tinidazole* or *ornidazole.* Such combinations are quite commonly used for 1 to 2 weeks to treat PID.

## Premenstrual Syndrome

It occurs in the second half of menstrual period. A variety of symptoms occur such as nervousness, irritation, mood changes, some pain in breasts and sometimes headache. These changes are due to hormones estrogen and progesterone. These symptoms last for a week or longer and are relieved by menstruation.

Assurance, salt restriction, calcium supplements are helpful. Some drugs which are beneficial:

1. Vitamin $B_6$ (*Pyridoxin,* B-LONG 10mg) alone, or along with other vitamins and minerals help correct nutritional factors.
2. Anti-inflammatory pain relievers (see chapter 'Pain Relievers') also help.
3. Evening *primrose* oil (PRIMOSA, SIMROSE cap. 500mg) 1 cap. twice a day and antioxidants (ANTOXID, LYCORED).
4. Some doctors prescribe *fluoxetine* (FLUDAC 20mg) for treatment of mood changes, but it is not required in all cases.

## Menorrhagia (Excessive Menstruation)

It is a cyclical bleeding at normal interval. The bleeding is excessive either in amount or duration or both which is diagnosed by passage of big clots, increased number of sanitary pad usage or soiling of clothes despite pads.

Level of hemoglobin can give an idea of magnitude of disease. Bleeding could be due to increased surface area of uterus like fibroids, hormonal imbalance, ovarian tumor or even IUCD in the uterus. When there is no discernible cause and irregular menstruation occurs it is called as dysfunctional uterine bleeding. This is related to excess of estrogen hormone. This diagnosis is made when biopsy of inner uterus is not abnormal. The treatment is of appropriate cause and haemostatics, hormones and antifibrinolytics are used as given below:

- To immediately stop the bleeding *Norethisterane* (REGISTRONE, PRIMOLUT-N) 5 to 15 mg/day is given. Withdrawal bleeding occurs after 3 to 5 days of stoppage.
- Later oral pills are given from 5 to 25th day for at least 3 cycles (periods).
- *Danazol* 200 to 400 mg/daily in 4 divided doses for 3 months.
- Prostaglandins inhibitors like *Mafenamic* acid 150 to 600mg/daily.
- Antifibrinolytic drugs like *Tranexamic* acid (TRAPE, TX) 1g four times a day.
- Other coagulants used are *Ethamsylate* (ETHAMSYL, SYLATE), *Bioflavonoids* (CVP GYNAE) and *Rutin* (KERUTIN-C).
- Surgery-Dilatation and curettage (D&C) for removal of hyperplastic endometrium.
- Endometrial ablation and resection – Laser ablation, roller ball ablation and transcervical resection (TCRE) are some of the methods. Overall success rate is 70 to 80 per cent.

## Scanty Menstruation

This is of two types: *Oligomenorrhoea*: When menstrual bleeding is more than 35 days apart with constant frequency, and

*Hypomenorrhoea:* When bleeding is unduly scanty and lasts for less than 2 days.

| | | |
|---|---|---|
| **Causes** | Age related | During adolescence, preceding menopause. |
| | Weight related | Obesity |
| | Stress related | Anorexia nervosa, stress of examination and psychogenic. |
| | Endocrinal | Thyroid dysfunction, Polycystic ovarian disease, Hyperprolactinemia. |
| | Infection | Tuberculosis |

The primary cause is taken care of and appropriate drugs used. Cyclic hormonal treatment is needed to restore normal menstruation.

## Menopause

This means permanent cessation of menstruation at the end of reproductive life due to follicular inactivity. Age of menopause is genetically predetermined, the average age being 50 years. Premature menopause is when menses stops at or below 40 years of age and delayed when menopause fails to occur even beyond 55 years. Diagnosis is from classic hot flushes, mood changes and confirmed by elevated FSH levels (Follicular Stimulating Hormone secreted by the pitiutary) and decreased oestadiol levels (a kind of estrogen).

**Hormonol Replacement Treatment (HRT)** ensures benefits and minimises risks, particularly in symptomatic women and also prevents osteoporosis, artherosclerosis, cardiovascular diseases, urogenital atrophy (thinning of inner layer of genital and urinary passage) etc. Oestrogen reduces the risk of Alzheimer's disease also.

### **Contraindications** (Condition under which HRT is not recommended)

Undiagnosed genital bleeding, oestrogen dependent tumors, history of venous thromboembolism and liver/gall bladder disease. HRT can be continued as long as the benefits are desired, provided treatment is monitored. The increased incidence of breast cancer is debatable (see chapter on Methods of Preventing Pregnancy).

## Urinary Stress Incontinence

In this condition there is leaking or flow of urine on coughing, sneezing or laughing. There is a rise in abdominal pressure during such stress. There is also laxity of muscles around vagina and

**Which Hormone to be used in HRT?**

(A) For woman without uterus

(B) For woman with uterus

*Oestrogens* only by mouth (orally), vaginal creams

*Oestrogens* with *progesterone* by mouth (orally), transdermal patch, implants and injectables, subsdermal implant, percutaneous gel.

weakening of muscle-rings (sphinctors). Stress incontinence causes extreme degree of embarassment and women avoid attending social functions. In addition, it leads to infections and must be treated. This disorder is more common in obese women and those who have sustained vaginal injuries due to repeated childbirths.

**Treatment:** General measures are weight reduction, treatment of cough and constipation. Pelvic floor exercises help in early cases. These are:

1. Drawing up of anus and tightening of vagina.
2. Stopping urine in between and squeezing the muscles (as if getting rid of last drops of urine)
3. Electrical stimulation of perineal muscles by physiotherapists.

If these measures fail then adrenergic drugs, hormones and implants around urinary tube (urethra) may help. Finally restorative surgery may be required.

# 15

# Drugs Used in Disorders of the Heart

The heart is a unique organ in our body. It pumps blood to all parts of body untiringly and continuously. Do you know how does it get energy? Not from the blood in its cavities but from special blood vessels which penetrate into its muscles and are called coronary arteries. As it beats regularly it has to repair the wear and tear while in action! Another peculiarity is that coronary arteries are more prone to narrowing and blockage by atherosclerosis, a process of deposition of fatty material which gets, hardened gradually. The resulting occlusion impairs the blood supply to heart muscle, a condition called ischaemia (thirst amongst plenty!). When occlusion is complete ischaemic necrosis (cell death) results and a clinical entity called acute myocardial infarction (heart attack) occurs. A condition in-between these two is called 'intermediate syndrome'.

Depending on the extent of occlusion there may be chest pain on exertion (stable or exertional angina pectoris) which gets relieved on rest, prolonged chest pain with sweating and marked ECG changes (acute myocardial infarction) or increasingly severe chest pain on minimal exertion (unstable angina). Occasionally, a person may be without chest pain and only on routine angiography, narrowing is detected. In rare cases sudden death may be the first (and last!) manifestation of the disease called coronary artery disease (CAD) or ischaemic heart disease (IHD).

In acute attack of angina (IHD) the patient experiences heaviness, pressure, tightness, or a squeezing type of pain in the chest lasting for a few minutes, and is relieved by nitroglycerin tablet placed under tongue. In the second form, the chest pain which is of an extremely severe squeezing or crushing type, often lasting for long periods, and associated with nausea, vomiting, giddiness, and sweating may be due to myocardial infarction. Although the pain in the chest and deficiency of oxygen supply are features common to both conditions, the pain in angina pectoris appears to be due to the narrowing of lumen of the coronary arteries, whereas in myocardial infarction, there is complete shut down of the blood supply to segment of heart muscle, leading to necrosis. Due to these differences, the treatment of these two conditions varies considerably and will be discussed separately.

**Causes of Coronary Artery Disease (Ischaemic Heart Disease):** Atherosclerosis is the most common cause. It starts at an early age and progresses with age. For this reason the incidence of heart attacks is greater during the 50s or later years. It is interesting to note that the incidence of atherosclerosis and heart attack is lower in women in child bearing age. It may be besides other factors, due to the protective effect of the naturally occurring hormone oestrogen in their body. There are various factors which may enhance the process of atherosclerosis, such as a fatty and high caloric diet, lack of physical activity, obesity, cigarette smoking and diabetes.

A study on Japanese and Asian immigrants showed that change in food habits — eating plenty of rich foods, was the main cause of higher (upto 8 times) incidence of heart disease. It is, therefore, necessary for patients of heart attack to exercise control over diet and eat food which is low in fat and calories (see chapters on high BP, Drugs for high blood lipids and Slimming agents.)

## Drugs Used in Angina Pectoris

There are three distinct aims of the treatment of angina pectoris: 1) treatment of an acute attack or prevention of an attack shortly before undergoing physical exertion; and 2) chronic prophylaxis (long-term prevention) of future attacks, and 3) changing life style of patient (non-drug treatment).

### Drugs Used in an Acute Attack

**Glyceryl Trinitrate or Nitroglycerine** (ANGISED, SORBITRATE)

This is frequently used for termination and immediate prevention of an acute attack. It has been found to be a very useful agent for short-term prophylaxis, allowing the patient to undertake essential chores, experience the normal pleasures of life, and save him from extreme anxiety due to the persistent fear of another possible attack. It provides the necessary psychological relief and raises the morale of the patient dramatically. *Glyceryl trinitrate* reduces the work of the heart by lowering the blood pressure. The reduced load leads to a lowering in the demand for oxygen by the heart muscle. In addition, there is some evidence that the drugs may improve the circulation by widening the blood vessels of the area of the heart where the oxygen supply is deficient.

***Dosage***

| *Drug* | *Peak effect* | *Duration* |
|---|---|---|
| Glyceryl Trinitrate (Sublingual) | 4 to 8 min | 10 to 30 min. |
| Glyceryl Trinitrate (Oral spray) | 4 to 10 min. | 20 to 300 min. |

*Glyceryl trinitrate* (GTN) is available in the form of a tablet of 0.5 mg which should be kept under the tongue to allow its absorption in the mouth. It should not be swallowed but chewed.

**Not All Chest Pains are Heart Attacks**

We must point out that all chest pains are not due to heart disease. Three common causes of chest pain are gastro-intestinal disorders (gastro-esòphageal acid reflux-GERD), diseases of the gall-bladder, liver, spleen, lungs, and the muscles of the chest wall (small rib-joints).

It is therefore, quite important to rule out these possibilities before labeling a person as a patient of heart disease. Such a verdict places a tremendous psychological burden on the patient and wrong diagnosis and treatment can sometimes produce a cardiac cripple. On the other hand, a patient of heart attack needs prompt care and treatment which may be started immediately.

Since *Glyceryl trinitrate* deteriorates very quickly, the patient should always keep a fresh supply in a sealed bottle. If active, the tablets should give rise to a tingling, burning, or stinging sensation on the tongue. Cotton should not be put in the container of tablets. The container should be made of glass and not of plastic.

During an acute attack, a tablet is kept under the tongue and spat out or swallowed as soon as the pain is relieved. To provide short-term prophylaxis, a tablet is chewed 3 minutes before the stressful activity or exertion. This kind of acute prophylactic effect may last for more than 30 minutes. *Isosorbide dinitrate* (ISORDIL, SORBITRATE 5 mg) is another effective drug used sublingually (1 to 2 tablets). A spray of 400 microgram per dose of *nitroglycerine* into the mouth and repeated after 15 minutes can also help.

***Adverse Effects:*** Nitrates do not cause any serious adverse effects. Headache is the commonest adverse effect which occurs in 25 to 40% of the patients. Other adverse effects are dizziness, weakness, and transient fall of blood pressure.

***Precautions:***

1. If there is no relief from chest pain with 3 doses of *nitroglycerine* taken at 3 minute intervals, no additional dose should be taken; the pain may be due to actual heart attack. Doctor should be consulted immediately.
2. The patient should take rest as soon as the attack occurs. Rest shortens the duration of the attack.
3. The drug can be chewed and should be spat out or swallowed as soon as the pain is relieved.
4. The patient should not be allowed to move suddenly as there may be a sudden fall in the blood pressure, resulting in fainting.
5. Alcoholic drinks should be avoided as the drug may interact to cause marked vasodilatation and faintness.

## Drugs for Long-Term Prevention

There are five groups of drugs used to prevent angina pectoris. These are : 1) Beta blockers, 2) Calcium entry blockers, 3) Nitrates, 4) Potassium channel openers, and 5) Heart muscle cell protectors.

**Tests for Finding out the Obstruction and Functional Heart Damage in Ischaemic Heart Disease (IHD)**

- Resting and exercise (treadmill) test
- Echocardiography
- Myocardioal perfusion studies (Thalium-201 Scintigraphy)
- Radionuceid angiography
- Heart CT and MRI
- Coronary Angiography
- Left ventricular Angiography

**Beta Blockers (Atenolol** 50-100 mg, **Metoprolol** 100-200 mg, **Celiprolol** 200-400 mg, **Carvedilol** 6.25 -25 mg, **Propranolol** 80-160 mg)

These drugs reduce work of the heart so oxygen need is lessened, particularly during exercise, thus increasing the exercise capacity. Continuous use lowers the risk of sudden death due to attacks. In unstable angina, betablockers are not preferred because some of them *(propranolol)* may increase the narrowing of coronaries. These drugs must be taken regularly unlike *nitroglycerine* (as and when needed) and should never be stopped abruptly.

***Adverse Effects:*** Tiredness, fatigue, slow pulse, leg pains, are common adverse effects. Some elderly persons complain of cold hands and feet, dreams or loss of sleep and worsening of asthma. Congestive heart failure (poor pumping of blood) and poor control of diabetes may occur by non selective betablockers *(propranolol).*

***Precautions:***

1. These drugs should not be stopped adruptly as this can cause heart attack.
2. Do not take *verapamil* or *diltiazem* (see later) along with these drugs.
3. The safety of these drugs has not been established in pregnancy.
4. Elderly patients may start with a smaller dose.

**Nitrates**

Various preparations and daily doses for prevention of angina are shown in the table:

| *Drugs* | *Brand Names/Potency* | *No. of doses/day* |
|---|---|---|
| 1. *Isosorbide dinitrate* | SORBITRATE 10 mg | 4 to 6/day |
| 2. *Isosorbide mononitrate* | VASOTRATE 10 mg<br>MONOTRATE 10 mg | 2 to 3/day |
| 3. *Nitroglycerine* | CAP. ANGISPAN TR<br>2.5 mg, 6.5 mg | 2 to 3/day |
| | NITRODERM TTS SKIN PATCH<br>5 mg, 10 mg | One patch for 14 to 16 hrs<br>Relief (at night) |
| | MYOVIN OINTMENT 2% | 1 to 2 inch length to be spread on chest or thigh without rubbing<br>3 to 6/day |
| 4. *Pentaerythrityl tetranitrate* | PERITRATE 10 mg<br>PERITRATE SA 80 mg | 3 to 4/day<br>1 to 2/day |
| 5. *Erythrityl tetranitrate* | CARDILATE 5 mg, 15 mg | 4 to 5/day |

**Calcium Entry Blockers**

**Drugs Blocking Calcium Channels in Heart Muscle: Verapamil** (ISOPTIN), **Nifedipine** (NICARDIA), **Diltiazem** (DILZEM), **Benidipine** (CARITEC 4 mg)

These drugs (except *nifedipine*) block the calcium channels in the cells of the heart muscles and blood vessels, causing decreased contraction of the heart muscles and dilation of the blood vessels in the body and heart. Of these, the first three are used widely in clinical practice. Although all four of them are potent coronary vasodilators, they differ in their action on the blood vessels and the contraction of the heart. *Nifedipine* is a more potent vasodilator than either *verapamil, diltiazem* or *benidipine.* Similarly, *verapamil* inhibits the contraction of the heart more than that of *nifedipine, diltiazem* or *benidipine.*

**Verapamil** (ISOPTIN)

It reduces anginal attacks by relieving the coronary artery spasm, increasing the oxygen supply, and reducing the oxygen demand by decreasing the heart rate and after-load (back pressure of blood from the body to the heart). *Verapamil* is effective in angina prevention in a dose of 40-80 mg, three times a day. It is also useful in slowing very rapid heart rates in Paoxysmal Atrial Tachycardia (PAT).

***Adverse Effects:*** Constipation is the most common adverse effect of *verapamil.* It may cause headache, vertigo, weakness, nervousness, gastric upsets, and allergy in the form of itching, flushing or rash, and decreased pumping action of the heart (congestive heart failure). Rebound angina may occur following a sudden withdrawal of *verapamil.* Heart blocks may occur, however, occurance of heart arrest is rare.

***Precautions:***

1. Do not use it with beta blockers.
2. *Digoxin* levels in the blood increase when *verapamil* is taken along with it. These drugs should be used cautiously if taken together.
3. It is found in human milk and should be avoided during pregnancy and after labour.
4. In patients with severely impaired liver function, its dose should be reduced to 30%.

**Nifedipine** (NICARDIA, NICARIA-CD, CALCIGARD RETARD)

This has a potent vasodilator property with little depressant effect on the heart. It prevents coronary artery spasms but may promote 'coronary steal' (diversion of blood flow from the occluded coronary artery to a healthy area of the heart. It may cause tachycardia and palpitations. Long acting preparations (NICARDIA-CD) are used twice a day as these do not cause that much tachycardia and are preferred. Many other longer acting alternatives such as *amlodipine* (2.5 mg, 5 mg), *S-amlodipine* (2.5 mg), *nitrendipine* (10 mg, 20 mg), *felodipine* (2.5, 5 mg), *Lacidipine* (SINOPIN tab. 2 mg, 4 mg given in a usual dose of 4 mg once a day) and *Lercanidipine* (LEREZ tab. 10 mg, 20 mg given in a usual dose of 10-20 mg. once a day are also available. These are mainly used in high BP.

***Adverse Effects:*** *Nifedipine* may cause headache, palpitation, dizziness, weakness, nausea, flushing, a transient decrease in blood pressure, and allergic skin reaction. Swelling over feet due to vasodilation is common.

***Precautions:***

1. If the attack continues to be frequent and severe, other anti-anginal drugs may be substituted.
2. Diabetic patients should get their blood sugar checked more frequently as the drug may at time elevate blood glucose levels.
3. The drug should not be withdrawn suddenly as this may cause a rebound attack of angina.

**Diltiazem** (DILZEM 30 mg DILZEM SR 90 mg)

Its action on the heart rate is less than *verapamil.* It decreases blood pressure to a lesser extent than *nifedipine.* It relieves spasms of coronary arteries. It is also useful in PAT.

***Dosage:*** Initially a dose of 30 to 60 mg, three times daily, before meals and at bedtime is advised. It should be increased gradually to the optimum dose of 60 mg, 3 or 4 times daily. Slow Release (SR) preparations are used twice a day.

***Adverse Effects:*** Constipation is the most common adverse effect. Headache, vertigo, weakness, nervousness, gastric upsets, and allergy in the form of itching, flushing or rash, and decreased pumping action of the heart (congestive heart failure) may occur. Rebound angina, heart blocks and rarely cardiac arrest may occur following a sudden withdrawal of *diltiazem.*

***Precautions:***

1. Do not use it with a beta blocker (it can be a dangerous combination).
2. *Digoxin* levels in the blood increase when *verapamil* is taken. These drugs should be used cautiously if taken together.
3. In patients with severely impaired liver function, its dose should be reduced to 30%.

### Potassium Channel Openers

**Nicorandil** (NICORAN 5 mg, 10 mg)

It acts like organic nitrates and is useful in stable angina, unstable angina and due to prevention of ischaemia (lack of oxygen supply). Blood flow to heart muscles increases. Usual dose is 5 to 10 mg, 3 times a day. Adverse effects are flushing and palpitation, weakness, mouth ulcer, nausea and vomiting. It should be avoided with *nitrates* or *nifedipine.*

### Myocardial Protector

**Trimetazidine** (CYTOGARD, FLAVEDON - 20 mg)

This drug does not change contractions, heart rate or blood pressure but reduces angina frequency and increases work capacity by improving metabolism and energy utilization in heart muscles. Adverse effects are mild-gastric upset, fatigue, giddiness and muscle pain. It is an expensive drug.

**Coronary Revascularization Procedures***

- Per Cutaneous interventions (PCIs)
- Balloon Angioplasty
- Balloon Angioplasty with Stents
- Concurrent use of newer active agents such as Abcixmab, Eptifibatide or Tirofiban during angioplasty to reduce chances of heart attacks.
- Coronary Bypass Grafting using Saphenous (leg) veins, Internal mammary (chest wall) artery or Radial (forearm) artery

**Coronary Revascularization Procedure:**

Open chest wall operation

Minimally invasive technique

Beating heart surgery

* The term Coronary Revascularization is the process of restoring the flow of oxygen and nutrients to the heart. In other words; bring blood to the heart by surgery, to bypass blockages/obstructions.

**Oxyfedrine** (ILDAMEN 8 mg)

This drug improves metabolism so that oxygen deprivation (ischaemia) does not occur. It is used in a dose of 8 mg, 3 times a day. Taste disturbance is a usual side effect of it.

## Drugs Used in Unstable angina

Since many cases with continuous chest pain in this condition may progress to real heart-attack, aggressive treatment is required. *Aspirin* 150-325 mg with *Clopidogrel*-75mg, intravenous *nitroglycerin* and *heparin* or low molecular weight *heparin* is also given. *Atenolol* or other betablocker is also used. If drugs are not effective, an angiography with opening of block vessels (angioplasty) or establishing circulation with a bypass is undertaken.

## Treatment of Myocardial Infarction

In myocardial infarction there is pain in the chest which may spread towards the stomach or left arm, similar to that caused in angina. It is more severe in intensity and lasts longer than anginal pain. It may be associated with a pain in the stomach region and is often confused with pain due to acute indigestion or gas formation. Myocardial infarction is usually associated with a feeling of weakness, sweating, nausea, vomiting, giddiness and impending doom.

Myocardial infarction is caused by occlusion or obstruction of a coronary artery by a thrombus (blood clot adhering to the wall of the artery). The part of the muscles to be prefused by the obstructed artery becomes ischaemic or deficient in blood supply and the cells of the muscles die. They are finally replaced by fibrous tissues in vessels. Myocardial infarction is a medical emergency and the patient must be warned to seek medical aid as soon as possible. In most cases it has been observed that the delay is not only because of the time taken in transporting the patient to the hospital or the arrival of the physician, but also due to the delayed decision to call for medical help after the realization of the pain. Early treatment with thrombolytics have changed the outlook of this disease. Remember the golden hours; the first 4 to 6 hours of the onset of chest pain when cell death could be prevented by thrombolytics. So rush!! Don't wait.

The treatment of myocardial infarction consists of: 1) immediate steps which should be taken; and 2) continued use of drugs to avoid further complications.

### Immediate Treatment and Drugs

**Relief from pain:** Sublingual *nitroglycerin* is given initially for pain relief. If it fails then, the most effective drug is *morphine.* It may cause some amount of nausea initially but the relief of pain soon gives a feeling of well-being. It may produce a slight fall in blood pressure which is helpful in decreasing the workload on the heart. It is advisable to give *morphine* in as small a dose as possible. In some cases it can produce a severe fall in blood pressure. A dose of 5 mg given intravenously or subcutaneously is usually sufficient in providing relief from pain. *Buprenorphine* can be given in place of *morphine.*

**Oxygen Inhalation:** Oxygen inhalation through nasal prongs or face mask is used if oxygen saturation is low.

**Rest:** Rest reduces the work of the heart and restricts the area of the muscle suffering from decreased oxygen supply. It has been found that about 6 to 8 weeks are required for the healing of the affected area. For this reason earlier doctors recommended complete bed rest for about 6 weeks. However, these days most cardiologists do not consider it necessary, but believe that early mobilization helps to improve muscle tone and the general body condition, and the complications are minimized. According to current practice a patient with an uncomplicated condition can sit in a chair on second day and walk upto toilet on 3rd day. He can return home in 5 to 7 days. The patient should not stand up suddenly as there may be a fall in blood pressure. After 4 to 6 weeks he is encouraged to gradually return to work. He should have adequate sleep at night and lie down for an hour both in the afternoon and evening. After 8 weeks the activity should be regulated according to the exercise tolerance. Driving is permitted at this time.

**Reperfusion of the Heart Muscle:** Dissolution of clot (clot-busting) is the most important step in the treatment of myocardial infarction. There are agents like *streptokinase, urokinase, alteplase, reteplase, tenecteplase* which dissolve the clot in the blocked coronary artery , open it and provide reperfusion. *Urokinase, alteplase, reteplase* and *tenecteplase* are very expensive. *Streptokinase* is less expensive but can cause allergy in patients with history of sore throat due to streptococal infection. High level of antibodies may render it ineffective. *Uronkinase* (DEBUNASE) has also become cheaper and it can be used in those who are allergic to *streptokinase.* Each of these drugs may cause bleeding. They are not used in very high BP, pregnancy and recent surgery. If hazards of thrombolytics are high, immediate angioplasty (opening by probes) of infarct related artery is done. The maximum amount of benefit occurs if the drug is given early. Even minutes count ('minutes mean muscle'). However, even when patients present themselves after 6 hours beneficial effects have been observed. With *tenecteplase* low-molar *heparin,* such as *enoxaparin* (CLEXANE,LOMORIN-NX) is used in a dose of 30 to 60 mg initially and then 1 mg/kg twice a day.

**Aspirin:** A dose of 75-300 mg daily improves survival (30% reduction in death). *Aspirin* in low doses prevents stickiness and formation of aggregates of platelets. *Clopidogrel* (CLOPEVAS, PLAGERIL) is another powerful drug which inhibits platelet function.

**Prevention of IHD**

Polypill is an emerging concept of use of statin, *aspirin* and blood pressure lowering drugs in a single pill form to treat and prevent heart disease. This could prevent heart attacks significantly. At present trials are going on.

- Use of Statins: patients with vascular involvement must reduce LDL-C to <100 mg(preferably 70 mg%) — 'Lower the better'.
- Smoking Cessation
- Maintaining ideal body weight
- Exercise not only improves physical power but also increases coronary new vessel formation in heart muscles.
- Homocysteine levels can be reduced by folic acid 1-2 mg/day along with Vitamin-B6 and B12 *(Methylcobalamin)*
- *Aspirin* 80-325 mg/day

**Diet:** Food increases the blood flow in the stomach and increases the work of the heart. Therefore, the quantity of each meal should be kept small. During the first 5 days a liquid diet divided into 6 small feedings, is preferred. The solids can be gradually added after a week or so. The diet should be restricted in calories and saturated fats.

**Bowels:** The patient may suffer from constipation due to the liquid diet, bedrest, and drugs he is taking. He should be reassured that it will not do any harm even if he does not pass stools for a few days but straining may prove to be very harmful. However, it has been found that the patient is often distressed and uncomfortable without a bowel movement. He may be permitted to use rectal suppositories or may be given 30 ml of liquid paraffin.

**Sedation:** Sedation is quite useful during the acute phase of the illness. *Diazepam* 5 mg, three times a day is useful.

**Emotional Problems:** Anxiety, depression and stress can upset the patient. Reassurance (to spouse also), explanation and counselling are required.

**Anti-coagulants:** Subcutaneous *heparin* in a dose of 25000 units per day further prevents thrombus (clots) formation. It is used after clot dissolution with *streptokinase/urokinase.* It is continued for three days along with tablets of *warfarin* or other anti-clot drugs which are continued for subsequent treatment. This treatment is must if there is irregularity of pulse due to atrial fibrillation. Chances of bleeding are increased but close monitoring with blood tests avoids use of excessive doses.

**Role of Betablockers:** They provide some benefit when given, following an acute heart attack. *Metoprolol* or *carvedilol* are commonly used.

***Role of ACE-inhibitors:*** *Enalapril, Ramipril* or other ACE-inhibitors is usually given following heart attack for 6 months or longer.

**Nitroglycerin:** Intravenous NTG is very useful in left heart failure to relieve persistent chest pain due to ischaemia.

**Treatment of Complications:** Ventricular rhythm disturbance is a serious problem and requires IV lignocaine and electrical shock (defibrillator used). Sometimes very slow pulse develops after a heart-attack. *Atropine* is used intravenously in this condition.

Pump failure (cardiogenic shock) is due to very large infarcts and is a bad prognostic indicator and requires treatment with *dopamine* and fluids. Mechanical devices may also be needed.

### Subsequent Treatment and Drugs

Those who improve are at the risk of further ischaemia. Indentifying those patients by exercise test (ECG) and echocardiography is necessary. This is done at the time of discharge from hospital and 4 weeks after heart attack. Some patients may require bypass or angioplasty. The preventive measures (secondary preventions) are also started. Antiplatelet drugs *(Aspirin, clopidegrel),* betablockers, ACE inhibitors (*Ramipril* 2-5 mg once or twice a day) and reduction of raised blood fats by statins are the main measures. *Ramipril* prevents heart failure, improves survival, reduces hospitalisation and improves quality of life. Giving up smoking is single most effective contribution from patient himself. In those who continue to smoke have double death rate in 5 years after a heart attack.

# 16

# Drugs Used in Heart Failure

The heart pumps blood, which supplies nourishment to all parts of the body, including itself. During each contraction, the heart pumps out a certain amount of blood but under certain circumstances, such as in severe anaemia, chronic infection of lungs, overactivity of the thyroid gland, rheumatic or bacterial heart disease, disease of heart muscles, after a larger myocardial infarction (heart attack) and high blood pressure, its pumping capacity is decreased and this condition is called heart failure or congestive heart failure. Heart failure does not mean stoppage of the heart as is generally believed. The decreased output of the blood leads to back pressure of blood, causing enlargement of the heart and engorgement of the veins. Due to this back pressure, some amount of fluid and sodium ions pass out of the capillaries and collect in the tissues, causing swelling (edema). There is also a congestion of blood in the lungs, which causes difficulty in breathing and induces coughing. There is a decrease in the working capacity and when severe, even walking may be difficult. An x-ray of chest, electrocardiogram and echocardiogram (ultrasonic examination of heart) usually reveals the cause of heart failure (CHF).

## Treatment and Drugs

The treatment of heart failure includes general measures and drug treatment.

**Bedrest:** The patient must take adequate bedrest, for 10 to 15 days. The rest decreases the work of the heart and helps in early recovery.

**Diet:** In congestive heart failure there is collection of fluid with sodium in the extracellular tissues. The intake of sodium chloride in the diet should be drastically reduced to 2-3 gm/day. That means no addition of salt in vegetable and chapatis intially.

Drugs which can contribute to the CHF such as *verapamil,* pain relievers, steroid hormones, *propranolol* should be stopped.

If anemia is detected, it should be vigorously treated.

**Drugs:** The aim of drug treatment is to increase the contractility of the heart muscle, control sodium and water retention, decrease the workload on the heart and improve heart performance.

## Drugs Increasing Contractility of the Heart

### Digoxin (LANOXIN 0.25 mg )

*Digoxin* increases the force of contraction of the heart to make it a more efficient pump and lowering the heart rate. It is, therefore, very important that the dosages should be regulated so that the heart rate does not fall below 60 beats per minute. With improvement in the efficiency of the pumping action, the size of the heart return to normal and the back pressure is relieved. The fluid collected in the tissues returns to the circulation and edema or swelling is relieved. Breathlessness and cough are also set at ease. It is less commonly used now a days because benefits are for a short term and eventually the underlying cause determines the progress of disease. Now a days doctors advise gradual reduction of dose and stop it completely after 2 to 3 months. Overall deaths due to CHF are not reduced by this drug.

**Adverse Effects:** The adverse effects occur because of an overdose. If the heart rate falls below 60 beats per minute, the dose should be reduced. Some times even the normal dose may cause minor adverse effects such as loss of appetite, nausea and vomiting. When these symptoms persist, the doses should be reduced. A dose slightly greater than the normal dose may cause a number of serious toxic effects like headache, nervous irritability, abdominal pain, and a tingling sensation. Visual adverse effects in the form of greenish-yellow vision and flickering sensations are also quite common. Overdosage may make the heart hyper-irritable and it may start beating irregularly.

***Precautions:***

1. It is ineffective in heart failure due to beriberi, hyperactivity of the thyroid, and severe anaemia and should, therefore, not be used in these conditions.
2. Most oral diuretic drugs which increase the urine flow cause excretion of potassium from the body. Loss of potassium may increase the risk of the adverse effects of *digoxin*. Such patients are advised to take plenty of fruit juices and leafy vegetables which are rich in potassium. Potassium chloride tablets 5 gm may also be given but they cause gastric irritations.
3. A patient on this drug should not be given *calcium gluconate* intravenously. Several deaths have occured because of these two drugs being given together.
4. Sodium chloride (common salt) intake should be drastically reduced. All the foodstuffs rich in salt, such as *namkins*, salted dry fruits and nuts, *papad, chutney,* pickles, should be

**Stages of Heart failure**

The American Heart Association classified heart failure as

Stage-A : Patients at high risk of developing CHF

Stage-B : Structural heart disease likely to cause CHF

Stage-C : Current or previous symptoms of CHF

Stage-D : Advanced structural disease with marked CHF

*It is clear that most patients seek advice very late when symptoms develop and therefore CHF has a poor prognosis and mortality (5 year mortality is 50%).*

avoided. Butter and *ghee* should be replaced with vegetable oils. If the patient is overweight, he should try to reduce his total caloric intake in order to reduce weight.

## Drugs to Control Sodium and Water Retention

### Diuretics

Drugs which increase urine formation are very useful in CHF. (See chapter 'Drugs Used in High Blood Pressure' also).

### Furosemide

It is a very potent drug used orally and intravenously to treat severe CHF and oedema in lungs due to Left Heart Failure. Usual dose is 40-80 mg/day. Drug causes loss of electrolytes particularly potassium. Therefore, it is absolutely necessary to get extra potassium (as potassium chloride) during its regular use. One way to obviate loss of potassium is by giving another variety of drugs along with *furosemide.* These drugs are called as Potassium-Sparing diuretics. These counteract the loss of potassium. Such drugs are:

*Spironolactone* (LASILACTONE, SPIROMIDE AND FRUSELAR-C) is a combination of *furosemide* 20 mg and *spironolactone.*

*Triamterene* (FRUSEMENE) is a combination of *furosemide* 20 mg and *triamterene* 50 mg.

*Torasemide* (DYTOR, TIDE 10 mg) is yet another potent diuretic. It is also available with *spironolactone* ( TORLACTONE).

### Thiazides

For mild to moderate CHF, *thiazides* act as good diuretics allowing loss of sodium, potassium and water in urine. The same problem exists with their use and therefore potassium supplementation is necessary. Addition of a potassium sparing diuretic along with a *thiazide* is quite common practice to reduce potassium loss. For examples, ALDACTIDE which is a combination of *hydroflumethiozide* 25 mg and *spironolactone* 25 mg. BIDURET which is a combination of *hydrochlorothiazide* 50 mg and *amiloride* 5 mg. In some cases longer use of *thiazide* may cause impotency, poor control of diabetes, rise in blood levels of uric acid (gouty pains may occur) and lipids. Allergy may occur, occasionally.

## Drugs that Provide Long Term Benefits in CHF

### ACE- inhibitors

**Captopril,** (CAPOTEN) **Enalapril** (ENACE), **Lisinopril** (LISTRIL) and **Ramipril** (RAMACE) are the drugs which decrease formation of chemicals (aldosterone and angiotensin-II) which are responsible for causing structural changes in the heart with CHF. Therefore, their use in low doses for a longer period alters the course of disease (unfortunately *digoxin* could not do so!). The size and thickness of heart muscles revert back to normal and pumping capacity improves without significant adverse effects! This has been proved in multicentric drug trials which show prolongation of a 'good quality' life in CHF. The chances of sudden death are reduced and episodes of CHF recurrences are less. Obviously, they are increasingly used now a days (See chapter 'Drugs Used in High Blood Pressure'). Patients who are unable to tolerate ACE-inhibitors due to dry hacking cough, *losartan* (LOSAR) *candesartan* (CANDESAR) or *valsartan* (VALENT) is given.

**Other Treatment Modalities**

Implatable cardioverter defibrillators, cardiomyoplasty, ventricular assist devices and heart transplantation are future treatment options for CHF.

**Role of Beta-blockers:** It is a parodox that a drug which worsens CHF has shown to be beneficial in long term for the some disorder, provided CHF is treated beforehand and very low doses of *metoprolol, carvedilol* and *bisoprolol* are used. After 2 or 3 months the pumping capacity of heart increases and episodes of hospitalisation reduce. In a large clinical study of over 2000 patients it was found that such medicines reduce mortality by over 35% and therefore the trial was prematurely terminated! The only caveat is that use should be judicious and systolic dysfunction (poor heart contractions) is the underlying problem and patient has mild to moderate CHF treated or compensated with routine drugs only. (See chapter 'Drugs Used in High Blood Pressure'). Very small doses are used initially and patients are instructed to take weight daily so as to know the status of fluid retention. If fluid retention is suspected the doses of betablockers are reduced.

**Role of other Drugs:** *Spironolactone* acts as a mild diuretic but more importantly prevents heart muscle damage (fibrotic changes) when added to ACE-inhibitors in low doses of 12.5 to 25 mg per day. Its benefits are slow but steady. It should never be taken if there is kidney damage. In poor relaxation (diastolic phase) of heart, calcium channel blockers are effective. *Nitrates* (*Isosorbide dinitrate* ISORDIL), *hydralazine,* blood thinning agents and rhythm regulating drugs are also needed in some cases.

# 17

# Drugs to Treat High Blood Pressure

High blood pressure or hypertension is a common disease affecting adult males and females. It has been estimated that beyond the age of 40, about one-third of men and one-fifth of women suffer from hypertension. It is called as a 'silent killer' because of its smothering effects on various organs of the body and that too without symptoms! Since all of us fear high blood pressure, let us first examine what blood pressure (B.P.) actually is and why blood should need a pressure at all.

**What Is Blood Pressure?** All the tissues and organs of the body need nourishment in the form of oxygen, glucose, and minerals for their normal functioning. This nourishment is carried by the blood to various sites through the blood vessels by the pumping action of the heart. With each contraction of the heart the blood is pushed into the arteries. In healthy persons this pressure is normal, but in others it may be more than normal and is then called high blood pressure or hypertension. In some cases it may be less than normal and is then termed low blood pressure or hypotension. Blood pressure has two components — Systolic (upper) and Diastolic (lower). It is written as 120/80 mm Hg which means 120 mm Hg systolic and 80 mm Hg diastolic. The abbreviations 'mm Hg' means millimeter of mercury.

***Types and Causes of Hypertension:*** Hypertension has been divided into two categories: essential or primary hypertension, the exact cause of which in not know but there is generally a narrowing of the blood vessels; and secondary hypertension, due to the involvement of some organs or systems such as the kidney, adrenal glands, and disorders like toxaemia of pregnancy.

**Role of Obesity and Smoking**

**Obesity:** 70% of hypertensive males and 61% of females are overweight. The Framingham study showed that for every 1.0 kg weight gain, the BP rises approximately by 1 mm Hg. A decrease in body weight by 1.0 kg reduces BP by 1.6/1.3 mm Hg.

***Smoking:*** Nicotine and carbon monoxide of smoke constrict blood vessels and thus raise BP. Estimates show that smoking 2 cigarettes a day causes a rise in BP by 16%. Other factors are early life events, emotional stress and late sleep hours (after 11 PM).

In secondary hypertension, the cause can be treated and blood pressure brought to normal. Primary hypertension lasts a lifetime and needs continuous treatment. The most frequently occurring hypertension (90% cases) is of primary variety. Syndrome-X is given to a constellation of obesity, high BP, insulin resistance and raised blood lipids. It is commonly seen in India.

## When Does Blood Pressure (BP) Become High?

**Normal and High Blood Pressure Readings**

| *Item* | *Systolic (mm Hg)* | | *Diastolic (mm Hg)* |
|---|---|---|---|
| Normal | Less than 120 | and | Less than 80 |
| Pre-hypertension | 120 to 139 | OR | 80 to 90 |
| Hypertension | | | |
| Stage 1 | 140 to 159 | OR | 90 to 99 |
| Stage 2 | 160 & above | OR | 100 and above |

The 7th report of the Joint National Committee on Prevention, detection, evaluation and treatment of High Blood Pressure. See JAMA May, 21 :289; 250-72.

The treatment of BP is generally determined by the rise of systolic and diastolic BP and their impact on the organs such as kidney, heart and brain.

**What Happens When the Blood Pressure Is High?** Many people who appear to be normal may be suffering from hypertension which is diagnosed only during a routine check-up. The symptoms of high blood pressure may be related to elevated pressure itself, a disease of the blood vessel, or some other underlying diseases responsible for elevation of blood pressure. The most common symptom of elevated blood pressure is headache, specially in the back portion of the head. This is usually more severe when the person wakes up in the morning. Other symptoms are dizziness, giddiness, palpitation, and easy fatigability. In more severe cases the symptoms are bleeding through the nose or blood in the urine, blurring of vision due to changes in the arteries of the retina (screen for vision in the eye), incidence of dizziness or fainting due to transient decrease in blood flow to the brain, pain in the chest, and breathlessness. When blood supply of brain is drastically reduced, paralysis or 'stroke' may occur.

It is a well-established fact that hypertension may be both the cause and effect of heart or kidney disorders and may decrease the life expectancy of a person. Statistics show that hypertension, if untreated, shortens the lifespan of a person. There is 2 to 4 fold increase in ischaemic heart disease. High blood pressure is the second commonest cause of kidney failure. It is, therefore, important to detect the cause early and start the treatment. The treatment consists of general measures and drugs therapy. Any BP above 140/90 mm Hg should be treated. New evidence shows that BP should be kept below 130/80 mm Hg in pregnancy, diabetes and kidney disease.

**Correct Way to Measure BP:** Routine office BP measurement is done in a sitting position. One has to sit quietly with back supported for 5 minutes and arm placed at the level of heart. Coffee, tea or smoking are not allowed in the preceding hour. For establishing hypertension at least three readings one week apart is must. At each sitting two readings should be taken to confirm diagnosis. Readings are taken in both arms and if there is a significant difference then the arm with higher reading is chosen for subsequent measurements.

In diabetics supine (in lying down position) BP is taken and then it is repeated 2 minutes after erect (upright) position. This is done to detect any fall in BP in upright position. This is very important in diabetics and elderly lest they may fall under the effect of medicines used to control hypertension. In a number of cases BP is higher in the physician's office (clinic) than at home. This is due to a stress in the presence of doctor (in white coat) and is called as 'white-coat hypertension'. This phenomenon is more common in females. Patients self-check provides information on response to treatment that may improve adherence to therapy and is useful in evaluating that 'white-coat' hypertension. Home measurements can be done by 'dial type' variant of BP instrument, electronic self-inflating sets or by miniature versions which are placed on wrists. These instruments are reasonably accurate. However, they must be calibrated from time to time.

## Treatment

The general measures for a patient of hypertension are: 1) relief from emotional stress; 2) control of diet; and 3) regular exercises. The relief from emotional stress and environmental changes help in controlling the blood pressure to some extent, although, keeping the patient away from internal stress is difficult.

In dietary management, three aspects should be considered:

1. **Reduction in sodium intake:** Sodium chloride or common salt is known to cause fluid retention, thereby increasing the blood volume in the body. This is particularly more important in diabetics and Afro Asians whose BP is 'salt-sensitive'. Hence, its restriction is useful in patients of hypertension. Based on this, the patients are instructed to curtail salt intake, but most patients are unable or unwilling to do so. It is advisable not to add additional salt in cooked food. Processed food containing a large amount of salt should be avoided. Salty foodstuffs such as pickles, *namkins, papad* should be avoided. The use of diuretics, which increase the formation of urine, in the treatment of hypertension, has provided an additional method of deceasing body sodium stores, and the most practical approach now is to advise mild dietary salt restriction to less than 5 g salt per day — a little less than a level teaspoon in conjunction with a diuretic drug.
2. **Caloric restriction:** This should be followed if the person is overweight. It has been found that in obese or overweight patients the reduction in weight helps in normalising the blood pressure in 75% cases even without the salt restriction. Foods to be eaten and avoided and the role of exercises are mentioned in the chapter on 'Slimming Drugs'.
3. **Restriction in the intake of saturated fat:** This is necessary in patients of hypertension as it is believed that this increases the risk of development of arteriosclerosis (see chapter on 'Drugs for Lowering Blood Fat Level').

   The table given on the next page gives guideline for dietary regulations and life style modifications.

**Lifestyle Modifications**

| *Lifestyle Modification* | *Recommendation* | *Reduction in SBP** (mm Hg) Range* |
|---|---|---|
| Weight reduction | Maintain normal weight | 5 to 20 mm Hg per 10 kg weight loss |
| DASH eating plan* | Diet rich in fruits, vegetables, low fats, high fibre | 8 to 14 mm Hg |
| Salt (sodium chloride) intake | Reduce less than 2.4 gm/day. Avoid APC (*Achar, papad, chatni*) | 2 to 8 mm Hg |
| Physical activity | Brisk walking (30 min. per day, most day, at least 5 days per week) | 4 to 9 mm Hg |
| Alcohol consumption | Not more than 2 drinks (30 ml or 30 ml ethanol, 670 ml beer, 280 ml wine, 90 ml whisky) | 2 to 4 mm Hg |

*Dietary Approaches to Stop Hypertension (DASH); **SBP = Systolic Blood Pressure

## Drugs

The first real drug to treat hypertension was given to the rest of the world by India's indigenous system of medicine, A*yurveda,* wherein the roots of the plant *'sarpgandha' (Rauwolfia serpentina)* were being used for various ailments. Subsequently in 1953, Swiss scientists isolated the pure chemical substance, and named it *reserpine* (SERPASIL), which remained in the forefront for the treatment of high blood pressure for almost 15 years. Now, it has been replaced by more modern drugs and is used only rarely.

The treatment of hypertension requires a careful approach, depending upon the response of the patient. Drugs are required for life long and regular use is a must.

### Thiazide Diuretics

**Hydrochlorothiazide-HCTZ** (HYDRAZIDE), **Polythiazide** (NEPHRIL), **Hydroflumethiazide** (DIADEMIL), **Chlorthalidone** (HYTHALTON), **Indapamide** (NATRILIX) and Xipamide

These drugs are slow acting but very effective in small doses. They reduce blood volume for a short period of time but their main effect is on the blood vessels which tend to relax with their use. These drugs increase the BP lowering effect of other drugs, and thus many BP lowering drugs are availablr in combination with a diuretic. It has been reported that with these oral diuretics, in 40% cases of mild to moderate hypertension, the BP returns to normal. In the remaining 60% cases, even if the response is not adequate, the action of other anti-hypertensive drugs is significantly enhanced. This enhancement of the effect is related to the control of sodium ions. The most popularly employed agents amongst these are *hydrochlorothiazide* (HYDRAZIDE 12.5 mg) and *Indapamide* (NATRILIX 2.5 mg). One advantage of thiazides is that they are effective in kidney stones. *Thiazides* also preserve mineral content of bones which is additional benefit in the elderly.

***Dosage:*** *Hydrochlorothiazide* is available in the form of tablets of 25 and 50 mg and its recommended dose is 12.5 to 50 mg daily, to be taken in the morning. *Indapamide* is used as 2.5 mg daily.

| Goals of treatment-How much to reduce? | |
|---|---|
| Low cardiovascular risk | Less than 140/90 mm Hg |
| High risk | Less than 130/80 mmHg |
| With Kidney disease | Less than 130/80 mmHg |
| With Diabete mellitus | Less than 130/80 mmHg |
| Pregnancy | Less than 130/80 mmHg |

***Adverse Effects of Diuretics:*** Diuretics are generally well tolerated drugs. Common adverse effects are dizziness and dryness of mouth. They can cause skin allergy. A number of metabolic changes are reported on long term use. These lower sodium and potassium in body. Reduction in potassium may cause muscle weakness and in very rare cases irregular heart activity. Therefore, supplementation of potassium (fruit juice, oral potassium chloride syrup) is a must with diuretics. They may worsen pre-existing diabetes, increase blood calcium *(thiazides)* or decrease calcium *(frusemide)* and most importantly may increase 'bad' lipid levels in blood. In some cases gout is worsened due to increased uric acid retention in the body. *Thiazides* lose efficacy in the presence of poor kidney function (if blood urea and serum creatinine levels are high). *Frusemide* is effective even if kidney function is impaired.

***Precautions:*** Careful use of diuretics can reduce the incidence of adverse events. These should be taken in the morning and not at night. Potassium supplementation is usually not required with low doses of diuretics. Diabetics, patients with high blood lipids and those with gouty arthritis should seek regular medical advice and get appropriate blood tests done regularly if they are taking diuretics.

## Adrenergic Beta-Blockers

**Propranolol** (BETASPAN, CIPLAR, INDERAL), **Metoprolol** (BETALOC), **Atenolol** (BETACARD, TENOLOL, TENSIMIN), **Acebutolol** (SECTRAL-400), **Oxprenolol** (TRASICOR)

These drugs result in slow and gradual reduction in blood pressure. However, they may be useful in patients with coronary artery disease like angina or after acute myocardial infarction or arrhythmias. These drugs reduce the rate of re-infarction. Elderly patients are less responsive to them than the young.

These drugs reduce the blood pressure by reducing both force and the rate of contraction of the heart. In patients who are also receiving diuretics, the total peripheral resistance (resistance against which blood flows) is reduced. They also inhibit release of the biogenic substances, renin and noradrenaline, which may contribute to their anti-hypertensive effect.

***Dosage:*** *Propranolol* is given in a dose of 20 to 40 mg two to four times daily. Its long-acting preparation BETACAPS TR is given in a dose of 40 to 80 mg once daily.

*Atenolol* is given in a dose of 25 mg once daily and increased to 100 mg once daily. It is presently the most commonly used drug. It is available in combination with a diuretic (TENORIC 25, 50). It is a preferred drug. *S-atenolol* (ADBETA and ADBETA-H) are also available.

*Metoprolol* is given in a dose of 50 mg and increased to 100 to 300 mg daily, if necessary. *Metoprolol* extended release (MEOLAR-XL,12.5, 25, 50 mg) is used once a day. It is also available with *hydrochlorothiazide* (METOLAR-H 100 mg+12.5 mg).

*Carvedilol* (CARLOC, ORICAR, 3.125mg, 12.5 mg, 25mg, 50mg) is used to treat high blood pressure in a dose of 12.5 mg twice a day and gradually increased upto 25 mg twice a day. It has additional antioxidant property also.

*Bisoprolol* (CORBIS 2.5mg, 5mg and 10 mg) is given in a dose of 2.5 to 10 mg once a day. CORBIS-H contains 6.25 mg of *hydrochlorothiaze* also.

*Nebivolol* (NEBICARD 2.5 mg, 5 mg) has blood vessel dilating effects. NEBICARD-H contains 12.5 mg *hydrochlorothiazide.*

***Adverse Effects:*** Some elderly patients develop cold hands and feet. The sudden stoppage of these drugs may precipitate an attack of angina or even myocardial infarction and in rare cases, sudden death.

These drugs increase airway resistance and may provoke asthmatic attacks in patients with a history of bronchial asthma, chronic bronchitis, or any other lung disease. Although the newer cardioselective beta-blockers like *metoprolol, atenolol* and *bisoprolol* may be safer in such patients, all of them should be used very cautiously.

These drugs prolong the blood sugar-lowering effects of anti-diabetic drugs and mask the symptoms of hypoglycaemia or low blood sugar. The adverse effects on the central nervous system include fatigue, lethargy, vivid dreams, depression, memory loss, hallucinations, delirium, psychotic reactions, and loss of sensation in the limbs or paresthesias. *Atenolol* which does not go to the brain, may be worth a trial in patients who experience such adverse effects with other beta-blockers. Blood lipids may increase by *propranolol* like drugs.

These drugs should be avoided during pregnancy as they may cross the placenta and produce adverse effects of low blood pressure and blood sugar in the newborn. These are also excreted in milk. Beta-blockers may cause sexual dysfunction such as decreased libido (sexual desire) and impotence.

***Precautions:***

1. *Propranolol* should not be used in patients suffering from respiratory diseases such as asthma, bronchitis, or emphysema.
2. They should be used with caution in patients of diabetes.
3. The prescribed drug should be withdrawn gradually over a period of 1 week as sudden discontinuation may cause a severe heart attack.
4. Doctor should be consulted if the heart rate (pulse rate) is less than 60 beats per minute.
5. If there are any adverse effects on the nervous system, the doctor should be consulted whether switching to *atenolol* or another drug is advisable.

### Alpha-Adrenergic Receptor Blockers

**Prazosin** (MINIPRESS-XL, PRAZOPRESS), **Terazosin** (TERAPRESS), **Doxazosin** (DOXACARD)

The main place of *prazosin* in the treatment of hypertension is as the third or fourth drug when *thiazides, propranolol and calcium blockers* fail to control the blood pressure. The first dose of this drug produces a curiously powerful effect and should be kept as low as 0.5 mg and preferably be given at bedtime. All of these drugs are effective in reducing obstruction to the urine flow in enlarged prostate. A major benefit is that these drugs do not change blood lipids and may increase good cholesterol (HDL-C).

***Dosage:*** Usual dose of MINIPRESS-XL is 2.5 mg to 5 mg depending upon the response, TERAZOSIN is usually given in a dose of 1 to 2 mg. It can be increased up to 40 mg, depending on the response.

***Adverse Effects:*** These can be postural hypotension, dizziness, and palpitation due to increase in the heart rate. Swelling of the feet and impotence may occur and may require a diuretic.

***Precautions:*** The dose should be kept as low as possible particularly if other diuretics are already being taken when this drug is started. It should be 0.5 mg or even 0.25 mg given at bedtime to avoid a sudden fall in the blood pressure in the elderly.

### **Methyldopa** (ALDOMET)

It is a drug which acts on certain areas of the brain like the medulla and hypothalamus which are known to control the blood pressure. It is considered to be the drug of choice for pregnancy associated hypertension. *Methyldopa* is administered orally in a dose of 250 mg, 3 to 4 times daily.

***Adverse Effects:*** *Methyldopa* causes sedation and drowsiness in almost all cases which disappear after a few days of therapy. Other adverse effects are quite rare: they include dryness of the mouth, nasal congestion, impotence, retention of fluids, drug allergy, and depression, it may cause derangement of the liver functions which return to normal when the drug is stopped. In rare circumstances it may cause anaemia (haemolytic anaemia) and depression of the bone marrow.

### **Clonidine** (ARKAMIN)

It acts like *methyldopa.* Its effects are enhanced by diuretics. Its usual dose is administered orally in a dose range of 50$\mu$g to 200$\mu$g in 2 to 3 divided parts in conjunction with *hydrochlorothiazide*, in case of mild to moderate hypertension.

***Adverse Effects and Precautions:*** It causes drowsiness and dryness of the mouth which may persist as long as the treatment is continued. Other adverse effects are constipation and impotence which may occur in 10% to 20% cases on prolonged use. Allergic reactions including skin rash and itching are not so serious. When the drug is suddenly stopped, restlessness, chills, nausca, swcating, and insomnia with a sharp rise in the blood pressure may occur. Due to these adverse effects its use is declining.

### **Angiotensin-Converting Enzyme (ACE) Inhibitors**

These drugs reduce the blood pressure by preventing the production of *angiotensin-II* which constricts blood vessels in the body. The anti-hypertensive effect is related to vasodilatation (decreased total peripheral resistance). The blood pressure falls within two hours, but several weeks are required for achieving a maximum therapeutic response. Diuretics enhance the anti-hypertensive effects. Currently these drugs are the most commonly used in diabetes when associated with hypertension.

**Captopril** (ACETEN, ANGIOPRIL, CAPTOPRIL)

*Captopril* is used in a dose of 12.5 mg, twice or thrice daily. It can be increased to 25 –50 mg three times daily.

***Adverse Effects:*** About 10 per cent patients develop skin rashes with this drug. Loss or disturbance of taste occurs in about 70 per cent patients. Gastro-intestinal symptoms like nausea, vomiting, abdominal pain, flatulence, and diarrhoea may occur. It may cause loss of protein in the urine in 2 per cent patients and affect the kidneys adversely. Anti-arthritis drugs like *indomethacin* and *aspirin* antagonize the anti-hypertensive effect of *captopril.* A dry hacking cough is troublesome side effect, occurring in about 30 per cent cases and may require change of drug.

**Commonly used ACE-Is**

| *Combinations* | *Brand Names* |
|---|---|
| *Enalapril* 2.5mg, 5mg, 10mg | ENAM, ENVAS,ENACE |
| *Enalapril* 10mg with HCTZ,25 mg | ENACE-D, NORMACE-D |
| *Imidapril* 5mg,10mg | TANATRIL |
| *Lisinopril* 2.5mg, 5mg, 10 mg | LISTRIL, LIPRIL, LISICARD |
| *Lisinopril* 5mg with HCTZ25 mg | LISTRIL Plus, CIPRIL-H |
| *Perindopril* 2mg, 4mg | COVERSYL |
| *Perindopril* 2mg with *Indapamide* 1.25 mg | PERIGARD-D |
| *Ramipril* 2.5mg, 5mg | RAMACE, CARDACE |
| *Ramipril* plus HCTZ | RAMACE-H, ZIPRIL-H |

***Beneficial effects of ACE-Is:***

A number of benefits accrue from their use. These are

1. Smooth reduction of BP in all cases of high blood pressure.
2. Protective effect on heart (reversal of remodeling and hypertrophy) resulting in better output.
3. Preservation of kidney function in diabetics.
4. Improvement in the quality of life
5. Prevention of vascular damage by their antiatherogenic effects.
6. Improvement in function of vascular inner coat (endothelium).
7. *Ramipril* is shown to decrease cardiovascular deaths by 25 percent, stroke by 31 percent and heart attacks by 20 percent.
8. No derangement of sexual function.

***Precautions***

1. *Captopril* and *enalapril* cause rapid fall in the blood pressure and may precipitate a fainting attack.
2. These should be used cautiously in patients with coronary artery disease.
3. Kidney function should be checked frequently with these drugs. The dose should be reduced in patients with impaired kidney function.
4. These drugs should never be used during pregnancy as they cause foetal growth retardation.

## Angiotensin Receptor blockers

This group of drugs are suitable for those who cannot tolerate ACE inhibitor. Antihypertensive effects are similar to those of ACE-Is.

| *Combinations* | *Brand Names* |
|---|---|
| *Losartan*<br>dose 50-100 mg daily | (LOSACOR, TOZAART 25 mg, 50 mg) |
| *Losartan* 50 mg with HCTZ, 12.5 mg | TOZAAR-H |
| *Losartan* 50mg with *Ramipril*,2.5 mg | TOZAAR-R |
| *Losartan* 50 mg with *Perindopril* 4mg | LOSAR-A |
| *Losartan* 50 mg with *Atenolol* 50 mg | LOSAR beta |
| *Candesartan* (CANTAR, CANDESAR 4 mg, 8 mg, 16 mg tablet) once a day | |
| *Candesartan* 4mg with HCTZ 12.5 mg | CANDESAR-H |
| *Irbesartan* once a day | (IROVEL 150 mg, 300 mg ) |
| *Telmisartan* once a day | (TELSAR,TELIMED 40mg, 80 mg tab) |
| *Telmisartan* with HCTZ | TELIMED-H,TELSAR-H |
| *Telmisartan* 40 mg with *Ramipril* 2.5 mg | TELMA- R |
| *Valsartan* (VALENT 40mg, 80mg, 160 mg) daily | |
| *Valsartan* with HCTZ | VALENT-R |

Drugs from both of these groups (Angiotensin receptor blockers and Angiotensin converting enzyme inhibitors) are increasingly used in hypertension to prevent damage on heart, brain and kidneys.

## Hydralazine

It is one of the safest drugs available for the treatment of high blood pressure in pregnancy. It is given in a smaller dose of 20 mg twice daily and the doses are gradually increased in order to avoid headache and flushing which are prominent at the start of the therapy. It may be combined with *propranolol.*

***Adverse Effects:*** *Hydralazine* causes headache, flushing, palpitation, and peripheral edema. Most of these adverse effects are counteracted by *thiazide* diuretics and *propranolol* which may have been already given to a patient before starting therapy with this drug. The systemic lupus reaction is rarely seen when the daily doses of *hydralazine* are kept below 200 mg.

***Precautions:***

1. Some people metabolize *hydralazine* slowly (slow acetylators) due to a deficient genetic make-up. For this reason the dose should be increased slowly. This minimizes the adverse effects of headache and flushing.
2. *Hydralazine* should not be taken by patients of angina or with any history of heart disease.

## Minoxidil (MINTOP 2% lotion)

This drug is used in the treatment of severe hypertension in emergency rooms. It increases hair growth and has been used for treatment of baldness as 2% lotion. It is used only in severe uncontrollable hypertension.

## Calcium Channel blockers

This group of drugs decrease inward movement of calcium ion in cells of heart and blood vessels. Therefore, heart rate and pumping action of heart are reduced directly by drugs such as *diltiazem* and *verapamil.* These drugs reduce blood pressure in a variety of ways and protect kidney function also.

**Commonly used Calcium Channel Blockers**

| *Combinations* | *Brand Names* |
|---|---|
| *Amlodipine* | (AMLODAC, AMLOKIND,STAMLO 2.5 mg, 5mg, 10 mg) once a day |
| *Amlodipine* 5mg with *Atenolol* 50mg | STAMLO-beta, AMLODAC-AT,AMLOVAS-AT |
| *Amlodipine* 5mg with *Enalapril* 5mg | AMACE |
| *Amlodipine* 5mg with *Lisinopril* 5mg | HIPRIL-A, NUMLO-L, LISTRIL-AM |
| *Amlodipine* 5mg with *Losartan* 50 mg | AMLOPRESS-Z, AMLOKIND-L |
| *Amlodipine* 5 mg with *Benazepril* 10 mg | AMACE-BP |
| *S-amlodipine* 2.5 mg | ESAM, ESLO |
| *S-amlodipine* 2.5 mg with *Ramipril* 2.5 mg | ESAM-R |
| *S-amlodipine* 2.5 mg with *Atenolol* 50 mg | ESAM-AT |
| *S-Amlodipine* 2.5 mg with *osartan* 50 mg | LOSARTA |
| *S-Amlodipine* 2.5 mg with *Nebivalol* 5mg | NEBICARD-S |
| OTHERS are | |
| *Felodipine* 2.5mg, 5mg, 10 mg | PLENDIL |
| *Lercanidipine* 10mg, 20mg | LERKA |
| *Lacidipine* 2mg, 4mg | SINOPRIL |
| *Nifedipine* 5mg,10mg,20mg | Cap CARDULE |
| *Nifedipine* extended release | CARDULE-R, NICARDIA-R,NICARDIA-CD 3 |
| *Nimodipine* 30 mg | NIMODIP in strokes |
| *Nitrendipine* 10mg, 20 mg | NITREPIN |

***Advantges:*** All CCBs are useful in angina, IHD and hypertension. Except *diltiazem* and *verapamil* all can be combined with beta-blockers (*Atenolol* commonly). They are also useful in migraine and peripheral vascular disease. Kidney blood flow is well maintained and *nifedipine* may increase urine output. The anthypertensive effect is not blunted by anti-inflammatory pain relievers which is its unique feature. These should be used with caution in angina to avoid alarming rise in pulse rate.

***Adverse effects and Precautions:*** As a group CCBs can cause sensation of vomiting, constipation, swelling over feet and hypotension. *Verapamil* and *diltazem* precipitate congestive heart failure and heart blocks. *Verapamil* and *diltiazem* are never used with betablockers. They are not safe in pregnancy. These drugs do not significantly alter blood lipids and may have some bronchodilatory effects, thus are very useful in asthmatic hypertensives. In this aspect they are better than nonselective beta-blockers.

## Drug combinations

Use of two to three drugs is common in the treatment of high BP and fixed dose combinations of them are available.

| *Combinations* | *Brand Names* |
|---|---|
| *Reserpine* 0.1 mg + *Dihydralazine* 10 mg + *Hydrochlorothiazide* 10 mg | SERPASiL |
| *Losartan* 50 mg + *Ramipril* 2.5 mg + *Hydrochlorothiazide* 12.5 mg | SARTACE-H |

## Factors Influencing the Treatment of Hypertension

Several factors may be responsible for the hypertension of a patient and we do not always know the cause in each one of them. The drugs described above do not cure hypertension, these only lower the BP and let the patient live a normal or near normal life with the treatment. A patient's response varies from drug to drug or the combination. After careful trial and selection a drug is selected which may have to be taken for a long time and perhaps for the whole life.

The following advice may be useful:

***Elderly patients:*** Multiple drug trials have shown even better protection against stroke and other complications by treatment of the elderly than in the middle-aged. In elderly group there is rise in systolic BP while diastolic may remain normal. This is called as Isolated Systolic Hypertension (ISH-SBP of 160 mm Hg or above). Old dictum of calculation of BP as 90+ age is no longer tenable. Non-drug treatment includes exercise, salt restriction, liberal potassium, weight reduction and control over fats. Walking sharpens cognitive skills in elderly. Low doses of thiazides are considered to be effective. *Nifedipine* and *amlodipine* are second alternatives. There are problems in the use of beta-blockers. ACE-Is are also used in elderly. One advantage is that these drugs improve insulin sensitivity in elderly diabetics so that diabetes is nicely controlled. As a precaution, low doses should be administered initially, to try to maintain diastolic BP below 80 mm Hg.

***Smokers:*** Smokers should quit smoking. It is an independent risk factor for heart disease and stroke. Smoking damages the inner layer of blood vessels, accelerates rise in BP and increases chances of occurrence of complications. Effects of certain drugs *(propranolol)* is reduced. Smokers should avoid beta-blockers.

***Overweight Patients:*** These patients have high cardiac output, low peripheral resistance and increased plasma volume. Apart from vigorous weight reduction, fat restricted low caloric diet should be given. Low dose diuretics are recommended for hypertension. ACE-Is do not have adverse effect of lipids and are able to improve left heart function. Therefore, this group is commonly prescribed in obese patients.

***Diabetic Patients:*** Association of diabetes with high BP is common in a large number of patients. The harmful effects of high BP are more along with diabetes. Therefore tight control of diabetes and hypertension requires use of multiple drugs. This may result in interactions some of which can be harmful to the patients. In diabetes BP goals are lower than for nondiabetic (as stated earlier). The aim is to be keep DBP 80 mm Hg or lower. High doses of diuretics and beta-blockers impair insulin action, therefore, best avoided. ACE-Is improve glucose tolerance and kidney function in diabetes and hence they are the logical choice.

***Asthmatic Patients:*** CCBs have some bronchodilator effect. Therefore, *nifedipine* and *amlodipine* should be used in asthmatics. Beta-blockers are best avoided. ACE-Is can increase cough.

***Patients with High Blood Lipid Levels:*** If given, the dose of diuretics should be as low as possible. Betablockers tend to increase triglyceride levels, decrease HDL (high is good) and impair insulin sensitivity, so is best avoided. In contrast, *prazosin* clearly improves the lipid profile and is the logical choice. As ACE-Is and CCBs are 'lipid neutral' they may be used.

***Cost-effectiveness:*** As the prevalence of high BP is increasing even in low socio-economic class, the cost of the therapy is becoming a major factor in drug selection. In general 'generic' drugs are very effective and relatively unexpensive. Sometimes fixed dose combinations (FDCs) are cheaper than two or three individual drugs. Newer drugs (not necessarily better) are always costlier than time tested older drugs. Diuretics, CCBs and ACE-Is are becoming cheaper and are costeffective too.

***Use of Other Drugs while on Treatment of Hypertension:*** This is very important. One may suffer from other disease during treatment and may take medicines which may interact adversely with each other. Remember that if extra medication is needed then the prescribing physician should be informed about drugs being taken for hypertension.

***In Cough and Cold:*** Do not self medicate with OTC formulas. These may have drugs like *phenylpropanolamine* and *ephedrine* which may oppose the BP lowering effects of antihypertensives. Those patients taking *propranolol* or *atenolol* may have severe rise in BP with such cough/ cold remedies. Some patients with depression are given 'Tricyclic antidepressants'. These drugs antagonize BP lowering effects of *clonidine.* A number of pain relievers may also oppose the BP lowering effects of drugs. Thus *aspirin, indomethacin, ibuprofen* should be used sparingly and the treating physician should be informed about using them.

# 18

# Drugs Used in Disorders of the Joints

••••••

During the evolution process the human being evolved from four-legged to a two legged being. We have to pay a price of it. The entire weight of our body now rests on two legs instead of four. The knees take the weight of the whole body and are more strained. Exercise keeps joints lubricated for their mobility. However, now a days there is hardly any time to do the exercises. The physical activities have reduced and one feels lazy to go for morning walk specially after a late night on the previous day. A few decades ago there were only a few cars and one had to walk a distance to fulfill his daily needs. There were no lifts or escalators. Drive-in restaurants and cinemas were non-existent. There was enough physical activity to keep the joints moving.

We are also paying a price of our changed life style. The Indian style toilets made us to sit in squatting position gave enough exercise to our knees. Our mother cooked the food on wood fire sitting on the ground and we circled around to eat. This made our joints more flexible. Now every one looks for more and more of comforts and do not make the joints exercise. For joints there is a famous saying, 'use it or loose it'.

## Arthritis

Disorders related to inflammation of the joints are called arthritis. In our body there are many joints but commonly afflicted are joints of the legs, arms, and back. There are several types of joints disorders like Rheumatoid arthritis, Osteoarthritis, Spondylosis, Spondylitis, lumbago, frozen shoulder, but pain, swelling and immobility of the affected joint are common in all disorders. The cause of most of these disorders is not known and usually, symptomatic treatment consisting of conventional pain relievers and anti-inflammatory drugs are given. In some cases the disorder may be due to a faulty posture. This can be treated by correcting the posture and physiotherapy. These will be discussed towards the end of this chapter. Conventional pain relievers have already been discussed (see chapter on 'Pain Relievers'). There are 3 common types of arthritide, Osteoarthritis, Rheumatoid arthritis and chronic gout.

## Drugs Used in the Treatment of Rheumatoid Arthritis

Rheumatoid arthritis (RA) affects females around 40 years of age. There is involvement of small joints of hand and feet on both sides along with systemic manifestations. The disease is diagnosed by a raised ESR, Positive RA* factor and elevated CCP titre. If not treated then crippling deformities and restriction of movements may occur. In order to prevent these complications now a days different kind of drugs are used. The treatment involves two group of drugs — Anti-inflammatory pain relievers for mild to moderately severe disease; and Disease modifying antirheumatic drugs(DMARDs)

***Anti-inflammatory pain relievers:*** The usual doses of anti-inflammatory drugs are given in table. Adverse effects of anti-inflammatory are on stomach, kidney and cardiovascular system (See chapter Pain Relievers).

| *Drug* | *Usual dose (mg)* | *Remarks* |
|---|---|---|
| *Ibuprofen* | 400 to 600 thrice a day | Comparatively safer |
| *Naproxen** | 125 to 250 Twice a day | Not with food, Safer |
| *Indomethacin** | 25 to 50 thrice a day | Headache, more toxic |
| *Aceclofenac* | 100 twice/thrice a day | Newer,helps in tissue repair |
| *Diclofenac* | 50 thrice;SR twice/once | Liver damage |
| *Ketoprofen* | 50 to 100 twice a day | Like other drugs |
| *Piroxicam* | 20 to 40 Once a day | Swelling feet |
| *Lornoxicam* | 4 to 8 twice a day | — |
| *Nimesulide* | 100 twice aday | Not recommned for children, liver toxicity |
| *Etoricoxib** | 6 to 120 once; alternate days | Stomach friendly |

Useful in Acute Gout also.

### Role of Disease Modifying Drugs in Rheumatoid arthritis

Anti-inflammatory pain relievers reduce inflammation and pain but do not alter the progress of disease, hence now a days early use of Disease Modifying Antirheumatic Drugs (DMARDs) is recommended. These agents are slower acting but produce a gradual improvement and reduce the disability in RA.

### **Methotrexate** (NEOTREXATE 2.5 mg)

It is frequently used to prevent joint damage in Rheumatoid arthritis in a dose of 7.5 mg per week. It should not be taken immediately after meals. It produces benefits in 3 to 6 weeks. Prolonged use of *methotrexate* may cause liver damage and recurrent infections of lungs. Folic acid follow up is usually needed to avoid deficiency of folic acid and macrocytic anemia (a type of anemia in which size of red cells is increased).

### **Leflunomide** (LEFRA, LEFUMIDE 100 mg, 10mg, 20mg)

It is a new drug which changes the function of special white blood cell (T lymphocyte) so that it does not make harmful chemicals against joint-membranes. It is used as 100mg daily for 3 days and then 20mg once a day. It may cause diarrhoea, skin rash and temporary hair loss.

---

* **Rheumatoid factor (RA factor) is an antibody (IgM) present in high quantity in the blood of patients with rheumatoid arthritis. The most specific test is presence of another antibody Cyclic Citrullinated Peptide (CCP) in the blood.**

### Hydroxychloroquine (HCQs 200 mg once a day)

It may be used alone once a day or along with other DMARDs. Regular eye tests should be done to detect retinal involvement.

### Sulfasalazine (SALAZOPYRINE, SALZA-500 mg)

It is second line drug given twice a day which achieves slow improvement in 2 to 3 months. Patients with 'sulpha' allergy should not be given this drug

**Minocycline** *Tetracycline* antibiotics *Minocycline* and *doxycycline* are found to be effective in rheumatoid arthritis.

### Gold Salts: Oral Gold (AURONOFFIN 3mg,6mg, RIDAURA)

It is effective in arresting the disease progress. Injectable gold (AUROTHIAMALTE) is given as 50mg deep intramuscularly once a week.

It has high toxicity such as fall in blood pressure, eczema, kidney damage, nerve and liver damage. Therefore it is to be taken under strict medical supervision.

*Azathioprine* and *D-penicillamine* are other drugs which are used in rheumatoid arthritis.

### Biological DMARDs

An interesting group of drugs* which inhibit TNF (tumor necrotic factor-alpha), a chemical responsible for joint damage.

*Etanercept* (EMBREL 25 mg injection). This is a costly drug given subcutaneously as 25 mg twice a week for 6 months. It may cause severe respiratory infections.

*Abatacept* is a fusion protein which has received USA-FDA approval for RA.

### Role of Steroids in Rheumatoid Arthritis

If there is involvement of single larger joint (intra-articular triamcinolone) or involvement of vital organ membranes (heart) then *prednisolone* in low dose 10 to 20 mg daily may be used.

## Osteoarthritis (Degenerative joint Disease)

Unlike rheumatoid arthritis, osteoarthritis (OA) is the disease of elderly affecting several joints. The knee and hip joints and the finger joints are commonly involved .The degeneration of joint cartilage results in narrowing of joint space, bone resorption and damage to the joint .There is

**Treatment**

- Use of anti-inflammatory pain relievers
- Use of disease modifying treatments
- Supportive agents
- Exercise strengthens muscle and movents are preserved. Quadriceps drill is a time tested exercise which reduces pain of knee joint. Overweight individuals should reduce weight to lessen burdern on knee joints. Use of wedge-insoles (shoes) may help in improving gait.

* *Infiximab* and *Adalimumab* are yet not available in our country.

limitation of movement which is painful. The aim of treatment is to reduce pain, maintain mobility and reduce disability. In severe cases joint replacement is the only option available.

### Pain Relievers

*Paracetamol* is the commonly used pain reliever and if it not effective then other NSAIDs may be used (See chapter on Pain Relievers).

### Diacerein (JOINCERIN, OSTOGARD, DYCERIN 50 mg cap)

*Diacerein* is a slower acting drug which reduces the rate of narrowing of joint space and reduces pain. It is given in a usual dose is 50 mg once a day then gradually increased to 50 mg twice a day. It is available along with *chondroitin sulphate* (DYCERIN-GM). It may cause loose stools.

### Role of Neutraceuticals

*Glucosamine* and *chondroitin* sulphate are increasingly tried in osteoarthritis. These protect the joint cartilage. A number of formulations are available. Some of these are-

| *Formulation* | *Glucosamine* | *Chondroitin* | *MSM** | *Other Ingredients* |
|---|---|---|---|---|
| CARTILLAMINE LUBRIJOINT | 500 mg | — | — | |
| CARTILLAMINE Forte | 250 mg | 200 mg | — | — |
| CARTIVIT | 250 mg | 400 mg | 250 mg | Vit C, E, Mn |
| REJOINT | 250 mg | 400 mg | — | Vit C, E Mn |
| CARTIGEN Plus | 250 mg | — | 250 mg | — |
| NEUKIND ORTHO | 250 mg | — | 750 mg | Methylcobalmin 750 μg |
| JOINACE | 750 mg | — | 200 mg | — |

Methyl sulfonyl Methane

### Viscosupplementation

It is another fascinating therapy in which *Hyaluronan* (Hyaluronic acid) is injected into joint space for adequate lubrication and viscosity. Interestingly, *hyaluronan* was used intravenous in race horses to reduce their joint pains! This treatment is given when drugs have failed. Once injected the effects last for a long time.

### Other agents

Removal of excessive joint fluid and use of steroids (*Intra-articular triamcinolone* 20 mg) into knee joint once in three months (Not more than 3 to 4 per year) may help.

Green tea (Camellia sinensis) has *polyphenols* which are anti-inflammatory and antioxidants. *Ginger extract* (170 mg) is also effective.

## Drug Treatment of Gout

Gout is a disease of metabolism. There is over production of uric acid in body which gets deposited in joints. The most common joint involved is big toe joint. Typically pain is very severe and associated with swelling. Patient is not able to sleep. The disease tends to recur and affects bigger joints.

### Drugs for Acute Gout

*Indomethacin, naproxen, proxicam* or *etoricoxib* can be used for pain relief. These drugs may take a few hours for a good effect. The drug of choice is *colchicine* an *alkaloid* from the plant *colchicum autumnale.* One mg of colchicine is taken initially and then ¼ mg is taken every 2 hours till 1 to 2 mg total dose is taken. The effect is dramatic and occurs quickly in 4 to 8 hours. The adverse effects include nausea, vomiting and diarrhoea.

*Glucocorticoids: Methylprednisolone IV* or *prednisolone* orally may provide dramatic improvement and pain relief in acute gout.

## Drugs for Chronic Gout

### Allopurinol (ZYLORIC, CIPLORIC100mg, 300 mg)

This drug decreases formation of uric acid so blood uric acid levels and their deposition on joint-membrances. Usual dose is 100mg three times a day.

***Adverse Effects and Precautions:*** Allergic reactions, headache, dizziness and muscle pains may occur. Fluid and water should be taken more during drug treatment. It should not be given during pregnancy and breast feeding. There are some drugs whose effects may be changed by *allopurinal* so inform your doctor about taking medicines.

### Probenecil (BENECID)

It acts on kidneys to increase removal of uric acid in urine. Its usual dose is 500mg two times a day. It is well tolerated but some times epigastric pain and allergy can occur. It may change the excretion of other drugs such as *penicillin, cephalosporin* and *indomethacin* (excretion reduced). It also decreases excretion of *Rifampicin* in bile. Other drugs used are *sulfunpyrazone* (ARTIRAN) and *oxypurinol.*

### To avoid

- Food items which are high in purine
- Red meat and gravies
- Yeast extracts
- Alcoholic beverages
- Sea food
- Beans, peas, lentils, spinach, cauliflower and mushrooms
- *Pyrazinamide, Thiazide-* diuretics, *Niacin,* Low dose *aspirin* (they elevate uric and therefore should be avoided).

# 19

# Drugs Used in Malaria

* * * * * *

About two decades ago it was thought that malaria had been eradicated from India but recently, there has been a resurgence of this disease. Malaria spreads through a mosquito bite (female anopheles prefers to bite at night!) and the common causative organisms in India are *plasmodium vivax* and *p. Falciparum.* Malaria is characterized by fever every alternate day, followed by rigor or shivering and accompanied by headache and muscle pain. In some cases, there may be enlargement of the liver and spleen. *P falciparum* causes brain malaria which requires intensive care or else death may occur.The final diagnosis can be made by examining the blood for the presence of the parasite. Lately, resistant strains have erupted in some areas of India. This has made the treatment more difficult since they are resistant to usual anti-malarial drugs.

***How Does the Disease Progress?*** The malarial parasite injected into the bloodstream by the bite of the female anopheles mosquito reaches the liver where it multiplies. The baby parasites are released from the liver into the bloodstream, where they enter the red blood cells (RBCs) or return to the liver. Those which enter the RBCs, grow and further multiply. This leads to distension and bursting of RBCs and releasing the toxic metabolites of these multiplied parasites, resulting in rigor and fever. The released parasite may re-enter into other RBCs to repeat the cycle of growth and multiplication, causing another attack of rigor and fever. This new cycle in RBCs takes about 48 hours and accounts for the occurrence of fever and rigor every alternate day. Those which enter the liver may be responsible for continuance of the disease as it takes about two weeks' time to complete the cycle of multiplication in the liver. The parasites can be attacked in the RBCs or in the liver.

## Drugs

### Chloroquine (LARIAGO, RESOCHIN-150 mg base)

This is the drug of choice for benign tertian malaria which is usually caused by *plasmodium vivax.* The oral dose is 600 mg of *chloroquine* (base), followed after 6 hours by 300 mg, then 150 mg twice daily, for the next two days. The other drug of this group is *amodiaquine*. However, some stains of *P. falciparum* are resistant to *chloroquine*. In such situation, *quinine* is given intravenously.

***Adverse Effects of Chloroquine:*** Nausea, vomiting and stomach pain are some adverse effects of this drug. Headache, itching and blurring of vision occur occasionally. It can be given during pregnancy. Parenteral choroquine injections should not be used in children.

### **Mefloquine** (MEFLOTAS,MEFLIAM)

It is used for treating an acute attack and curing malaria due to resistant strains of parasites. It is a reserve drug. Its usual dose is 1.5g. once a week. Its adverse effects are irritation in the stomach, fatigue, headache, dizziness, visual disturbances, vertigo, tinnitus, insomnia, restlessness, anxiety psychosis, or seizures and heart-rate irregularities.

***Precautions:***

1. It should not be used in patients with a history of epilepsy or any psychiatric disorder.
2. It should not be used in children below two years.
3. Avoid its use in *quinine,* quinodine or any other drugs which may cause disturbance of heart beat before or after *mefloquine.*
4. It should not be used in pregnancy.
5. Driving or operating any machinery should be avoided.

### **Quinine** (QUINARSOL-300, SULQUIN, ZEQUIN)

This drug is obtained from the bark of the plant *cinchona* which is cultivated in Eastern India. The plant originated in South America where it grew wild. For almost a century, until the forties, the drug enjoyed an unrivalled role in the treatment of malaria. Its value declined gradually with the discovery of newer drugs, during the Second World War, which were more effective and less toxic. Its actions are similar to *chloroquine.* It is still a valuable drug for the treatment of certain multi resistant strains of the malarial parasites causing brain fever (cerebral malaria).

***Dosage:*** It is given in a dose of 300 to 600 mg orally, three to four times a day for 7 to 10 days. In cerebral malaria drug has to be given by intravenous route with glucose and saline.

***Adverse Effects:*** The adverse effects of large doses of *quinine* are quite serious and in some hypersensitive individuals may be caused even by small doses. These include ringing sounds in the ears, loss of hearing, vertigo, blurring of vision, skin rashes, nausea, vomiting, diarrhoea, abdominal pain, fever, convulsions, fall in blood pressure, and depression of respiration. It may also cause destruction of red blood cells (haemolytic anaemia). *Quinine* when administered intravenously in cerebral malaria may cause marked fall in blood sugar.

***Precautions***

1. Stop the drug immediately if allergy or palor of the skin (due to haemolytic anaemia) occur.
2. Avoid its use if you suffer from ringing in the ear or visual disturbances (optic neuritis).
3. Take the drug after meals.
4. Avoid its use during the first few months of pregnancy as it may cause abortion.

**Primaquine** (MALARID, PRIMACIP-7.5mg, 15 mg)
It is used for a complete cure. It is usually given along with or after *chloroquine.* Although it has prophylactic properties, it is not used for this purpose because of its toxic nature. *Primaquine* is given in a dose of 15 mg per day for 2 weeks, for a complete cure.

***Adverse Effects:*** In therapeutic doses it may cause abdominal discomfort and anaemia. Large doses may cause marked discomfort and alteration in blood (methaemoglobinaemia) and destruction of red blood cells (haemolytic anaemia) in individuals who have low level of an enzyme called as G-6 PD. Spot tests are available for testing of G-6-PD deficiency state. If G-6 PD deficiency is detected, *bulaquin* (AABLAQUIN) is available which is claimed to be tolerated well in a dose of 25 mg/ day for 5 days. The drug should be taken under medical supervision.

**Note:** Due to its toxic side-effects the drug is not allowed to be sold in regular chemist shops and is available only through the public health department.

### Combination Drugs

These drugs originate from a Chinese plant and are effective in cerebral malaria and in *chloroquine*-resistant *falciparum* malaria. These drugs are potent and rapidly acting and their use is increasing.

*Artesunate* (FALCIGO, FALSICARE, FALSIQUIN, ARTESTAR) is given in a oral dose of 100 mg twice a day on the first day, then 100 mg once a day for 4 days. Inj *artesunate* (60 mg/ml) is used in severe cases.

*Artemether* (LARITHER, PALUTHER) is given intramuscularly 80 mg, twice a day on the first day then 80 mg once a day for 4 days. *Artemether* is also available in combination with *Lumefantrine* (COMBITHER, FALCIRID).

*Arteether* (E-MALMALTHER, PALTHER 150 mg inj) is given intramuscular 150 mg once a day for 3 days.

***Adverse Effects:*** Bowel disturbance, irregularity of heart, fall in white blood cell count and abdominal pain have been reported. One should avoid drugs which aggravate these changes on heart-rhythm. These should not be used for prevention of malaria.

### Other Drugs

*Doxycycline* is commonly used with *pyrimethamine* and *quinine* for resistant falciparum malaria. *Atovaquone, Halofantrine, Lumefantine* and fixed dose combination of *chloroproguanil* with *dapsone* are yet to be available in India.

**Drug Combinations:** These are used for prevention of resistant malaria.

| *Combinations* | *Brand Names* |
|---|---|
| *Pyrimethamine* (25 mg) with *Sulfadoxine* (500 mg) | MALOCIDE, REZIZ, MALAPRIM |
| *Pyrimethamine* (25 mg) with *Sulfamethoxypyrazine* (500 mg) | METAKELFIN |
| *Pyrimethamine* (*Pyrimethamine* 25 mg with *Sulfamethoxazole* 500 mg | MALARWIN |

These combinations are used both for prophylaxis and treatment of *chloroquine* resistant malaria. For the treatment of an acute attack, 2 to 3 tablets are taken as a single dose. Patients who are allergic to 'sulfa' drugs and in infants this should not be used. Now a days *falciparum* parasites have developed resistance to this combination also.

WHO recommends following combinations in resistant malaria —

| *Regime* | *Comments* |
|---|---|
| *Artemether+ Lumefantrine* | Resistant malaria |
| *Artesunate+Amodiaquine* | Commonly used in Africa |
| *Artesunate+Sulfadoxine+Pyrimethamine* | - |
| *Artesunate+Mefloquine* | Usual treatment |
| *Amodiaquine+sulfadixine+pyrimethamine* | Low cost |

## Malaria while Travelling

Malaria can be prevented by *chloroquin* 500 mg (2 tab) to be taken once a week, starting from the time of entering, the infected region continued weekly till there, and for 4 weeks after leaving. If resistance is reported, *mefloquin* 250 mg tablet is taken as above. If it is not tolerated then *Doxycyline* 100 mg in a day for 2 days before entering the region continued while staying there, and for 4 weeks after leaving should be taken.

## Anti-mosquito remedies

Mosquito repellants are used to provide protection. Citronella oil can be applied as vanishing cream. Synthetic pyrethroids are available as mats, coils and volatile liquids for continuous use. These should be kept away from children and infants. Indian plant *neem* containing limonoids in its leaves that have a mosquito repellant property and have been used traditionally for this purpose.

# 20

# Drugs Used in Mental Depression

All of us go through cyclic variations in moods — sometimes happy and cheerful, and at other times, sad and depressed. Do we always need drugs when we are depressed? No, we don't. Drugs may be needed only when the depression becomes persistent in the form of a disease called Endogenous (mental) depression, interfering with our capacity to cope with everyday life.

**Symptoms of Mental Depression:** A patient of mental depression suffers from a slow down of physical and mental processes. There is lack of interest in immediate surroundings. The thinking capacity and ability to concentrate is greatly impaired. There may be complete or partial loss of memory, with only unhappy experiences being recalled. The appetite is inhibited or even augmented, and the person suffers from a lack of energy and loss of weight. Sexual desire diminishes and the person may suffer from insomnia or early morning awakening. As the disease advances, the patient shows behavioural abnormalities and may complain of various mental and physical symptoms. He may become extremely tense and anxious as if something dreadful is about to happen, or may develop a fear of meeting people. In some patients there may be a feeling of self-deprecation, guilt, or unworthiness. Such patients are prone to committing suicide if not treated properly. Alcohol addiction is associated with severe depression.

**Types of Mental Depression:** There are three broad types of mental depression — reactive, endogenous, and drug-induced. When it is associated with marked dejection, such as following the death of a near relative or friend, some major illness, failure in business or loss of job, or due to any other episode causing severe and persistent psychic trauma, it is called reactive depression, also called as Transient situational disturbance, i.e. a reaction to a particular event. Another type of depression found in many cases is endogenous depression, which means that it is not due to any obvious external reason but comes from within the patient. Certain drugs may cause mental depression. This kind of mental depression is called drug-induced or iatrogenic depression. These drugs are *propranolol, methyldopa, reserpine, oral contraceptives, cimetidine, indomethacin,* long term use of *corticosteroids* and withdrawal of *amphetamines*.

## Treatment and Drugs

The extent of illness should be carefully evaluated before starting therapy with antidepressant drugs. These drugs take 2 to 3 weeks' time to take effect, and the patient should be duly informed. Timely antidepressive therapy prevents the development of suicidal or homicidal tendencies. If drugs fail, then electroconvulsive therapy (ECT) may provide quick relief in severe depression.

### Tricyclic Group

**Imipramine** (DEPSONIL), **Amitriptyline** (SAROTENA), **Trimipramine** (SURMONTIL), **Clomipramine** (CLOFRANIL), **Amoxapine**, (DEMOLOX), **Doxepin** (SPECTRA)

Tricyclic antidepressants are commonly used in the treatment of mental depression. Of all tricyclics, *imipramine* has been most extensively used. These drugs raise the spirits or improve the mood of depressed patient. In a normal person these may cause drowsiness, fatigue, and uneasiness. The onset of the antidepressant action of these drugs is very slow, and usually take 2 to 3 weeks' time, although the side-effect appear much earlier. It is during this period that the patient needs reassurance. These agents are ineffective in controlling violent symptoms which are sometimes associated with mental depression. In such cases *phenothiazines* can be used simultaneously to overcome these symptoms. If the patient also has insomnia, *amitriptyline,* or *trimipramine,* which cause some sedation may be helpful. *Imipramine* is also useful in preventing bedwetting by children. For this, it is given at bedtime.

**Other uses of Antidepressants**

| *Drugs* | *Uses* |
|---|---|
| *Amitriptyline* | Migraine prevention |
| *Bupropion* | Smoking cessation (A chewing gum is available) |
| *Fluoxetine* | Obsessive compulsive disease, Bulimia |
| *Clomipramine* | Obsessive compulsive disease, Bulimia |
| *Imipramine* | Bed-wetting in children, Neuropathic pain |
| *Doxepin* | Atopic Eczema (Noctaderm 5% cream) |
| *Trazodone* | Sexual inadequacies |
| *Venlafaxine* | Generalised anxiety disorder |

***Dosage:*** The tricyclic antidepressants are given orally in small doses initially for a week or so, and then gradually increased. The doses of *imipramime, amitriptyline,* and *trimipramine* are nearly the same. These are usually given in a dose of 50 to 100 mg during the first week and then gradually increased upto 300 mg. The dose can be further increased or decreased, depending upon the response of the patient.

***Adverse Effects:*** These drugs cause dry mouth,urinary disturbance, constipation,blurred vision and heart rate disturbing potential (so are found unsuitable in heart disease) and erectile dysfunction in young adults (*trazodone* may cause painful erections) and increase chances of fits. These have very low safety margin. For these reasons their use is declining.

***Precautions***

1. These drugs should be administered only to an established patient of mental depression. Once the treatment starts, it must be continued for at least a few months.
2. These drugs should not be given to a patient receiving *monoamine oxidase inhibitors* (such as *nialamide*), as their interaction may cause high fever, depression of respiration, and

marked excitement. a gap of at least two weeks should be allowed before switching from one group of drugs to another.

3. The action of sedatives like *phenobarbitone, meprobamate, diazepam,* alcohol is enhanced, and may lead to a dangerous depression of the central nervous system.
4. These drugs interfere with the actions of *some BP lowering drugs.*
5. Drugs like *phenothiazines* or thyroid preparation enhance the action of tricyclic antidepressants; their doses must, therefore, be regulated.
6. Pregnant and lactating mothers should avoid these drugs as they may cause interference with the development of the foetus.
7. Depressed patients have suicidal tendencies. Therefore, a close watch on the intake of the drug should be kept.

### New Generation Antidepressant

Due to a large number of side-effects caused by the tricyclic antidepressants and the *monoamine oxidase* inhibitors, efforts have been made by pharmaceutical research groups to bring out newer and safer drugs. The drugs which have been introduced in India are shown in page 121.

### Selective Serotonin Reuptake Inhibitors (SRIs)

The major drawback of conventional tricyclic antidepressants are unacceptable effects on heart (fall in BP, rhythm disturbances) anticholinergic and neurological adverse effects. Low safety margin, as fatalities are common. Slow onset of action. Propensity to precipitate fits; sedation; incomplete/poor response in some patients. Advent of selective serotonin reuptake inhibitors (SSRIs) and serotonine noradrenaline reuptake inhibitors (SNRIs) have overcome above limitations to a greater extent. Such drugs are shown in the table given on page 121. These are becoming preferred drugs for the treatment of endogenous depression because of their merits, which are:

- Quick onset of action (*fluoxetine*-2-6 weeks)
- Little or no sedation.
- No interference with mental functions.
- No postural fall in blood pressure so appropriate in elderly.
- No precipitation of convulsions.
- Little chance of overdose and heart rhythm disturbance.
- Antidepressant efficacy equal to tricyclics.
- Utility in anxiety, phobia and obsessive compulsive neurosis.

***Adverse Effects:*** Nausea, interference with ejaculation, orgasm nervousness, restlessness, insomnia, loss of appetite, mild abnormal movements, headache and diarrhoea may occur importantly. These drugs may adversely interact with antihistaminics, antipsychotics, *propranolol, carbamazepine* and *diazepam*. Therefore, patients on such medications should have appropriate dose adjustments. Sometimes discontinuation of SSRIs result in bowel upset, pins-needles sensations, bodyache and sleep disturbance.

**Newer SSRIs/SNRIs**

| Drug | Adverse Effects: Sedation | Fall in BP | Fits | Heart Rhythm Disturbance | Usual Dose mg/day |
|---|---|---|---|---|---|
| *Fluoxetine* (FLUDAC, FLUNIL) | Negligible | No | No | No | 20 to 60 |
| *Fluoxamine* (Tab. FLUVOXIN 50 mg) | -do- | No | No | No | 50 to 200 |
| *Paroxetine* (Tab. PAROTIN, RAXIT 10, 20 mg) | -do- | No | No | No | 20 to 50 |
| *Sertraline* (SERLIFT 25-50 mg, SERENATA) | -do- | No | No | No | 50 to 200 |
| *Citolapram* (Tab. CETADEP, CELICA 10 mg, 20 mg) | No | No | No | No | 20 to 40 |
| *S-citalopram* (ESDEP, S-CETADEP, TOPDIP-S) | No | No | No | No | 10 to 20 |
| *Amineptine* (SURVECTOR 100mg Tab.) | -do- | Yes | No | Yes | 100 to 200 |
| *Trazodone* (TRAZONIL 25 mg, 50 mg) | Marked | Yes | No | Sometimes | 50 to 200 |
| **Minaserin* (TETRADEP 10 mg, 20 mg or DEPNON) | Moderate | Often | may precipitate | May occur | 30 to 100 |
| *Bupropion* (SMOQUIT 150 mg) | No | No | Moderate chances | No | 150 to 300 |
| *Mirtazapine* (Tab. MIRTAZ,MIRT 15-45 mg) | Marked | Sometimes | No | No | 15 to 45 |
| *Tinepline* (STABLON 12.5 mg) | Negligible | — | — | — | 12.5, 37 |
| *Venlafaxine* (Cap. VENLAROR VENLIFT 37.5, 75 mg) | No | No | No | sometimes | 75 to 150 |
| *Duloxetine** (DULOJOY, SYMBAL, SYMBAL-M) | Minimal | No | No | No | 40 to 60 |

* Some anticholinergic side effects present.

## St John's Wort (HYPERICIN, HYLAX)

*Hypericin* is an active ingredient of aerial parts of St John's Wart. It is an effective mood elevator and antidepressant in mild to moderate depression in a dose of 1 capsule three times twice a day. It is particularly used when depression is due to a serious medical illness, concurrent medications (*amitryptyline,* anti HIV drugs, *Theophylline* and *warfarin*) interact with it.

## Mono-amine oxidase inhibitors (MAO-Is)

These are older drugs effective in depression but show a lot of adverse interactions with drugs and food. The cheese reaction occurs when foods/beverages such as cheese, bean, red wine, over ripe fruits, broad beans, yeast and soya sauce (all contain a chemical tyramine) are taken by patients on MAO-Is.

# 21

# Drugs Used in Major Mental Illnesses

Mental illness is one of the most complicated disorders about which very little is known. No one likes to be labelled as mentally sick. Few of these patients are subjected to medical treatment. In some cases, it is considered that the illness is due to the entrance of some evil spirit into the body, and to get rid of it, prayers are offered.

Recent findings have shown that there are definite biochemical aberrations in the brain which cause mental illness. Since the 1950s, several drugs have been introduced which can effectively control the symptoms in most cases. These drugs allow a patient to live a fairly normal life and also prevent further deterioration of mental state.

**Types of Mental Disorders:** Depending upon the symptoms, mental disorders have been broadly divided into three groups: major mental illnesses (psychosis, schizophrenia — literally means 'split mind'and mania); minor mental illness (neurosis, anxiety reaction); and mental depression (affective disorder). In this chapter we shall consider the drugs used for the treatment of major mental illnesses. The drugs used in the treatment of anxiety reaction and mental depression are described in separate chapters.

In general, a major mental illness is characterized by such mental symptoms which cannot be reconciled with. The patient may have violent and uncontrollable instances of destructive behaviour; or he may suffer from illusion which is a false perception of reality: for example, a rope lying on the floor may appear to be a crawling snake; or delusion; which is a false sense of interpretation: for example, he may feel that he is a rich person and people around him are trying to conspire to cheat him and drive him to poverty; or hallucination; which is a false perception not accounted for by any external stimulus: for example, a person may imagine he is sitting in a garden full of trees and flowers with a kaleidoscopic play of colours, or walking around a lake, or that he can hear melodious music, when none of these really exists. Such symptoms have been reported to be caused by psychotomimetic drugs, hallucinogens like LSD, *mescaline,* and cannabis (*bhang, charas or ganja*), which have been widely abused by the younger generation. There is a disorganised thinking and abnormal behaviour including self neglect. The most important negative symptoms include flattening of emotions, poor verbalization, little interest in surroundings and relationships.

## Treatment and Drugs

Anti-psychotics (major tranquillizers) are used for the treatment of serious mental disorders. These agents bring about tranquility, peace and calmness of mind. These drugs are also called neuroleptic agents. Their contribution towards the well-being of humanity is praiseworthy. These relatively new substances were not known until the beginning of 1950s when the doctors had practically no equivalents to treat psychosis. Such patients were a problem for the doctor and more so for the family, who in most cases wrote them off, even while they were alive. The patients were often a source of embarrassment to the family, neighbours and distant relatives. Thanks to these drugs, the situation has altered dramatically. Millions of families have been saved from disruption and ultimate ruin. Many patients are living a near-normal lives and even neighbours have not discovered their true mental state. These drugs have saved the careers of many scientists, writers, artists and even politicians. Inspite of organic mental derailment, international celebrities have successfully retained their positions with the help of these drugs.

### Phenothiazines

**Chlorpromazine** (LARGACTIL), **Fluphenazine** (ANATENSOL), **Trifluoperazine** (ESKAZINE), **Thioridazine** (MELLERIL)

These anti-psychotic drugs modify the thought disorder and control violent symptoms. The selection of a particular medication often depends upon its side-effects. If a patient has responded well to a drug in the past, the same drug should be tried again.

*Chloropromazine,* the first drug of this group, has been most extensively studied, and in all cases where it is difficult to choose a drug, therapy can be started with this one. *Fluphenazine* and *Trifluoperazine* cause more muscle rigidity, although they have a weaker sedative effect than *Chlorpromazine. Thioridazine,* on the other hand, causes the least amount of muscle rigidity but produces moderate sedation. Although *Haloperidol* (discussed later) causes muscle rigidity, it is the safer drug for a patient with heart disease or compromised liver function.

***Dosage:*** In general, for the treatment of acute psychosis, the therapy is started with low doses which may be increased rapidly within 2 to 3 days to achieve control of the symptoms. The doses are then adjusted to maintenance level after a month or so. The usual range of doses are given in the table on the next page.

***Adverse Effects:*** The most common side-effect experienced by the patient is extrapyramidal syndrome (EPS) in the form of muscular rigidity; tremors and difficulty in walking, a situation which resembles Parkinson's disease. Addition of anticholinergic drug (PACITANE) may reduce EPS. The most serious side-effect, although quite rare, is allergic reaction, especially in the form of depression of the bone marrow, that is, the blood-forming system of the body. These drugs may cause orthostatic or postural hypotension which is not a serious problem unless the drug is given by injection. Other adverse effects are faintness, palipitation, dryness of the mouth, difficulty of urination and semen ejaculation, constipation, and nasal stuffiness. There may be slight fall in the body temperature and the patient may feel cold, drowsy, and weak. These drugs may also cause obstructive jaundice in 2 to 4% of the cases. They also cause increase in weight due to increase in appetite and in women they cause increased secretion of milk. They may precipitate convulsions also.

**Some Commonly Used Drugs in Mental Disorders**

| Drugs | Trade Names | Daily Usual Dose/mg | Daily Extreme Dose/mg |
|---|---|---|---|
| Cholpromazine | LARGACTIL, EMETIL | 200-800 | 25-2500 |
| Fluphenazine | FLUDECAN | 2-10 | 1-25 |
| Trifluoperazine | NEOCALM | 4-15 | 2-64 |
| Thioridazine | MELLERIL, THIORIL | 100-600 | 50-800 |
| Haloperidol | SERENACE, DEPIDOL | 2-6 | 1-30 |
| Trifluperidol | TRIPERIDOL | 0.5 | 8 |
| Pimozide | ORAP, MOZEP | 2-5 | 10 |

**Butyrophenones**

**Haloperidol** (SERENACE), **Trifluperidol** (TRIPERIDOL), **Pimozide** (ORAP, MOZEP)

These are some drugs of this class which are used in the treatment of major mental illnesses. They cause a higher incidence of extrapyramidal symptoms than *phenothiazines,* but the fall in blood pressure is less common. In rare cases, they may affect the bone marrow to cause a decrease in white blood cells. The toxicity to the liver is also considerably less. Some reports have indicated that the drug may convert a manic reaction into depression. *Pimozide* (MOZEP), a sister drug which has similar actions is given in doses of 2 to 5 mg. It has longer duration of action therefore, is good in maintenance therapy. It may cause a disturbance of heart rhythm. The usual oral dose of *haloperidol* is 2 to 6 mg per day and of *Trifluperidol* 0.5 mg per day.

***Precautions***

1. It has been reported that most psychotic patients fail to take the drugs regularly. In such cases, *fluphenazine decanoate,* a long-acting preparation, can be injected weekly.
2. Anti-psychotic drugs enhance the effect of respiratory depressant drugs and therefore, sleeping tablets or potent pain relievers like *morphine* and *pethidine* should be given cautiously to patients taking these drugs.
3. These drugs should be used very cautiously in patients with heart or liver diseases.
4. If the muscle rigidity is troublesome, the dose may be reduced or anti-parkinsonian drugs may be administered.
5. If the treatment is to be stopped, the dose should be reduced gradually to prevent precipitation of severe psychotic reaction due to the drug withdrawal.
6. If there is any evidence of allergic reactions as characterized by sore throat or fever, the particular drug should be stopped and another substituted.
7. Those patients who are taking blood pressure lowering agents, antihistaminic and *levodopa* concurrently should be monitored closely to avoid adverse interactions.

**Clozapine** (CLOPAZ, LOZAPINE, SIZAPEN, Tab. 25, 100 mg)

It is effective in resistant cases and does not cause extrapyramidal symptoms (abnormal movements). It does not raise prolactin level also. It may decrease white blood cell count (Agranulocytosis in 0.8% cases) weekly white cell count are done to detect early change. It may precipitate convulsions.

**Resperidone** (RESPIDON, ROZIDOL, ZISPER 1 mg, 2 mg, 4 mg)

A potent antipsychotic useful in acute psychosis. It is least likely to precipitate convulsions. Usual dose is 1 to 4 mg/day. It can, sometimes, cause postural fall in blood pressures.

**Olanzapine** (LOZAP, OLIZA, OLAPIN Tab. 2.5-20 mg)
It is a broad spectrum antipsychotic and improves positive and negative symptoms in schizophrenia. It can be combined with lithium/sodium valproate for mania.

It causes dry mouth, constipation, sleepiness, nervousness and weight gain. It is epileptogenic but rise in prolactin level does not occur.

**Quetiapine** (QUEL, QUITICOOL, SEROQUIN 25-200 mg)
It is as effective as *haloperidol* on negative and positive symptoms,causes less EPS. It causes dizziness, metabolic changes sleep disturbance and fall in BP on standing. Eye lens change requires regular eye examination.

**Ziprasidone** (AZONA, ZIPSYDON-20mg, 40mg, 60 mg)
It is as effective as quetiapine and does not cause metabolic changes but may precipitate heart rhythm disturbance.

*Loxapine* (LOXAPAC 10 to 50 mg cap.) and *Aripiprazole* (ASPRITO, ARIDUS 10 mg, 20 mg Tab., REAL ONE 10 to 30 mg Tab.) are other agents.

**Metabolic effects of Newer antipsychotics drugs:** Rise in blood sugar, lipids and weight gain is found with the use of *Clozapine, Olanzapine, Resperidone* and *Quetiapine.*

***Precautions:***

1. These drugs should be used very cautiously in patients with heart or liver diseases.
2. If the treatment is to be stopped, the dose should be reduced gradually to prevent precipitation of severe psychotic reaction due to the drug withdrawal.
3. If there is any evidence of allergic reactions as characterized by sore throat or fever, the particular drug should be stopped and another substituted.
4. Patients who are taking blood pressure lowering agents, antihistaminic and *levodopa* concurrently should have close monitoring to avoid adverse interactions.
5. Lactation and irregular menstruations may occur, therefore should be avoided in patients with breast diseases cancer.
6. Regular blood lipid and sugar levels should be measured.

The anti-psychotic agents should improve the acute symptoms within 48 hours. A demonstrable positive response may take about 3 weeks and the full effect may require 6 weeks to 6 months. It may be necessary to continue the treatment for several years. It has been found that the relapse rate after stopping treatment is about 30 to 40 per cent. Resistant cases may require use of other agents such as *Lithium, valproate* and *carbazepine.* In catatonic type of disease Electro Convulsive Therapy (ECT) may be useful.

Divided doses may be needed initially but maintenance doses are given once at night. Patients who do not take these medicines regularly are given longer acting injectable drugs like *fluphenazine decanoate,* a long-acting preparation, can be injected at 2 weeks intervals. A twice monthly injection of resperidone 25-50 mg IM is also available.

## Mania and Manic Depressive Illness

### Lithium Carbonate

A simple inorganic salt, *lithium carbonate* is effective in the treatment of manic phase of manic depression as a mood-stabilizing agent, prevention of mania in manic depressive illness, recurrent unipolar depression, and as an antidepressant in all patients who do not fall into a definite group. It does not produce any depressant or stimulant effect in a normal man. The efficacy and safety of lithium salts for acute mania and for the prevention of recurrent attacks of manic depressive illness is now highly impressive.

***Dosage:*** During an acute attack, *lithium carbonate* is given orally in a dose of 400 to 450 mg, 4 times a day. The maintenance dose is 300 mg, 4 times a day.

***Adverse Effects:*** Fatigue, muscular weakness, slurred speech, ataxia, tremors of the hands, excessive urination and thirst may occur. Nausea, vomiting, and diarrhoea may also occur, but these are not serious and can be minimized by giving the drug with food or in smaller doses at specified intervals. Higher doses may cause muscular twitchings and convulsions.

***Precautions:***

1. The total daily dose should be given in several divided portions at fixed intervals.
2. The drug should not be administered on an empty stomach.
3. Salt intake should be increased as *lithium* increase excretion of sodium from the body.
4. Anti-psychotic and tricyclic antidepressants can be given with *lithium,* but the doses should be as low as possible, as their combination may cause difficulty in passing urine.
5. Proper treatment necessitates estimation of blood levels of lithium periodically.

During acute phase, *Inj haloperidol* (SERENACE-5-10 mg) is needed. Alternatively, *resperidone, aripiprazole* or *olanzepine,* may be given orally. A few cases requires *Lorazepam* (2 to 3 mg) or *clonazepam* 1 to 2 mg for rapid control of mood. Lithium is started to stabilize the mood. Alternatives to *lithium* for maintenance therapy are *valproic acid, carbamazepine, topiramate* (See drugs for Epilepsy) and *verapamil.* It is a safer alternative during pregnancy. Among the other treatments are *phototherapy* and *psychotherapy*. In *phototherapy* the patient is placed in a room lit by light to simulate the season. It is most effective in mild seasonal depression.

# 22

# Drugs Used in Migraine

••••••

When the first edition of this book was published 30 years back we thought that in a few years there will be clear cut knowledge on the cause of migraine and specific treatment will be found out. Our hopes have been belied and today we know it a little better but have not fully understood it. The drugs used in the treatment are more effective but no cure has been found out.

It is a natural phenomenon that we suffer more from disease as we grow older, but migraine is a peculiar disease in the sense that it occurs at a young age (20-40 years) and wears off at old age. Another peculiarity is that it is more common in females (18% females suffer as against 6% of males). Does it mean that it has some relation to female sex hormones or to menstruation? We do not know yet. Let us see what this much talked about disease means. What is its cause? Is it a hereditary disease? What can we do about it?

**Symptoms:** Migraine is a recurring and intense headache which may not be relieved by conventional pain relievers. Does this mean that any severe type of headache which is not relieved by conventional pain relievers is migraine? No, migraine is a disease characterized by a pulsating or throbbing pain usually on one side of the head, and associated with one or more of the following symptoms: nausea, giddiness, vomiting, abdominal cramps, visual disturbances such as flashing of light, speech disturbances, sensory disturbances, or changes in mood. It is generally preceded by a peculiar warning signal (prodromal symptoms) known as sensory aura, which gives an indication of the onset of the attack. It may occur at any age and has been reported that over half of the migraine patients have close relatives who also have headache. Migrainous headache is more severe than tension headache.

**Causes:** The exact cause of migraine is not known. It is generally believed to be due to the pulsating dilation of the arteries of the head which activate pain percepting nerve twigs. It is uncommon in old age because of the narrowing of the arteries. Drugs which constrict blood vessels provide relief in migraine. A neurochemical substance, serotonin, has also been implicated as a causative factor of migraine. Most patients can know about an impending attack and should start treatment early to avail greater benefit.

**Precipitating Factors:** The various factors which may trigger off an attack are given below. Every possible effort should be made to avoid these.

*Psychological Factors:* Prolonged emotional strain due to fear, frustration, isolation, and rejection, or physical stress such as fatigue or excessive heat may trigger an attack of migraine. A migraine personality is characterized by compulsive perfectionism, achievement orientation.

*Foods:* Contrary to the belief that periodic fasting improves health, missing meals for more than 5 hours during the day or 13 hours at night may precipitate an attack of migraine. Certain foods such as cheese, chocolate, alcohol, citrus fruits, flavouring agents like ajinomoto (*monosodium glutamate*) used in Chinese foods, instant and canned soups, roasted nuts, processed meat, and instant gravies, may be the precipitating factors. An excessive amount of coffee or its sudden withdrawal may trigger an attack.

*Alcoholic Beverage:* Alcoholic beverages may show a periodic vulnerability to migraine.

The hormone estrogen has an influence on migraine. An attack may return during pregnancy. When the estrogen is high, though, there may have been a remission since childhood or adolescence . It may also occur soon after delivery.

Estrogen therapy or estrogen-containing oral contraceptives may worsen a migraine. If you prefer to use oral contraceptives, use the one which has the smallest amount of estrogen, such as OVRAL-L or PRIMOVLAR-30.

*Diseases:* Hypertension, cervical spondylosis, mental depression or anxiety may produce migraine like headaches. Migrainous headache is different than the 'Cluster headache'.

*Miscellaneous Factors:* Change in weather, barometric conditions, and exposure to glaring light may trigger a migraine too.

'Weekend migraine', more common in the West, is caused by the 'let down' phenomenon. Alcoholic overindulgence, increased social demands, or late sleeping are the contributing factors.

## Drugs

An attack of migraine may last for several hours and varies in severity. In some, attack is mild and require simple pain relievers such as *paracetamol* or *aspirin.* In others, it is severe and disabling and, therefore, needs to be treated with specific anti-migraine drugs. The drugs for treatment of migraine are of two types: 1) those used for relief in an acute attack; 2) those used for prevention of future attacks.

## Drugs Used in Acute Attack

### Ergotamine Tartrate (ERGOPHEN, VASOGRAIN)

*Ergotamine* is the drug of choice in the treatment of an acute attack of migraine. It causes constriction of blood vessels of the head which are dilated during an attack of migraine. It is most effective if taken before the attack starts, that is, when prodromal symptoms appear.

**Dosage:** It is generally used in a dose of 2 mg at the onset of attack, followed by 1 mg every hour until the headache is relieved, or a total dosage of 6 mg has been reached. It can be given sublingually also. In some people who have severe nausea or vomiting due to migraine, it can be given by inhalation, as rectal suppository or by intramuscularly (best avoided).

***Adverse Effects:*** *Ergotamine* may produce nausea, vomiting, abdominal, discomfort, diarrhoea, increased thirst, and drowsiness. More serious adverse reactions include weakness, pain or cramps in the leg and neck muscles, chest distress or pain, and an increase or a decrease in the heart rate. In sensitive individuals it may cause localized swelling and itching. In rare cases prolonged use may result in decaying of the fingers and toes (gangrene) due to constriction of blood vessels.

***Precautions:***

1. If *ergotamine* has been taken for a prolonged period of time, it should be discontinued gradually to avoid rebound headaches due to vasodilation.
2. It should not be taken by patients having high blood pressure , anginal pain of IHD andperipheral vascular disease
3. It should be avoided in cases of peptic ulcer, kidney or liver disease, and infection.
4. It should not be given to pregnant women as it stimulates the uterus and may cause abortion.
5. It should be used cautiously in children. A pain-relieving product without *ergotamine* may be preferred.

### **Dihydroergotamine Mesylate** (DIHYDERGOT, DHE 45)

This can be used by the intramuscular or intravenous route. Its effect is less pronounced than *ergotamine.* Only a small percentage of persons respond to this drug. The adverse effects and precautions for *dihydroergotamine* are the same as those for *ergotamine.*

### **Triptans** (SUMATRIPTAN, SUMITREX, MIGRATAN, 50, 100 mg tab; 60 mg/5 ml amp.)

These are newer drugs and are very effective in acute migraine. These are better tolerated than *ergotamine.* About three-fourths of the patients get complete relief within 2-3 hours. However, in some cases the pain may recur in 24 hours, due to short duration of action of the drug.

*Sumatriptan* constricts dilated blood vessels and reduces swelling and inflammation which causes pain. Usual dose is 50-100 mg orally at the onset of pain and repeated after 24 hours. It can be used by subcutaneous injection (3 to 6 mg). This injection is painful. These should not be used in children.

### **Rizatriptan** (RIZACT 5mh, 10 mg)

It is better absorbed and more potent than and is used in a dose of 10 mg as soon as possible and repeated after 2 hours.

***Precautions and Adverse Effects:*** Tightness of head and chest, abnormal sensations (paraesthesia) in arms and legs, weakness and dizziness are common short lasting adverse effects. Serious effects are slow pulse (bradycardia), precipitation of heart attack (acute myocardial infarction). In rare cases it may cause sudden death. Some cases of fits and drug allergy are also reported. Therefore, *sumatriptan* should never be taken by patients suffering from heart disease (coronary artery disease), epilepsy and high blood pressure. Other contra-indications are pregnancy, liver and kidney diseases. Patients should not drive to avoid any casualty. It is never combined with *ergotamine.*

## Drugs for Prevention of Future Attacks

Preventive treatment is needed if the attacks occur more than 2 to 3 times a month. Before starting this kind of treatment one must try to avoid or treat the above-mentioned precipitating factors. In most cases, it occurs unpredictably or develops in relation to such provoking factors as the work situation, which cannot be avoided or modified. The drugs for the prevention of attacks of migraine are described in the order in which they might be useful for this purpose.

### Beta-Adrenergic Receptor Blockers

**Propranolol** (INDERAL, BETASPAN)

This is moderately effective in preventing attacks of migraine and remains the most commonly used drug in this condition. *Metoprolol, timolol* and *atenolol* are effective in some cases.

***Dosage:*** In the beginning low doses of 20 mg are given 2 to 3 times daily; these are increased every 2 to 3 weeks until either the migraine attacks become significantly less frequent and/or dose of 160 mg/day is reached.

***Adverse Effects:*** It may decrease the working capacity of the heart, specially if large doses are used. In asthmatic patients it aggravates the disease. Some patients experience a feeling of weakness or lassitude and leg pains.

***Precautions:***

1. It should be used with great caution if the heart is weak.
2. It should not be used in patients suffering from asthma or related lung disease like bronchitis and emphysema (enlargement of the air sacs of the lungs, causing breathlessness).
3. Diabetes patients should get their blood sugar checked regularly while taking this drug.
4. It should never be stopped abruptly as it may precipitate a heart attack. Always consult a doctor if you want to stop this drug.
5. Do not increase the dose if a feeling of weakness or lassitude develops.

### Anti-Serotonin Drugs

**Cyproheptadine** (PERITOL, CIPLACTIN)

This drug blocks the receptors for the neurochemical serotonin in the brain and prevents dilatation of the blood vessels which cause a headache — most important factors in preventing migraine. It also has antihistamine and anti-acetylcholine effects. *Cyproheptadine* has an anti-bradykinin effect on reducing pain. Its efficacy is low. Treatment with *cyproheptadine* is begun with 2 to 4 mg tablet 2 to 3 times daily.

***Adverse Effects:*** The main adverse effects are drowsiness, dry mouth and appetite stimulation. It is often used in children for increasing their weight.

***Precautions:***

1. Restrict the food intake to minimize weight gain.
2. There may be drowsiness in the beginning. This becomes less and less as the treatment is continued.

**Amitriptyline** (SAROTENA, TRYPTOMER tab. 10 mg, 25 mg)
This is a mood-elevating drug used in the treatment of mental depression. It inhibits the uptake of serotonin in the brain and is moderately effective in preventing attacks of migraine. It is given in a usual dose of 50-200 mg single or divided thrice daily.

***Adverse Effects:*** Adverse effects are mild if small doses used in migraine. It has an anti-acetylcholine effect, causing dryness of the mouth and blurring in vision. The sedation caused by it is not troublesome if it is taken at bedtime.

***Precautions:***

1. Take the drug at bedtime as it reduces sedation.
2. Avoid its use if you are taking sedatives and tranquillizers.

**Calcium Antagonists**
**Flunarizine** ( NOMIGRAIN, FLUNARIL 5 mg tab./cap.)
Regular intake of calcium antagonists prevents attacks of migraine. Recent studies have confirmed this finding. Of these drugs *flunarizine* is the most effective. *Flunarizine* is commonly used for prevention of migraine and is found to be as effective as *propranolol.* It has selective action on brain blood vessels. It is to be given once daily in a 10 to 20 mg dose at bedtime for the first 15 days, and then the dose can be reduced to 10 mg gradually.

***Adverse Effects:*** Sedation, constipation, dry mouth, weight gain, flushing and fall in blood pressure are some of the adverse effects.

**Clonidine** (ARKAMIN)
This is another anti-hypertensive drug for migraine which is taken in a dose of one-eighth of that in hypertension. It is effective in only a small proportion of patients. Doses range from 0.025 mg to 0.05 mg, 2 to 3 times a day.

***Adverse Effects:*** Adverse effects such as drowsiness, fall in blood pressure and dryness of the mouth are rare. Controlled clinical studies conducted in recent years have indicated that it does not produce any significant benefit.

*Divalproex Sodium* (DIPROEX, VALANCE 125 to 250 mg) and *Sodium Valproate* (VALPARIN 200 mg) are anticonvulsants and are found to be effective antimigraine drugs. Long term use is associated with loss of hair, weakness and liver damage.

*Topiramate* (TOPIVAL, TOPIRAIN 25, 50 mg) an anticonulsant is also found to be useful. Its long term use is associated with kidney stone formation so take plenty of fluids with it. The drug should never be stopped abruptly. The doctor should be consulted if visual disturbance occurs.

## Other Drugs

Natural products such as *feverfew* — a medicinal herb and *butterbur*-a perennial shrub (75 mg extract) have also been tried. *Feverfew* has active substance (parthenolide) that reduces serotonin release and the benefit is found to be substantial.

Botulinum toxin type-A is a newer treatment which has shown 50% reduction in mean frequency of headache. It is investigational and costly.

# 23

# Drugs that Prevent Nausea and Vomiting

Nausea is a desire to vomit, which may or may not culminate in vomiting. Vomiting sometimes serves a useful purpose by getting rid of noxious substances from the stomach, but often leads to troublesome and deleterious consequences. In some, nausea and vomiting may be mild and short-lasting, requiring no treatment, but in others there may be prolonged vomiting resulting in excessive loss of salts and water from the body, leading to dehydration. Dehydration is more common if the vomiting is associated with diarrhoea. Vomiting is sometimes induced as a measure to remove poison from stomach.

**Causes:** Nausea and vomiting may occur even in a healthy person due to indigestion, an unpleasant smell, unpalatable food, drugs and chemicals, travel sickness, and pregnancy. These may also be caused by food poisoning; acute abdominal emergencies like appendicitis; obstruction of the intestines; disease of the stomach, gall-bladder and pancreas, liver, or peritoneum; acute infective illnesses like hepatitis, cholera, meningitis, malaria; heart disease like myocardial infarction.

The treatment of nausea and vomiting varies according to the cause. If it is due to any underlying disease, measures must be taken to treat the disease. If it is frequent and prolonged, causing dehydration, fluids should be administered intravenously. In most cases symptomatic treatment with drugs is effective in controlling the vomiting. Nausea and vomiting during motion sickness and pregnancy requires a different treatment.

## Drugs in Symptomatic Treatment

### Phenothiazines and Other Dopamine Agonists

**Prochlorperazine** (STEMETIL,STEMETIL-MD, WESTEL 5 mg), **Triflupromazine** (SIQUIL), **Promethazine** (PHENERGAN, AVOMINE), **Trifluoperazine** (NEOCALM, TRAZINE)

These agents are very effective in preventing vomiting due to almost any causes. The adverse effects, and precautions to be observed during their use, are the same as those of other *phenothiazines* described under 'Drugs Used in Major Mental Illnesses.' *Promethazine theoclate* (AVOMINE) is very often given in vomiting due to motion sickness.

***Dosage:*** These can be given by mouth, or if not retained by the mouth due to vomiting by intramuscular injection. The average dose of *prochlorperazine* is 5 to 10 mg; *triflupromazine,* 10 to 25 mg; and *promethazine,* 10 to 20 mg, twice a day.

### Antihistaminics

### Cyclizine (MARZINE), Meclizine (ANCOLAN), Dimenhydrinate (DRAMAMINE), Cinnarizine (STUGERON), Doxylamine (DOXINATE)

These drugs are reported to be less effective in preventing nausea and vomiting than *phenothiazines* and are used less often for this purpose. However all of them are very effective in the treatment of giddiness and vertigo due to various diseases such as Labyrinthitis, Meniere's disease and disease of brain-stem.

**Some Antihistaminics Used for Nausea and Vomiting**

| *Drugs* | *Dose/mg* | *Onset of Effect/min* | *Duration of Effect/hrs* | *Common Adverse Effects* |
|---|---|---|---|---|
| *Cinnarizine CINZAN* | 25-50 | 30 | 8 | Drowsiness, lethargy, visual disturbances, dry mouth and skin reaction |
| *Dimenhydrinate DRAMAMINE* | 50-100 | 30-60 | 4-6 | Sleepiness, dizziness, dry mouth visual Disturbances |
| *Meclizine DILIGAN* | 25 | 30-60 | 24 | Dry mouth, drowsiness, visual disturbances |

### Metoclopramide (REGLAN, PERINORM)

This drug prevents vomiting by a double mechanism, i.e. by a central action on the brain and by a direct action on the stomach. It is of specific benefit in: 1) vomiting during anaesthesia; and 2) vomiting after surgery. It is used in nursing mothers to improve lactation. Since it increases movements of stomach and intestines, it is also used in dyspepsia, reflux esophagitis (heart-burn) and post meal distension in diabetics. The usual dose is 5 to 10 mg, three times daily, by oral or intramuscular route.

***Adverse Effects and Precautions:*** It may cause sedation, diarrhoea and skin rash, and promote lactation. In some patients it may cause dystonia (abnormal jerky movements of face specially in children). It should be taken 15 to 30 minutes before a meal. It should not be given in bleeding ulcers.

### Domperidone (DOMSTAL, ENDOPACE)

This acts both on the stomach and the vomiting centre in the brain. It has less side-effects, especially on movement, than the commonly used *metoclopramide.* It is safe for patients suffering from Parkinsonism. It is combined with *omeprazole* or *rabeprazole* (DOMSTAL-O, ROLES-D) for the treatment of reflux disease. The usual dose of this drug is 20 to 40 mg, three to four times a day.

***Adverse Effects:*** It causes headache, dryness of the mouth, drowsiness, and breast engorgement and pain.

**Levosulpiride** (LESURIDE 25 mg tab): This is useful to prevent nausea and vomiting in a dose of 25 mg 2 to 3 times a day. It may cause dry mouth abnormal movements and sometimes fall in blood pressure. It may cause loss of sleep so do not take after 4 pm. Avoid alcohol while taking this drug.

**Cisapride** (CIZA, SYSPRIDE, UNIPRIDE- 10 mg, Tab; 5 mg/5 ml Syrup)
This drug has less antiemetic effect but promotes emptying of stomach and increases movements of large bowel which are needed for easier passage of stool. Hence this drug is used in chronic constipation (10 mg three times a day for at least two weeks) and heart-burn. Unfortunately, its use is associated with irregularity of heart beat so its use has declined. It is no longer available in USA.

A derivative of *cisapride* is *mosapride* (MOSID 5 mg, 10 mg tab.) which does not produce irregular heart beat. *Mosapride* is also available as a chewable tablet containing methyl polysiloxasane (125 mg) for the purpose of heart burn. Its anti vomiting effects are less.

**Itopride** (ITOKINE, ITONORM,TONATE 50 mg,150 mg tab)
It is mainly used to improve movement of sluggish bowels which results in constipation. It is available in combination with *rabeprazole* (VELOZ-I) for heart burn.

**Ondansetron** (EMSET, VOMISET 4 mg, 8 mg Tab; 2 mg/ ml injection)
This has fewer side-effects than *metoclopramide*. In doses of 8 mg, twice a day, it is very effective for nausea and vomiting due to radiotherapy or anticancer drugs and for postoperative nausea and vomiting. It can cause headache, constipation and allergic reactions. *Tropesetron* and *palonasetron* (PALZEN 0.25 mg/ml inj) are like *ondansetron* in actions.

**Granesetron** (GRANICIP, GRANISET 1mg, 2mg)
It is 10 to 15 times stronger in suppressing vomiting due to anticancer drugs.

Corticosteroids (*Dexamethasone* 8 to 10 mg given IV also suppresses nausea and vomiting due to *cisplatin* (anticancer drug).

*Dronabinol* is a synthetic drug from cannabis and has been found to have good anti vomiting effect.

## Drugs Used in Nausea and Vomiting during Pregnancy

Nausea and vomiting commonly occur during the first 3 months of pregnancy. The exact cause of these symptoms is not known. It is believed that certain psychological, hormonal, and nutritional factors may be involved. In some, the symptoms are mild and last only for a short period and can be corrected by psychological support. There are no absolutely safe drugs which can be used comfortably. You may find it interesting to know that *thalidomide,* a sedative, once extensively used in Europe by pregnant women, resulted in the malformation of the hands and legs in thousands of foetuses.

Vitamin-$B_6$ (*pyridoxine* 50 mg per day), and taking small frequent meals containing carbohydrates are helpful. If these measures fail, certain drugs can be given in as small a dose as possible, keeping in the mind the risk of adverse effects on the foetus (unborn child).

If the vomiting is very severe and incapacitating, *cyclizine* 50 mg, or *doxylamine*– (DOXINATE, E-PREG, FEELGOOD, VOMINATE 10 mg) be given for a few days.

Meclozine (DILIGAN, PNV, PREGNIDOXIN tab 25 mg with $B_6$) is commonly used drug. A preparation containing glucose, laevulose and phosphoric acid (REGURNIL SYRUP) may be used in 'morning sickness'. It should be given in a dose of 15 to 30 ml 3 to 5 times a day. It acts locally in stomach.

## Drugs Used in Nausea and Vomiting Due to Motion Sickness

The cause of nausea and vomiting in motion sickness is not known. It is believed to be due to the imbalance in the autonomic nervous system. The most effective agents in this situation are *belladonna* alkaloids, *scopolamine,* or *hyoscine.* Alternative drugs are *cyclizine, meclizine* or *promethazine* in the doses described earlier.

### **Scopolamine** (HYOSCINE tab. 0.25 mg)

*Scopolamine,* also known as *hyoscine,* is very effective in controlling nausea, vomiting, and giddiness experienced by some people while travelling by land, sea, or air. A long acting skin 'patch' is also available to provide relief for about 72 hours. The usual dose is 0.6 to 1.2 mg.

*Betahistine* (VERTIN, BETAVERT, VERTSTAR 8 mg, 16 mg tab) *Cinnarizine* (CINZAN, STUGERON, VERTIGON 25 mg) and *Promethazine theoclate* (AVOMINE 25 mg) are also useful.

***Adverse Effects and precautions:*** *Scopolamine* may cause drowsiness, dryness of the mouth, blurring of vision, constipation, and difficulty in passing urine. It should not be taken by patients with an enlarged prostate.

# 24

# Drugs Used in Osteoporosis

Bones always imply hardness. What would happen if bones are no longer hard and tough? The term osteoporosis means 'porosity of bones'. It is more common as age advances, in post-menopausal females, chronic smokers and alcoholics, those taking corticosteroids or have blood cancer. The bones become weak and easily break with minor injuries and falls. The spongy bones (backbone and leg bones) are commonly affected. A diet low in calcium also is a contributing factor.

**Bone Mineral Density (BMD)** is done to diagnose osteoporosis by Dual energy X-ray absorption method and its unit is T-score. A T-score less than 2.5 is considered to be significant. Individuals who have systemic and endocrine disorders, fractures with trivial injuries, perimenopausal females, loss of height, kyphosis (forward bending) and those taking oral contraceptives and steroids should get the BMD done.

T score of > minus 1.0 Normal

T score of -1.0 to - 2.5 low bone density

T score of < minus 2.5 Osteoporosis

**Daily Calcium Requirements at Different Age**

| *Age* | *Required Calcium per day* |
|---|---|
| Birth to 6 months | 400 mg |
| 6 months to 1 year | 600 mg |
| 1 to 10 years | 800 to 1200 mg |
| 11 to 24 years | 1200 to 1500 mg |
| 25 to 50 (women and men) | 1000 mg |
| 51 to 64 (women on HRT* and men) | 1000 mg |
| 51 to 64 (women not on HRT) | 1500 mg |
| 65 or older | 1500 mg |

* HRT — Hormone Replacement Therapy.

**Non-drug Treatment:** A diet rich in calcium such as mutton, fish, fenugreek, beetroot, dairy products, milk, Seetaphal, soyabean and ragi having about 1000-1500 mg of calcium should be taken. Simultaneously protein intake is increased, but put a limit on salt, meat and coffee/tea. These increase calcium excretion! Regular exercises which strengthen muscles also reduce the risk of fractures due to falls. In overweight patient weight reduction is needed. *Avoid smoking and chewing tobacco.* Reduced alcohol intake and cessation of smoking are important life style changes for the health of bones.

## Drugs and Supplements

### Calcium supplements

Regular calcium use partly reduces the rate of bone loss in post menopausal women. Various preparations available are :

| *Calcium Salt* | *Brand Names* | *% Calcium* |
|---|---|---|
| Calcium Carbonate | CALPLUS, CALCIUM SANDOZ<br>CALCIPLUS (OYSTER SHELL)<br>SHELCAL (OYSTER SHELL) | 40% |
| Calcium Phosphate | CALPOVIT, OSTEOCALCIUM | 30% |
| Calcium Citrate | CLINICAL, MILICAL | 21% |
| Calcium Lactate | OMILCAL | 13% |
| Calcium Hydroxy apatite | NATCAL OSEX FORTE | — |

This means that if 1g of calcium carbonate is taken, 400mg elemental calcium is available. One important fact is that foods high in phytate and oxalate (wheatbran, spinach, rhubarb, almonds, beans and peas) reduce absorption of calcium. Therefore, calcium salts should not be taken with these food items. Calcium from oyster shell may contain unacceptably higher lead levels. Most of calcium preparations are well tolerated but constipation and gaseousness can occur.

### Vitamin-D

About 800 IU of vitamin-D taken along with 1.0 to 1.5 gm of calcium supplements reduces the risk of hip-fracture significantly. A number of formulations have vitamin-$D_3$ 100 to 400 IU along with calcium salts. In other preparations (ALPHABON) active form of vitamin (ALPHA CALCIDOL 250 $\mu$g) is incorporated. In these doses they are considered to cause no harm.

### Biphosphonates

These increases BMD by reducing resorption (removal) of calcium from bones. Those available in India are

### Alendronate (OSTEOPHOS, DENFOS 5mg)

It should be taken (5mg to 10 mg) in the morning, swallowed with full glass of water and nothing is taken (food or other medicines, coffee, tea, juice) for 30 to 60 minutes. The person should stand or sit up right (without lying down) for half an hour. Instead of taking it daily it can be taken 70 mg once a week.

### Risedonate (RISOWEEK, RISOPHOS-35mg)

It can be used in place of *alendronate* in a dose of 35 mg once a week.

**Zolendronate** (ZOLDRO, ZOLEDRON 4mg)

It is used intravenously well diluted and infused in 15 mins. Single dose is effective for one year.

*Ibandronate* (150 mg once a month) and *pamidronate* are other alternatives

***Adverse Effects:*** Epigastric pain and heart burn abdominal distension and pain, diarrhea or constipation, headache and muscle pains. It should be avoided in peptic ulcer.

**Raloxifene** (RALISTA, BONMAX, GYNISTA 60 mg)

It is a 'designer-drug'. That is it is designed to act on estrogen-receptors of bones and prevent osteoporosis. Its elder sister *Tamoxifen* (MAMOFEN) is designed to act on breast rather than on bones. While its younger sister *ormeloxifene* (SEVISTA) is designed to be used in uterine bleeding. *Raloxifene* may be used in postmenopausal osteoporosis (60 mg/day). It should not be used if there is a past history of leg-vein thrombosis and jaundice and undiagnosed uterine bleeding. It should not be used in males.

*Sodium Fluoride* (NAF tab) increases formation of bone.

*Calcitonin* (CALSYNAR) is a hormone produced by 'C' cells of thyroid gland. It has been used as nasal spray (200 IU) in osteoporosis. Its cost is prohibitive.

**K-vion** is a natural vitamin $K_2$ 7 derivative available as 50 $\mu$g tablet. It improves BMD by increasing bone forming cellular activity in osteoporosis.

*Teriparatide* is parathormone derivative which increases bone matrix. We should take adequate calcium and vitamin-D with it. Its dose is 20 $\mu$g daily to be given by subcutaneous injection for upto 2 years

*Thiazide* diuretics in low doses retain calcium by reducing its excretion.

**Role of Estrogen (Hormone Replacement Therapy) in Postmenopausal Women**

Low doses of estrogen as Hormone Replacement Therapy in women who have undergone hysterectomy (uterus removed) or estrogen and progesterone for women with intact uterus is given cyclically to prevent bone loss. Estrogens *reduce loss* of calcium in bones and increase BMD. They are also prevent ischaemic heart disease, Alzheimer disease and relieve's menopausal symptoms but these benefits must be weighted against risk of vaginal bleeding, venous thrombi in legs, chances of breast and uterine cancer before starting HRT.

# 25

# Pain Relievers

Everyone experiences pain at one time or another, although the capacity to tolerate pain differs substantially from individual to individual. Pain, whether severe or mild, is an unpleasant symptom which warns of some disturbance or disease in the body. In *Paradise Lost,* Milton declares, 'Pain is a perfect misery, the worst of evils; and excessive, overturns all patience'. There can be various reasons for pain. But we rarely try to find out the cause of pain, and run for a pain reliever. For example, we often take a pain reliever for a headache, without knowing the cause, which may be due to smoking or worrying; something the diet like aminoacid rich foods such as cheese, nuts, pork, and fish; heavy deterioration of vision; fever; inflammation; and other causes. A pain reliever does provide temporary relief, but unless the cause is removed, the headache will reappear. This does not mean that whenever there is pain, the cause should be discovered first. We agree that unbearable pain should be relieved immediately for allaying emotional distress. But when it is too frequent or the pain persists and is not relieved by ordinary pain relievers, a doctor should be consulted.

Pain is broadly divided into two categories: superficial and deep. Superficial pain is of mild to moderate type, such as a headache, toothache, muscular, joint or nerve pain, a cut in the skin and a small boil on the surface of the body. Such pain arises from the superficial structures of the body and is well localised. This pain is due to inflammation. Inflammation is body's response to an injury or infection. There is swelling of injured area due to formation of fluid and accumulation of white blood cells (defence cells). Swelling is associated with redness, heat, pain and the area aches on touch (tenderness). For type, pain-relievers (analgesics) like *paracetamol, aspirin, or Ibuprofen* are used.

Severe deep-seated pain originating from organs like the heart, kidneys, lungs, or other important organs requires a strong narcotic (opioid) pain reliever like *morphine, pethidine, Fentanyl or buprenorphine.* These drugs are potentially dangerous and may cause addiction, and should be taken only under the direct supervision of a doctor. Other narcotic pain relievers, such as *codeine, dextropropoxyphene, pentazocine, or Tramadol* have less addicting liability. These are also used for mild to moderate pain. Abdominal pain due to spasms of the intestines, gall-bladder, or ureter requires anti-spasmodic drugs, sometimes, along with a narcotic pain reliever (see chapter on 'Drugs Used in Abdominal Pain'). When the pain is due to hyperacidity, antacids are useful (see chapter on 'Drugs Used in Peptic Ulcer'). When the headache is very severe and of a pulsating type (migraine), vasoconstrictors are used (see chapter on 'Drugs Used in Migraine').

### Treatment: Non-narcotic and Narcotic Drugs

Narcotic pain relievers (opioid/analgesics) act on the brain to reduce the reaction to pain, whereas, non-narcotic drugs acts peripherally to reduce the sensitivity of the pain receptors to the chemical mediator, *prostaglandin*, by reducing its synthesis. The later group is called anti inflammatory drugs.

### Non-Narcotic Pain Relievers (Non-Steroidal Anti inflammatory Analgesics)

**Aspirin** (DISPRIN, MAJORAL, DYNASPIRIN)

*Aspirin (acetylsalicylic acid),* which has been in use for so many years now, is an inexpensive drug, commonly employed for the relief of pain and fever. However, it is often available in combination with *caffeine* and other non-narcotic pain relievers like *dextropropoxyphene*. These combinations do not offer any advantage over the use of *aspirin* alone and, on the contrary, increase the adverse effects and cost.

*Aspirin* is also used in the treatment of rheumatic fever and rheumatoid arthritis for which high doses are prescribed by the doctor. In smaller doses of 75 to 325 mg this is used to prevent or reduce the recurrence of myocardial infarction (heart attack) and reduce suffering in patients who have had an attack of stroke. The small dose of *aspirin acts* by inhibiting platelet (sticky disc-like blood cells) stickiness and glueing together and allows blood to remain fluid and prevents blockage of blood vessels in heart and brain. For this purpose doctors prescribe it along with another drug called as *clopidogrel.*

***Dosage:*** For relief of pain and fever a dose of 600 mg (2 tablets of 300 mg), 3 to 4 times a day is adequate.

***Adverse Effects:*** In adults, adverse effects of *aspirin* are rare except in those who have gastric trouble. It has an irritant action on the stomach, which causes heart burn or epigastric pain but bufferred aspirin may be better tolerated. Prolonged use may cause a small amount of blood loss in the stools (occult blood loss) which is normally harmless. Severe bleeding can occur in patients with a peptic ulcer (see chapter on 'Drugs Used in Peptic Ulcer'). Allergic reactions in the form of skin rashes and breathing difficulty (asthma) are rare.

Recently, an association of *aspirin* with Reye's syndrome in children below 15 years of age has been reported although there is no direct evidence of it. In this syndrome swelling in the brain (cerebral edema), vomiting, and enlargement of the liver occurs. It may be fatal in 50% of cases.

The Drug Controller General, Government of India, has recommended that *aspirin* should no longer be given to children under twelve years of age. It is, therefore, very important to study the contents of a pain-relieving mixture and avoid *aspirin* in children.

***Precautions:***

1. Do not take *aspirin* on an empty stomach.
2. If an allergic reaction such as skin rashes or difficulty in breathing, develops *aspirin* should be stopped and doctor consulted immediately.
3. Patients of hyperacidity or peptic ulcer should avoid it.
4. The drug should be stopped if there is blood in stool or the colour of the stool is black.
5. Those taking a drug for preventing clotting of the blood, should not take *aspirin* without consulting the doctor. *Aspirin* increases chances of bleeding if taken along with these drugs.
6. Its use in children below 12 years of age should be avoided.
7. It should be taken with caution during pregnancy as it may cause birth defects, and delay onset of labour.

**Paracetamol** (CALPOL, CROCIN, MELIDENS, PARACIN, METACIN)

*Paracetamol,* also called *acetaminophen,* gained popularity in the early 1950s, because of its being free from irritant action on the stomach. Like *aspirin* it lowers the body temperature and also relieves pain, but has little anti-inflammatory activity. However, several deaths reported in England due to its heavy consumption (about 10 g daily) caused concern among professionals. It was soon discovered that a large quantity of a toxic metabolite of this drug damaged the liver. With normal doses, the quantity of this metabolite is very small and the body can take care of it without any adverse effects. It is available as tablets, syrups, suppository (ANAMOL) and injections and is useful for pain and fever in children and to those who want to avoid *aspirin* due to gastric trouble. It is currently the most commonly used pain reliever and fever reducing drug and is available as a single drug as well as in combination with other drugs, such as *ibuprofen* (BUFEX PLUS, FLEXON, MAGADOL, ZUPAR), *aceclofenac* (ZERODOL-P), *pentazocine* (DYMIC, FORACET) and *dextropropoxyphene* (PROXYVON, PROXYTAB).

**Dosage**

| Age | Dose |
|---|---|
| 1 to 3 years | 80 mg to 120 mg, 3 to 4 times daily. |
| 3 to 6 years | 120 mg, 3 to 4 times daily. |
| 7 to 12 years | 162 mg to 325 mg, 3 to 4 times daily. |
| 12 and above | 500 mg to 650 mg, taken 3 to 4 times (upto a maximum 4g) a day |

***Adverse Effect:*** *Paracetamol* is a safe drug unless used in a daily dose of more than 4 g. Such overdosage damages the liver cells; this can be fatal. Allergic reactions in the form of skin rashes, itching, and drug fever are very rare. Rarely, it can promote an asthmatic attack in patients allergic to *aspirin.*

***Precautions:***

1. Those suffering from or have suffered, liver disease should avoid it.
2. Alcoholics with a weak liver should avoid its frequent use.
3. Adults should never take more than 4 g (8 tablets) of it in a day.
4. Stop the drug and consult the doctor if you develop any symptoms of allergy.
5. Avoid its continous use for more than 10 days except on the advice of a physician.

**Analgin** (NOVALGIN)

*Analgin* has various other names like *metamizol, dipyrone,* and *noramidopyrine.* The general belief that *analgin* is a more powerful pain reliever than others is far from true. We discourage its use as it can cause serious adverse reactions. However, it is a pity that general shops sell it freely.

*Analgin* depresses the bone marrow, which is the blood-forming organ, due to an allergic reaction which is life-threatening.

In most western countries, it has virtually disappeared from the therapeutic scene but continues to be sold in some East European and most developing countries. In India, a ban has been put on the use of *amidopyrine* due to its adverse effects, but the closely related drug, *analgin*, which is nothing but *nor-amidopyrine* and produces similar adverse effects, continues. The argument that it is available in injection form and can be used in emergencies in unconscious patients, is not acceptable, as the safer drug, *paracetamol,* is also available in this form.

**Opiod Analgesics For Cancer Pain**

| *Drug* | *Length of Effectiveness* | *Other Information* |
|---|---|---|
| *Morphine* | Intravenous or Intramuscular: 2 to 3 hrs. By Mouth: 3 to 4 hrs. Sustained release: 8 to 10 hrs. | Starts to work quickly; can be very effective for cancer pain |
| *Codeine* | By Mouth: 3 to 4 hrs. | Less potent than *morphine.* Sometimes taken with *aspirin* or *paracetamol.* |
| *Pethidine* | Intravenous or Intramuscular: about 3 hrs. By Mouth: not very effective | Can cause seizures, tremors & muscle spasms. |
| *Methadone* | By Mouth: 4 to 6 hrs., sometimes longer | Also used for treating heroin withdrawal. |
| *D-Propoxyphene* | By Mouth: 3 to 4 hrs. | Generally taken with aspirin or *acetaminophen* to treat mild pain. |
| *Levorphanol* | Intravenous or Intramuscular: 4 hrs. By Mouth: about 4 hrs. | Oral form is strong and can be used instead of *morphine.* |
| *Hydromorphone* | Intravenous or Intramuscular: 2 to 4 hrs. By Mouth: 2 to 4 hrs. Rectal suppository: 4 hrs. | Begins to work quickly can be used insted of *morphine;* helpful for cancer pain. |
| *Oxymorphone* | Intravenous or Intramuscular: 3 to 4 hrs. Rectal suppository : 4 hrs. | Starts to work quickly |
| *Oxycodone* | By Mouth: 3 to 4 hrs. | Usually combined with *aspirin* or *paracetamol.* |
| *Pentazocine* | By Mouth: upto 4 hrs. | Can block pain killing action of other opioids; about as strong as *codeine;* can cause confusion & anxiety specially in the elderly. |
| *Buprenorphine* | By Mouth: 6 to 8 hrs. Intramuscularly: 6 to 8 hrs. | Can block pain killing action of other drugs. It is 25 times more potent to *morphine.* It can cause fall in BP |
| *Fentanyl* | Skin Patch: releases 25-75 mcg/hr. | Intractable cancer pain. Change the area on reapplication. |

**Ibuproben** (BRUFEN)

It has pain relieving and anti-inflammatory effects and also reduces raised body temperature. It is perhaps the most commonly used pain relieving drug and available as an over-the-counter analgesic in India. The drug is also used in arthritis and soft tissue injuries and swelling such as cellulitis, vasectomy wounds, tooth extraction and after operations. It is considered to be the safest anti-inflammatory analgesic (except *paracetamol*) today. Its usual dose is Tab. 400 to 800 mg 3 times daily in adults and as suspension of 100 mg per 5 ml for children (10 to 15 mg per kg body weight).

Other drugs which have *ibuprofen* like actions are *neproxen* (ARTAGEN, NAPROSYN 250 mg tab.), *Ketoprofen* (OSTOFEN 50 mg tab.) and *Flurbiprofen* (ARFLUR 100 mg tab.). A number of fixed dose combinations of *ibuprofen* and *paracetamol* are available and are commonly used. These are no more effective than adequate doses of *ibuprofen* alone.

***Precautions***

1. *Ibuprofen* can cause gastric upset.
2. It should be avoided by pregnant women.
3. It suppresses platelet function so avoided in those taking low dose of *aspirin.*
4. Patient of high blood pressure may have a reduced BP lowering effect of antihypertensive drugs if full doses of *ibuprofen* are given.

### **Indomethacin** (INDOCAP)

It is a strong anti-inflammatory drug and thus alleviates injury related pain. It is used in *aspirin* resistant ankylosing spondylitis, rheumatoid arthritis and fever in cancers. It is especially useful to close the patent ductus (a birth effect of heart) in a dose of 0.1 to 0.2mg per kg. Usual dose is 25 to 50 mg three times a day. A suppository can be inserted in rectum to reduce morning stiffness in rheumatoid arthritis.

***Adverse Effects and Precautions:*** In 50 per cent users, it may cause gastric upset, nausea, vomiting, diaorrhea. Ironically it can cause headache. White blood cell count may decrease and allergic reactions may occur. *Indomethacin* reduces alertness so drivers, machine operators, epileptics and psychiatric patients should avoid its use. It is contraindicated in pregnancy. It may also lead to kidney damage.

### **Mephenamic Acid** (MEFTAL)

This drug has been used to reduce the pain during menstruation (dysmenorrhea). It shares many actions with *ibuprofen.* Usual dose of 250 to 500 mg is given three times a day. It is also available as a combination with *dicyclomine* (MEFTAL-SPAS for colics).

***Adverse Effects and Precautions:*** It may causes diarrhoea and kidney damage. Same precautions should be observed as for above drugs.

### **Diclofenac Sodium/ Potassium** (VOVERAN)

It has anti-inflammatory effect and is another commonly used drug in arthritis. It is used in a dose of 50 mg twice or three times a day. It is available as local gel or cream and injection for intramuscular use. A FDC with *paracetamol* is used as a strong analgesic.

***Adverse Effects:*** It may cause gastric upset, nausea, dizziness and liver toxicity.

### **Piroxicam** (Cap. PIROX, TOLDIN, DOLONEX DT-10 mg tablet)

It is given once a day. It may cause swelling (edema) of feet. Its adverse effects are like those of *diclofenac.* It is not given to children. *Meloxicam* (Tab. MELO, M-CAM 7.5mg, 15mg) and *tenoxicam* (TOBITIL 20mg) are related agents.

**Lornoxicam** (Cap. NYOX, LONOXI tab, FLEXILOR 8 mg inj)
It is a newer drug which acts like *piroxicam* and is considered to be safer. It is usually given as a tablet of 4 to 8 mg twice a day. Injectable *lornoxicam* quickly relieves severe pain. For sustained effect *lornoxicam* should be given orally.

***Adverse Effects Common to Anti-Inflammatory Analgesics:*** They may aggravate peptic ulcer, high B.P. (reduce effects of BP lowering drugs), congestive cardiac failure, kidney disease (blood urea, serum creatinine may rise) and bleeding disorder (Not given in haemophilia).

## Newer Non-narcotic Pain Relieving Drugs

In order to avoid/reduce the adverse effects of these drugs particularly on stomach (bleeding from existing ulcers, erosion of stomach lining), a number of drugs are developed which have analgesic activity equal to existing drugs but are friendly to stomach. This group of drugs is called COX-2 inhibitors. Some are less selective than others. These drugs are:

### How to choose the Right Pain-Relieving Tablet

The manufacture and sale of 'painkillers' is a big business. When in pain, most people rush to buy their favourite pain-relieving tablet. Painkiller often forms a part of the monthly grocery shopping list, just like the favourtie soap or toothpaste.

Tablets sold under different brand names have different constituents. It is advisable to check these constituents. The market if flooded with a variety of pain-relieving tablets comprising either a single drug containing *aspirin, paracetamol, codeine, pentazocine, dextropropoxyphene,* or a combination of drugs comprising the pain-reliever with a tranquillizer, an anti-vomiting drug, antacid, etc. as the other ingredient.

We think that a 600 mg dose of *aspirin* (two tablets of DISPRIN, DYNASPIRIN) or 500-1000 mg of *paracetamol* (one /two tablets of CROCIN, MELIDENS, PARACIN, CALPOL, METACIN) or *ibuprofen* 400-600 mg are enough to reduce pain in most cases. If the pain reappears or is of a severe nature and not relieved by these, a doctor should be consulted who may investigate the underlying cause and treat it. *A common mistake is to avoid consulting physician in the event of severe headache and later end up with finding brain haemorrhage as a cause of headache!*

It is advisable to avoid the use of multiple drugs containing pain relievers. These are not only expensive but may produce adverse effects like unwanted sedation, or drug dependence. Mixtures containing both tranquillizers and narcotic analgesics have no justification (ZOFLAM, WALAGESIC). *Analgin* and mixtures containing this drug (ALGESIN-O, BARALGAN, KILPANE, TRIGAN) should be avoided in view of the availability of safer drugs.

Newer drugs may be used when above drugs are not tolerated and adverse effects are unacceptable.

It is advisable to use Paracetamol for mild to moderate pain, *Ibuprofen, nimesulide* or *diclofenac* for musculoskeletal pains such as myalgia and arthralgia. For arthritis and its *flares naproxen, ibuprofen* or *aceclofenac* will suffice. In patients with history of acidity, ulcers and asthma it will be prudent to use *etoricoxib, nabumetone* (NIBUFLAM) or *nimesulide.* Arthritis in children is usually treated with safe anti-inflammatory drugs like *ibuprofen* and *naproxyn.* In them avoid longer use of *aspirin* and *paracetamol.*

A word of caution: patients with diseases of heart and kidney usually take multiple drugs. Use of pain relievers may adversely affect the overall benefits of these medicines. There is loss of BP reducing effect and worsening of kidney function with use of anti-inflammatory pain relievers. Loss of blood thining effect of low dose *aspirin* is reported with concurrent use of *ibuprofen!*

### Nimesulide (NISE, ORTHOBID, NIMEGESIC)

It is very commonly used drug for relieving pain and fever in adults and children. Its usual doses are 100 mg twice a day in adults. Several reports of severe liver damage in children have come from various countries. It is now not considered to be the first drug to be used in children. It does not precipitate asthma in susceptible patients. Therefore, *aspirin* sensitive individuals can take it. *Nimesulide* is available as tablet 100 mg oral and mouth dissolving-MD, Inj 75 mg/ml, Syp. 50 mg/5ml and gel for local use. It is also available as combination containing *serratiopeptide* and *paracetamol. It should not be used in young children.*

Some common combinations are (WILLGO-200 MG, NIMSAID-P, SUMOFLAM, NIMUPAIN PLUS, NOBEL-SPAS (has *dicyclomine*) and *Zolandin-MR* (has *tizanidine* as muscle relaxant).

### Nefopam (NEOMAX tab.)

It is a strong pain reliever (dose 30 mg) and can be used in place of *codeine* or *morphine.* It does not cause respiratory depression.

### Ketorolac (KETOROL, KENALFIN tab. 10 mg, 30 mg/ml Injection)

It is a strong analgesic but weak anti-inflammatory drug. It can be given by intramuscular injection in post operative pain. Dose by mouth is 10 mg thrice a day. It should not be used in children.

### Thiocolchicoside (THIOGESIC 4 mg, 8 mg tab)

It is used in painful muscle spasms in a dose of 8 to 16 mg. It may cause drowsiness, fall in blood pressure, stomach pain, vomitting and diarrhoea.

### Coxibs*

The COXIBs as a group are interesting pain relievers because of there safety on stomach lining. These are good for pain relief and are effective in osteoarthritis, dental pain, menstrual pain and low back pain. These are less likely to cause stomach problems and precipitation of asthma. But lack beneficial effects of low dose *aspirin* in heart attacks and other adverse effects of conventional drugs may also be seen (see *Aspirin/ Ibuprofen* )

*Celecoxib* (CELECT, CELIB Cap.100mg, 200mg) is given in a dose of 100 mg twice daily.

*Etoricoxib* (ETROBAX,TORCOXIA 60 mg, 90 mg) is given in a dose of 60-120 mg once a day.

*Parecoxib* (Injection PAROXIB, VALSAFE,VALERON 40 mg in 2 to 5 ml)

*Lumiraxocib* (LUMIRAXOCIB) is a newer drug not available in India.

Most of these agents (except *etoricoxib*) have sulpha-drug like structure. Therefore, those allergic to sulpha-drugs may develop skin allergy. These drugs should not be used if there is liver damage.

---

* In October 2004, E. Merck, the originator and manufacturer of *Rofecoxib* has withdrawn the drug from the USA market and has advised against its use since it could lead to heart attacks and strokes. So, *Rofecoxib* and *valdecoxib* should not be used. *Diclofenac* like safety profile is reported for *etoricoxib.*

***A Word About Analgesic Combinations:*** A large number of branded preparations contain an analgesic with a muscle relaxant, another analgesic, a sedative or an enzyme. At present it is not yet proved that such combinations are superior to single drug. Their cost is certainly more and therefore, such combinations should not be preferred.

## Narcotic Pain Relievers

Also called opiate pain relievers as their action is similar to that of *opium.* The most potent narcotic pain relievers are *morphine, pethidine,* and *methadone.* However, due to their high addicting liability, these are reserved for acute emergencies and prescribed for short durations. Other opiates like *codeine, dextropropoxyphene, pentazocine,* or *ethoheptazine* are less addictive and also less potent. When used in combination with the non-narcotic pain relievers mentioned earlier, they provide greater relief of pain than the individual drugs as these two acts by different mechanism. However, a full dose of each type of drugs is necessary. Unfortunately, the majority of such combinations do not have an adequate quantity of each of the drugs and for moderate pain, 2 to 3 tablets are required to be taken every 4 to 6 hours and not one tablet as sometimes suggested by the manufacturer.

### Codeine Phosphate

A constituent of *opium*, this is used as a cough suppressant in a dose range of 8 to 15 mg, and as a pain reliever from 15 to 60 mg, it is given 4 times a day as its action lasts for 6 to 7 hours. It is available in combination with *aspirin* (APIDIN) and *paracetamol* (CODOMOLINDON) for relieving pain. The small quantity of *codeine* in these mixtures does not provide adequate relief for pain unless 2 to 3 tablets are taken 4 times a day, making the cost high.

***Adverse Effects:*** *Codeine* occasionally causes constipation. Drowsiness and dizziness occur when it is taken repeatedly to relieve moderate pain.

***Precautions***

1. *Codeine* causes constipation. Take a high roughage diet while taking this drug.
2. Alcohol and anti-allergic drugs enhance its sedative effect. Avoid them while taking a formulation containing *codeine.*
3. Avoid its use in children, especially below one year of age, as they are more susceptible to its adverse effects.
4. It should be avoided by patients of bronchial asthma and other breathing problems.

### Dextropropoxyphene

Commonly called *propoxyphene, dextropropoxyphene* is about half to one-third as potent as *codeine* for the relief of pain. however, its action lasts for more than 24 hours. Its is available in the form of *dextropropoxyphene hydrochloride* salt of which a 65 mg dose is equal to 600 mg of *aspirin* or *paracetamol* for the relief of pain. Most of the drug combinations available contain 32.5 mg to 65 mg of the above-mentioned salt and 325 to 500 mg of *paracetamol* (WYGESIC, PROXYVON). It is also available with *ibuprofen* (SUBDU, IBUPROXYVON). For relief of pain, 2 to 3 tablets or capsules per day are required. The cost of these combinations is quite high.

***Adverse Effects:*** The most common effects are dizziness, drowsiness, nausea, and vomiting. The less common adverse effects include constipation, abdominal pain, and headache, although it is a pain reliever. A false sense of well-being (euphoria) or hopelessness (dysphoria) and some visual disturbances have been reported in rare cases.

The addiction liability of *propoxyphene* is less than that of *codeine*, but incidence of *propoxyphene* misuse has increased in recent years.

***Precautions:***

1. To avoid constipation, take a high roughage diet.
2. Avoid alcohol and other sedatives with it as it produces an addictive effect.
3. Avoid its use during pregnancy as it causes withdrawal symptoms in the newborn baby.
4. Avoid its use if you have suffered from liver, disease, as impairment of liver functions has been reported with this drug.

**Pentazocine** (FORTWIN, PENTAWIN, SOSEGON)

This drug is available in combination with *paracetamol* (FORACET, FORTAGESIC) and has a short duration of action. The dose of *pentazocine* required for pain relief is 5 to 100 mg every 3 to 4 hours. However, the small quantity of *pentazocine* (15 mg) available in the above-mentioned preparations is unlikely to provide any greater pain relief than that of *paracetamol* alone.

***Adverse Effects:*** The most common adverse effects of *pentazocine* are light-headedness, dizziness, nausea, vomiting, sedation, and sweating. It may also cause constipation, a dry mouth, flushing of the skin, palpitations, high blood pressure, mood changes, nightmares, and decreased sensation in the limbs, pruritis, and urinary retention. Muscle tremors, sleeplessness, disorientation, hallucinations, disturbances of vision, and allergic reactions can also occur.

***Precautions:***

1. It is a weak opioid antagonist and should be avoided if other narcotic pain relievers have been taken recently as it may precipitate withdrawal symptoms in the form of convulsions.
2. Those suffering from epilepsy should avoid this drug as it may increase the frequency of attack. In heart patient, it may precipitate an attack.
3. Do not operate machinery or drive any vehicle if you are taking this drug as it causes dizziness and an accident may occur.
4. It should not be used continuously by patients suffering from kidney, gall-bladder, or liver disorders.
5. Avoid alcohol and sedatives as marked sedation and respiratory depression may occur.

**Tramadol** (TRAMAZAC, CONTRAMAL, DOMADOL tab and Inj)

This is a more potent drug used for severe post operative and cancer pain and also in surgery. It is given in doses of 50 to 100 mg twice or thrice daily, but never more than 400 mg in a single day. It is also available in combination with *paracetamol* (DOMADOL PLUS, REVODOL). It does not cause respiratory depression or dependence (addiction). No alcohol should be taken with this drug.

**Fentanyl** (DURAGESIC 25, 50 and 75 μg skin patch; 50 mcg/ml inj)

It is used intravenously as an adjunct for anesthesia and for relief of cancer pain. One patch is effective for about 3 days and is found to be very useful in suppression of intractable cancer pain.

### Local pain relieving preparations

A number of drugs are now available as local gels, creams, ointments and liniments (need rubbing) for relief of sport injuries, sprains and joints paints. Some of these are:

| | |
|---|---|
| Diclofenac 1% gel | VOVERAN EMUGEL, RELAXYL gel, DICLORIL gel (contains methyl salicylate and menthol also) |
| Ibuprofen 10% gel | RIBUFEN gel |
| Nimesulide 1% gel | NIMULID gel |
| Piroxicam 0.5% gel | DOLONEX gel |
| Naproxen 10% gel | NAPROSYN gel |
| Flurbiprofen 5% gel | FROBEN gel |
| Capsicum oleoresin 5% | ALGIPAN (contains Histamine, methyl nicotinate and glycol Salicylate also) |
| Methyl-Salicylate cream 4 to 5% | MEFTAL FORTE gel |
| | AXANE cream (contains menthol & camphor) |
| | ETHNORUB (contains Mephensin 5% and Iodine 0.5%) |
| Alphalinoleic acid 3% | XEROFLAM gel (contains diclofenac, methyl-salicylate menthol). |
| Ketoprofen 2.5% gel | RHOFENID gel |

It is believed that these preparations have local effects and lack significant effects on other body organs. It appears that tall claims are made for their effects by manufacturers. A simple oil of winter green (methyl salicylate), camphor in oil or warm/hot fomentation may also provide comparably equal relief. A slight massage done increases warmth and blood flow that also contributes relief. Nevertheless they are useful in common joint disorders such as osteoarthritis, sprains, backache and pains arising from soft tissues such as muscles and tendons. These should never be applied on broken skins, abrasions or tears.

# 26

# Drugs Used in Parkinson's Disease

••••••

You only have to see a patient of Parkinson's disease once to be able to make an instantaneous diagnosis of this disease in another patient. The symptoms are so distinct that you cannot make a mistake. James Parkinson, after whom the disease is named, was the first to give a complete account of this disease in 1817. He described it thus:

> 'Involuntary tremulous motion, with lessened muscular power, in part not in action and even when supported; with a propensity to bend the trunk forward and to pass from a walking to running pace, the senses and intellects being uninjured.'

Parkinson's disease ( Parkinsonism) is chronic malady of the central nervous system, more common amongst the elderly, and characterized by muscle rigidity, rhythmic tremor, akinesia or immobility, loss of associated movements, and postural instability. The presence of these signs impairs the ability of the patient to make proper voluntary movements and to maintain posture through reflexes. The patient presents a characteristic feature of an expressionless or a 'mask-life' face, and has tremors of the hands. It is called as 'shaking palsy.'

***Causes:*** The real cause of this disease is not known. It is a disease of old age, but may also occur in middle age. It has a sporadic onset which is very gradual and prolonged. It is not considered to be a hereditary disease, although in about 6% cases, it has been found to run in families. The disease effects 1 in 250 persons after the age of 40 years. It is degenerative disease in which the centres of brain which normally maintain stance and movements lose functional nerve cells. Parkinsonism can sometimes be due to a known cause such as a late complication of viral encephalitis, injury to brain or arteriosclerosis but such cases are not common. Certain anti-psychotic drugs like *reserpine, chlorpromazine,* and *haloperidol* may cause symptoms similar to Parkinson's disease, but not the actual disease itself.

Although we do not know the cause of this disease, recent biochemical researches suggest that it may be due to a deficiency of a neurohormone *(dopamine)* and/or abundance of another neurohormone *(acetylcholine)* in the areas of brain. With this knowledge, it has now become possible to control the symptoms by using specific drugs to correct the neurochemical imbalance, if not to provide a complete cure. Besides drug therapy, it is very important for a patient to undertake suitable regular physical exercises to avoid permanent stiffness of the joints.

## Treatment and Drugs

The drugs used in the treatment of Parkinson's disease can be divided into those which correct: 1) the deficiency of dopamine; and 2) the effects caused by excessive acetylcholine.

## Drugs for Correcting Deficiency of Dopamine

**Levodopa** (LARODOPA)

*Levodopa* is the drug of first preference in the treatment of Parkinson's disease. It is a precursor of dopamine, a neurochemical, which is deficient in the brain of patients of this disease. *Dopamine* is not used orally, as it does not travel easily to the brain, whereas *levodopa* travels easily to the brain reaches this area and gets converted into *dopamine*. There is significant improvement in muscle rigidity and akinesia but not necessarily in tremors.

***Dosage:*** The average oral dose of *levodopa* is 4 g per day. It is usually started in a smaller dose of 250 mg twice daily, which is increased by 250 to 500 mg every week. It has been found that relief sets in 4 to 8 weeks when the daily dose has reached 2 to 2.5 g. These increases in the dose are continued till the maximum benefit is achieved or adverse effects appear. Once the adequate dose is found, it can be taken for several years without losing its value.

***Adverse Effects:*** During prolonged treatment with *levodopa,* a distressing complication of 'on-off phenomenon' may occur, in which a person who has been showing continued improvement by taking this drug, suddenly starts behaving as though no drug is being given to him. This period ranges from an hour to half a day. The adverse effects of *levodopa* are common and include nausea, vomiting, orthostatic hypotension (a fall in blood pressure on sudden standing from a lying-down position), choreoathetoid movements (lip smacking, grimacing, head turning or abnormal involuntary movements of the upper or lower limbs), and occasionally toxic delirium, confusion, depression, restlessness, agitation, and hallucinations.

It is quite important to keep the doses as low as possible to avoid the occurrence of the adverse effects of choreoathetoid movements.

***Precautions:***

1. The drug should not be taken on an empty stomach.
2. Patients who show a pronounced decrease in blood pressure on standing after a lying-down position should be protected from the possibility of fainting, by being made to wear tight long socks and occasionally being given small amounts of *ephedrine.*
3. Vitamin $B_6$ reverses the effects of *levodopa.* Avoid use of B complex preparations which invariably contain Vitamin $B_6$ (pyridoxine).

**Levodopa + Carbidopa** (TIDOMET-LS (100+10), TIDOMET FORTE (250+25), TIDOMET PLUS (100+25))

One of the problems with the use of *levodopa* is its high dose. Only 1% of this drug goes to the brain and the remaining 99% remains in the peripheral region, going waste and also causing unwanted adverse effects. *Carbidopa* inhibits the metabolic break down of *levodopa* in the intestines and thus allows greater penetration of this drug to the brain. This allows considerable economy in the use of *levodopa* and also reduces the distressing adverse effects like nausea and vomiting. This combination is, therefore, positively superior to the single drug. In fact, it is used in all most all of the patients requiring *levodopa*. The combination is available in three strengths and this allows selection of appropriate doses required for a patient. An advantage with this combination is that Vitamin $B_6$ or multivitamins can be given together. *Levodopa* is also available in combination with *benserzide* and this has the same effect as the combination with *carbidopa* and is sold under the trade name BENSPAR.

## Drugs for Correcting the Effects of Excess Acetylcholine

Prior to the introduction of *levodopa*, various drugs were used in the treatment of Parkinson's disease. Of these the most effective were *belladonna* alkaloids (anti-cholinergic drugs), obtained from the plant *Atropa belladonna,* and some synthetic drugs. These drugs rarely produced more than 10-25% improvement in the signs and symptoms, and the disease invariably progressed. One thing is certain though: these caused greater improvement in tremor than hypokinesia. These are the only drugs effective in drug-induced movement disorder particularly acute dystonia/ dyskinesia. They have a role in early and mild form of Parkinsonism disease also. All these drugs had adverse effects like dryness of the mouth, blurring of vision, constipation, urinary retention, and delirium. *Orphenadrine* has some stimulating effect. Other are sedating. The trade names and doses of some of these drugs are given in the following table:

**Drugs that Improve Tremors**

| *Drugs* | *Brand Names* | *Dose Range/mg* |
|---|---|---|
| *Trihexyphenidyl* | PACITANE, PARKIN, MANOHEXY (Tab, Inj.) | 2-20; injection 2 mg/ml |
| *Procyclidine* | KEMADRIN (Tab., Inj.) | 5-40; injection 5 mg/ml |
| *Orphenadrine* | DISIPAL, ORPHIPAL | 50-150 |

***Precautions:***

1. These drugs should not be administered to patients having difficulty in passing urine due to enlargement of the prostate or stone in the urinary tract.
2. These agents should be avoided in patients suffering from glaucoma (raised pressure in the eyes).
3. The medication is withdrawn gradually. Sudden stopping of the drug may cause an increase in the symptoms of parkinsonism.

## Other Drugs

***Amanatadine*** (AMANATREL) It brings about beneficial effects by releasing dopamine from the storage site. It is effective in 66% cases but the effect lasts only for 2 to 3 weeks, after which it declines.

***Bromocriptine*** (PROCTINAL 1.25 mg, 2.5 mg) intially it is given in a dose of ½ tablet daily with meals and gradually the dose is increased to 5 mg three times daily. The main value of this drug is to facilitate control of symptoms which appear as the effect of *levodopa* wears off ('end of dose' effects). Some patients show waxing and waning of symptoms with *levodopa* ('on-off' phenomenon) and in them smooth improvement can be achieved with addition of *bromocriptine*.

***Piribedil*** (TRIVASTAL-LA) is also like *levodopa* in action and is given in doses of 50-200 mg daily. It should not be given in pregnancy or heart disease.

***Pramipexole*** (PRAMIPREX, MIRAPREX 0.125 mg, 0.25 mg,1.0 mg) is used alone or along with *levodopa* to increase efficacy.

***Ropinirole*** (ROPITOR, PARKITOP 0.5 mg,1 mg, 2 mg tab) a useful drug in advanced cases and reduces the 'on-off' effects of *levodopa.*

***Citicoline*** (SOMAZINA,CITINOVA) 200 mg, 500 mg) is a newer drug useful to improve brain function in Parkinson's disease and in strokes.

***Entacapone*** and ***Tolcapone*** reduce fluctuations in the response due to *levodopa+carbidopa* and enhance the effect of latter. They are useful in advance disease only. A combination of *levodopa+carbidopa* and *entacapone* (STALEVO) is available in three strengths as a single pill.

***Selegiline*** (L-DEPRENYL, SELGIN 5 mg Tab.) is used as an adjunct to *levodopa+carbidopa* in a dose 5 mg in the morning and 5 mg at lunch. Additional doses are not beneficial. Because *selegiline* causes loss of sleep, it should not be taken at night. It is an interesting drug because there is some evidence to show that it may slow the process of neurodegeneration. It allows reduction in the dose of *carbidopa+levodopa.* It should not be given to epileptics and in chronic tardive dyskinesia. It may cause anxiety, confusion, restlessness, sexual dysfunction, tachycardia, hypertension and syncope.

***Rasagiline*** (AZILECT tab. 0.5 mg) is taken in a dose of 0.5 mg once daily. It is a newer drug like *seligiline.*

**Impact of Drugs** : Despite good initial response, the benefit with *Co-levodopa* progressively decreases. It is at this time that the addition of other drugs may offer further benefit. However, after a few year (5-7 years), there is a loss of benefit from dopaminergic drugs probably due to decrease in critical number of nerve cells (degeneration is ongoing) in the basal nuclei. Physical and social rehabilitation remain the last options for advanced cases.

27

# Drugs Used in Peptic Ulcers

India is known for its wide variety of cuisine. A large number of condiments and many varieties of chillies are used to titillate the palate, and so, we often tend to overeat. This gives rise to sour eructations, indigestion, and a stomach upset, and we look for an antacid, to set it right. Antacids counteract the excess of acid to prevent sour eructations but frequent use is unjustified as they hamper the digestion in the stomach.

Hydrochloric acid is the natural constituent of the secretions from the stomach, meant to make the digestive enzymes active. Why then should anybody work against this useful phenomenon provided by nature? Well, we may have to react when it is in excess and associated with a disease called peptic ulcer. Peptic ulcer is the term designated to localized destruction of the inner wall or mucosa of the stomach (gastric ulcer) or the upper part of the small intestine (duodenal ulcer). In other words, it is a wound (sore) inside the stomach or duodenum. A peptic ulcer is usually associated with hyperacidity; however, there are some people who have 6 to 8 times more acid than normal, yet do not suffer from the disease. On the other hand, there are others who have low acidity and may have peptic ulcers. A condition related to acidity is gastro esophageal reflux disorder (GERD) also called as reflux esophagitis or heartburn. Its cause and treatment is similar to peptic ulcer.

***Symptoms:*** Peptic ulcers are of two types: Duodenal and Gastric. A duodenal ulcer is associated with a sharp, penetrating, and burning type of pain in the upper part of the abdomen which occurs on empty stomach and is relieved by food.

Patients with duodenal ulcer tend to eat more and gain weight. In gastric ulcers the pain is increased immediately or soon after the meal and bloating nausea or vomiting may occur after meals. The pain experienced after meals is due to the stimulation of acid secretion which flows over the gastric ulcer, stimulating the pain receptor. Patients with gastric ulcer are thin and lean. The final diagnosis is made by examination of the stomach and its contents, X-ray after a barium meal (an X-ray of the abdominal region and digestive tract taken after the patient swallows an opaque contrast medium called barium sulphate) and by endoscopy in which a flexible fibre optic tube is passed through mouth into stomach and its end is illuminated to see changes in the inner lining. If the need be, the endoscopist can cut a tiny piece of tissue for minute or biopsy examination.

***Causes:*** The causes of peptic ulcers are complex, involving constitutional, emotional, neurogenic, and biochemical factors. Constitutionally, a person having a lean and thin physique, being highly emotional, and belonging to blood group 'O' is more prone to suffer from a peptic ulcer. Besides, hot and spicy food, excessive smoking and excessive use of alcohol, tea, coffee, and certain drugs like *corticosteroids, aspirin, indomethacin, caffeine*, and *theophylline* may also be responsible for peptic ulcers. All of us produce acid in stomach but only a few develop the ulcers because defensive factors in them are weakened. Amount of mucus production, irritants which break the continuity of stomach lining are such factors.

The treatment of peptic ulcer consists of general measures and use of specific drugs. If complications like bleeding or perforation at the site of the ulcer occur, surgical intervention may become necessary.

### Treatment and Drugs

General measures consist of physical and mental rest and control of diet. The diet should be bland in nature, and comprise small and frequent meals. In an acute peptic ulcer a meal mainly consists of milk given frequently. Milk not only counteracts acidity but also delays the emptying time of the stomach. Avoidance of too much coffee, tea and spicy foods and cessation of smoking are recommended. Avoid self use of NSAIDs which are ulcer promoting.

The drugs used in the treatment of a peptic ulcer include antacids, those which inhibit gastric secretion, anti-cholinergics, and those which promote healing. In persons suffering from anxiety reaction (see chapter on 'Drugs Used in Anxiety'), anti-anxiety drugs may be helpful. Of these, *diazepam* and *alprazolam* are used for their beneficial effects.

## Antacids

These drugs are basic in nature and thus neutralize the acid secreted in the stomach, and reduce bad effects of pepsin by inactivating it. They provide symptomatic relief and to a lesser extent, promote healing. Since stomach keeps on emptying itself and the action of the antacid lasts only for a short while, therefore, it is important to take antacids at frequent intervals.

Antacids can be divided into two major groups: those absorbable from the intestines, and those which are non-absorbable. Since absorbable antacids produce actions all over the body (systemic effects) they are not preferred. Non-absorbable antacids act in the stomach cavity only and do not cause blood acid base imbalance.

### Non-Absorbable Antacids

The ability of antacids to neutralize stomach acid is called as acid-neutralizing capacity (ANC) and varies from antacid to antacid. These are available as tablets and liquids, liquids are preferred to tablets because of their variable effects.

### Aluminium Hydroxide

It is slow acting and its ANC is variable. Food reduces its ANC. It causes constipation. It binds phosphates in the intestine and therefore is useful in phosphate stones, but causes weakness and loss of appetite. Small amount of aluminium may be absorbed particularly in kidney failure and may cause brain damage (encephalopathy). Commonly used preparation is ALUDROX 840mg tab. and 600mg/10ml syp. suspension.

**Megaldrate** (ULGEL 400mg)

It is a complex form of magnesium and aluminium and acts quickly and for longer time. It is commonly used in combination with *simethicone* which is defoaming agent. *Simethicone* is activated *dimethicone*. It helps expulsion of gasses by making a big bubble from tiny bubbles in stomach. This improves heart burn.

**Alginic acid**

It facilitates sticking of active drugs in antacid combinations over the raw ulcer area and thus provides a protection. It is found in many antcid formulations.

**Magnesium Hydroxide**

This watery suspension is called milk of magnesia. *Magnesium hydroxide* is more effective than *aluminium hydroxide*. Its full dose causes diarrhoea. Small amounts which are absorbed can not be removed efficiently in persons with impaired kidney function. Therefore, small doses are used. Because of opposite effects of aluminium and magnesium salts on bowel movements, these two are usually combined.

**Calcium Carbonate**

Although it is a strong and quick acting antacid it liberates carbon dioxide gas causing a marked discomfort and stomach distension. The rebound acid production (acid rebound) is highest with it. It may cause constipation. Milk-alkali syndrome occurred in those persons who took calcium carbonate and a lot of milk. Symptoms are headache, vomiting, weakness, abnormal calcium deposits and kidney stones. Therefore, now a days it is not preferred.

**Antacid Combinations** (DIGENE, GELUSIL, POLYCROL FORTE, MUCAINE and TRICAINE)

A number of antacid preparations have two or more antacids. They are considered better than single drug formulation because of their following merits:

1. Quick onset *(magnesium salt)* and longer duration *(aluminium salt)* of action.
2. Avoidance of constipation *(aluminium)* or diarrhoea *(magnesium)*.
3. Stomach emptying is undisturbed (*aluminium salts* delay while *magnesium salts*-hasten.
4. Reduction of dose of individual drug thus reduces systemic affects further.
5. In many preparations *methyl polysiloxane* (MPS) is added as it collapses froth and improves dispersion of antacids in the stomach cavity.

Liquid DIGENE is a combination of *magnesium hydroxide* 185mg, *aluminium hydroxide* 830mg, *carboxymethylcellulose* 100mg and *methyl polysilosane* 25mg in 10ml.

GELUSIL Liquid is a combination of *magnesium trisilicate* 6.25mg, *aluminium hydroxide* gel 312mg in 5ml.

POLYCROL FORTE Gel is a combination of *magnesium hydroxide* 100mg, *aluminium hydroxide* 250 mg and *dimethicone* 125 mg liquid.

MUCAINE and TRICAINE gel Liquid is a combination of *oxethazaine* 10 mg, *aluminium hydroxide,* 291 mg, *magnesium hydroxide* 98 mg liquid. *Oxethazaine* is local acting pain reliever.

Antacids are available as over-the-counter drugs for the relief from pain and heart burn. They are rarely used for healing of ulcers; they would be needed in very large dosages which would be inconvenient to take and would also upset bowel movement and cause acid rebound. Liquids are better than tablets. If taken, tablets must be chewed and gulped down with water. Availability of better drugs has also reduced their utility.

## $H_2$ Receptor blockers

General effects of these drugs are marked reduction in stomach acid production in response to meals and other stimuli is observed. Usually ulcers heal with adequate doses and there is no disturbance of the bowel activity. Any of the four drugs given below produce healing in 4 to 8 weeks when adequate doses are taken to suppress acid by 70% (in 24 hours). The doses used and preparation available are shown in the table:

**$H_2$ Blockers Used in Peptic Ulcer**

| *Drug* | *Preparation* | *Initial dose 6-8 weeks* | *Maintain thereafter* | *Important features* |
|---|---|---|---|---|
| *Cimetidine* | Tab. CIMETIGET 200 and 400mg | 400mg twice a day or 800mg Tab. ULCIBAN | 400 mg at night | Produces endocrine and nervous system adverse effects. Interacts with other drugs. Less preferred nowadays. |
| *Ranitidine* | Tab. RANTAC 150mg, 300mg Tab. ZINETAC, HISTAC (Inj. RANITIN 50mg/2ml) | 150mg twice a day or 300mg at night | 150 mg | Less adverse effects. Less drug interactions. No endocrine effects. |
| *Famotidine* | Tab. FAMTAC 20mg, 40mg Tab. TOPCID 20mg, 40mg | 20mg twice a day or 40mg at night | 20 mg | No endocrine effects. No drug interactions. Longer action. |
| *Roxatidine* | Tab. ROTANE 75mg, 150 mg Tab. ZORPEX | 75mg twice a day or 150mg at night | 75 mg | Like *Famotidine*. |

***Adverse effects*** (Mostly with *cimetidine*): The drug may cause headache, bowel upset, dry mouth, dizziness, skin rash. Confusion, delirium, fits and heart rhythm changes occur when used intravenously. Enlargement of male breast, loss of sex desire, impotence and temporary disease in sperm counts may occur. White cell count (polymorphs) falls on longer use of *cimetidine.*

### Drug Interaction (Mostly with *cimetidine*)

Toxicity of *theophylline, phenytoin,* anti diabetic drugs, *nifedipine, quinidine, propranolol, warfarin* is increased because *cimetidine* decreases their metabolic inactivation by liver. Antacids reduce absorption of $H_2$ blockers and thus they should be taken after a gap of 2 to 3 hours. Because of these interactions *cimetidine* is not popular drug.

## Anti-Cholinergic Drugs

*Pirenzpine* and *Telezepine* are two drugs which reduce volume of stomach juice without causing much adverse effects of other anticholinergic drugs. These have limited role in the management of peptic ulcer because they decrease the activity of stomach. The acid stays there for a longer time and may cause damage to ulcerated surface. Systemic side effects such as dry mouth, constipation and urinary retention may occur in the elderly.

**Inhibitors of Acid Pump: Omeprazole** (LOMAC, LOKIT, OMEZAC, OMEZ, OMEZOL, PROTOLOC)
It is the single most sold drug in the world. This inhibits the so-called proton pump situated in the secretory cells of the stomach. Thus, the final phase of acid secretion is inhibited by this drug. It is more potent and longer acting than histamine blockers. A dose of 20 to 40mg acts for more than 24 hours and produces complete inhibition of acid secretion. The ulcer heals within 2 to 4 weeks, that is, twice as fast as with *ranitidine*. The healing rate is almost 100%. Its profound and long-lasting effect may make it a drug of choice in peptic ulcers and reflux esophagitis. It inhibits H pylori organism also and therefore it is used along with other antibiotics for eradication of H pylori.

***Dosage:*** A 20 to 40 mg/day dose is given before breakfast.

***Adverse Effects:*** It causes infrequent adverse effects like nausea, diarrhoea, pain in the abdomen, dizziness, headache and skin rash. These are generally mild and do not require reduction in dosages. It reduces disposal of *diazepam, phenytoin* and *warfarin* from the body and therefore at times dose adjustments of these drugs need to be done.

**Lansoprazole** (LANZOL, LANZAP)
It acts rapidly and for a longer time than *omeprazole.* It is given in doses of 30mg per day for 4 to 12 weeks. Its dose should be decreased in liver disease.

**Pentoprazole** (PANTOCID, PANTODAC 40mg tab, 40mg inj.)
It is similar to *omeprazole* in action but is available as injectable iv preparation to be used in bleeding peptic ulcer and acute stress ulcers.

**Rabeprazole** (ROLES, VELOZ, 10mg, 20mg)
It is quickest and longer acting drug which increase mucus formation in stomach also. *Rabeprazole* is also available in combination with *domperidone* 30 mg (VELOZ-D, ROLES-D) and with *Itopride* 150 mg (RABETO PLUS, VELOZ-IT).

**Esomeprazole** (NEXPRO, ESOZ, 20mg, 40mg)
It has greater efficacy in GERD and equally effective to *omeprazole*. It is also available with *Domperidone* 30 mg (ESOFAG-D, RECIPER-D).

## Drugs Providing Protection to Mucosa

**Sucralfate** (ULCEKON, ULCERFATE, MUCOGARD)
This drug consists of *aluminum* and contains the salt of sucrose. It becomes a viscous paste in the acid of the stomach, which gets selectively adhered to the ulcer base and provides protection

from acid and enzyme pepsin to the ulcer. It also has a protective effect on the cells through local release of prostaglandin*.

***Dosage:*** The healing dose is 1g taken one hour before main meals and 1g at bedtime. A suspension is recommended for the treatment of oral ulcers (aphthous stomatitis). A gel preparation (PEPSIGARD GEL) can be used on bedsores, diabetic foot ulcers and burns.

***Adverse Effects:*** Constipation occurs in 2-3% of the patients. Other adverse effects are nausea, dyspepsia, dry mouth, headache, and itching.

***Note:*** It reduces blood phosphate levels so this effect is used in the treatment of kidney phosphate stones.

### **Misoprostol** (CYTOLOG, MISOPROST TAB)

It has both, an inhibitory effect on the acid secretion in the stomach and a protective effect on the cells of the stomach. It increases the protective mucus and strengthens the barrier with reduction of the back diffusion of acid. It accelerates ulcer healing. It has been mainly used for treatment of ulcers caused by *aspirin* and related drugs with low acid.

***Dosage:*** It is given in a dose of 200μg, 4 times a day.

***Adverse Effects:*** It produces nausea, dyspepsia, diarrhoea, and abdominal pain. It stimulates the uterus and should be avoided during pregnancy.

### **Carbenoxolone** (GASTRILCER)

This is extracted from the roots of the plant liquorice. It increases mucus and promotes healing, but because of its serious adverse effect of retaining salt and water, thus causing high blood pressure, this drug has little or no place in the treatment of gastric ulcers.

### **Colloidal Bismuth or Tripotassium Dicitrato Bismuthate TDB** (TRYMO, DENOL)

This is also used for the same purpose as *sucralfate.* It causes blackening of the stools and tongue, dizzines diarrhoea and bismuth toxicity. The dose is 240mg, twice daily, half an hour before meals. It detaches H pylori and kills them. So it is used in eradication regime also.

$H_2$ blockers or proton pump inhibitors produce healing of ulcers easily in almost 80% to 100% cases but on stopping them recurrence occurs and therefore continuous use of them in low doses for longer time (duration is uncertain, may be 1 to 2 years) for acid suppression is needed. To cure the ulcer one needs to identify the presence of H Pylori and use 1 to 2 week eradication regimes

## Eradication of H. Pylori infection in peptic ulcer

H-pylori (screw like bug) is responsible for causing chronic gastritis dyspepsia, peptic ulcer and stomach tumor in many cases. 90% cases of gastric and duodenal ulcers have H. pylori in their stomachs. Eradication of this organism is difficult with single drug. Therefore a combination of two or three drugs is used. Various combination used are —

*Part of a group of naturally occurring, chemically related hydroxy fatty acids that regulate acid secretion of the stomach.

*One week regime* (For antibiotics see the relevant chapter)

1. *Amoxycillin* 750mg twice a day + *Tinidazole* 500mg twice a day + *Omeprazole* 20mg twice a day (HP KIT, HELIBACT, HELIKIT)
2. *Clarithromycin* 250mg twice a day + *Tinidazole* 500mg twice a day + *Omeprazole* 20mg twice a day (PYLOBACT KIT, L-COT KIT)
3. *Amoxicillin* 750mg twice a day + *Tinidazole* 500mg twice a day + *Lansoprazole* 15mg cap twice a day (PYLOMAX KIT)
4. *Clarithromycin* 250mg twice a day + *Tinidazole* 500mg twice a day + *Lansoprazole* 30mg twice a day (HELIGO, PYLOKIT).
5. *Amoxicillin* 750 mg (2 tabs)+ *Clarithromycin* 250 mg(2 tab) + *Omeprazole* 20 mg (2 tab) (GI KIT)
6. *Amoxicillin* 750 mg(2tab) + *Tinidazole* 500 mg(2 tab) + *pantoprazole* 40 mg (2 tab) (ZOVANTA KIT)

In some countries these drugs are given for two weeks to achieve better cure rates. This is followed by *Omeprazole* 20 mg per day for 4-8 weeks.

## Reflux Esophagitis

It is a very common problem presenting as sour eructations, heartburn and water brash. The symptoms occur particularly after a large meal and increase on lying down. In this disorder the acid contents of stomach rise in the lower part of food pipe (esophagus). The lower end of food pipe has a valve like mechanism to prevent reguritation of acid contents. When this valve (Called as sphincter) becomes lax or weak, the acid burns the lining of food pipe causing erosions, ulcers and heartburns. In many cases of night time attacks of asthma, reflux is found to be a common problem. If untreated the food pipe is ultimately narrowed not allowing hard food to pass down (dysphagia). There is risk of cancer development. Therefore, it should be treated vigorously.

Persons suffering from reflux esophagitis should take light early dinner. The foot end of the bed should be raised to provide much relief. Weight reduction can also help.

***Dosage:*** *Omeprazole* 20mg twice a day or *lansoprazole* (15 to 30mg daily) for 4 to 8 weeks are better than $H_2$ blockers *(ranitidine* or *famotidine).* These are often combined with prokinetic drugs (See chapter on constipation). Common formulation are —

| | |
|---|---|
| OMIDOM, DOMSTAL-O | *Omeprazole + Domperidone* |
| PANTADOM | *Pantoprazole + Domperidone* |
| GANATON-TOTAL | *Pantoprazole + Itopride* |
| ZEROCID | *Lansoprazole + Domperidone* |
| VELOZ-D | *Rabeprazole + Domperidone* |
| VELOZ-M | *Rabeprazole + Mosapride* |
| VELOZ-IT | *Rabeprazole + Itopride* |

**Sodium alginate**: It forms thick frothy layer on the gastric juice and thus prevents acid regurgitation. It is combined with antacids (Reflux liquid, reflux forte tab.)

28

# Methods of Preventing Pregnancy

••••••

In one of his inaugural speeches, when he was Union Health Minister, Dr Karan Singh, remarked that the surest contraceptive was a glass of water. After a moment of silence someone asked, 'Before or after?' His reply was, 'Instead'. Indeed, in olden days the surest contraceptive method was abstinence. At present a number of methods for preventing pregnancy are available.

One may find different methods suitable at different stages of life. Information on various birth control methods available to couples today, is given below. Prior to that the human reproductive system is explained so that the working of the contraceptive methods can be understood properly.

## How Conception Takes Place

The sex glands of the man, the testes, produce seeds or sperms while the sex glands of the woman, the ovaries, produce eggs or ova. When the male seed (sperm) and the woman's egg (ovum) join together inside the woman's womb, a new life begins to grow.

**About the Woman:** The woman produces an egg cell once every month and this process is called ovulation. It usually occurs on 14$^{th}$ (12$^{th}$ to 16$^{th}$) day of menstrual cycle. The egg cell passes through the woman's egg-tubes (fallopian tubes) towards the womb (uterus). If about this time, the egg cell is met by a male sperm as a result of sexual intercourse, it can be fertilized and a pregnancy can take place. If the egg is not fertilized, it just passes out of the woman's body unnoticed.

**About the Man:** The male seeds produced by the testes passes through the spermatic duct and mix with fluids produced by seminal vesicles and prostate glands. This fluid is called semen. At the time of sexual climax, the semen which contains sperms, is ejaculated from the penis into the vagina. The sperms from the semen swim up to the womb, where one of them possibly meets the female egg and fertilizes it. This fertilized egg grows into a baby.

## Method of Preventing Pregnancy

Contraceptive methods seek to prevent this meeting of the egg cell and the sperm to avoid pregnancy. These methods have been divided into three broad categories: 1) natural methods, 2) spacing methods, and 3) terminal methods.

## Natural Methods

Natural methods are those which do not involve the use of any device or drug. They are Coitus Interruptus and the Rhythm Method.

### Coitus Interruptus

If the penis is withdrawn from the vagina before ejaculation or discharge, the semen is prevented from entering the woman's genital tract and no pregnancy takes place. This is called coitus interruptus or withdrawal method. It is perhaps the oldest method practiced by man to prevent conception from taking place.

***Merits:*** No artificial device is required to be used. With proper care and self-discipline, this method can be fairly effective.

***Drawbacks:*** This method may fail due to the escape of semen before climax or delayed withdrawal. It can be quite risky since even a single drop of semen contains thousands of sperms which are not visible to the naked eye. Pregnancy can still occur if the sperms enter the female genital tract. Therefore, a high degree of self-control is needed to practice this method successfully. Also, some males feel a lack of sexual satisfaction with this method.

### Rhythm Method (Safe Period)

The safe period or rhythm method is based on avoidance of sexual intercourse during the 'unsafe period' or the days when there is a possibility of the female egg and the male seed meeting. The woman normally produces one egg cell every month. If the male sperms do not enter the vagina at that time she cannot become pregnant. The egg (ovum) is released at about 14th day before menstrual date in most of the females and can live for almost 1 to 2 days. The male seed can remain alive in the female body for at least 3 to 4 days. That means an intercourse done 4 days before and at least upto 1 to 2 days after release of egg can result in pregnancy. This is the most unsafe period. The safe period varies from woman to woman but general guidelines can be given for calculations. One needs to follow the steps given below: For example, if the menses are expected to commence on the 28th of a month, then:

1. Count back 11 days (including the day of the start of menses i.e. 28th to 17th.
2. Count back additional 5 days, including the 17th i.e. to 12th.
3. Count back 4 days (including 12th) for the life of sperm and ovum i.e. to 8th.

### Result

1. Unsafe dates (i.e. conception can take place) are 9, 10, 11, 12, 13, 14, 15, 16, 17 i.e. 9 days.
2. Safe dates (no conception) are 1, 2, 3, 4, 5, 6, 7, 8 (8 days) and (18, 19, 20, 21, 22, 23, 24, 25, 26, 27, 28) 11 days i.e. (8+11) 19 days.

**How to Find Safe Period (From Your menstrual cycle)**

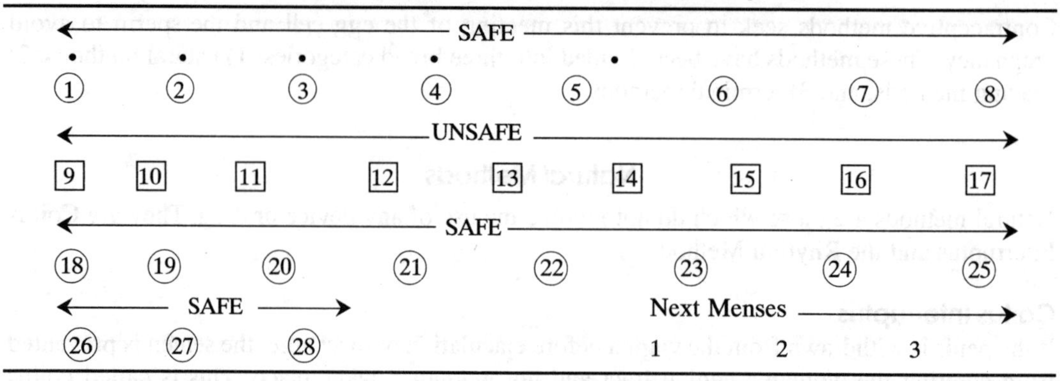


*Note:* Day 1 is Ist day of menstruation and may be any calendar date.
o Denotes 'Safe days' □ Denotes 'Unsafe days'. • Denotes Days of Menses

Woman can actually find out the day of egg release by noting morning temperature (before taking hot tea!) before getting out of bed. There is ½ -1°F rise in temperature after the egg is released. some times there is cramp like pain in the womb at the time of egg-release but not all can note it.

***Merits:*** This method requires no artificial device to be used. It is the only method approved of by the Roman Catholic Church.

***Drawbacks:*** It greatly reduces the opportunity for sexual relations and is unsuitable for women with irregular periods. Practice of the rhythm method requires considerable self-control and cooperation between the spouses. There is a likelihood of errors in recording the menstrual history which may result in a pregnancy even during the safe period. It is specially difficult to calculate the safe days during 'change of life' (menopause) when the periods become irregular. Emotional disturbances, diet, and travel can also upset the regularity of periods. Therefore, 'safe period is not always safe'.

## Spacing or Barrier Methods

There are several methods available which provide effective protection against pregnancy during the period they are used. These methods are the use of condoms, a diaphragm, an IUD, oral contraceptive pills, and spermicides. All these methods are good for delaying or spacing out the birth of children as they are easily reversed simply by stopping their use.

### Condom

The condom is an extremely thin rubber sheath used by the man. The condom is unrolled on the erect male organ before having sex. As it covers the penis, the sperms cannot go inside the woman's body. While unrolling the condom on the male sex organ, a little space should be left at the end so that the fluid, after the discharge, can spill into it.

A new condom should be used every time. At the end of the sexual act, the man must make sure to carefully withdraw his sex organ with the condom still in place to avoid spilling of the semen into the vagina. A spermicide (sperm killer) is added into lubricant of the condom in some varieties. A female condom is also introduced recently, but acceptance rate is lower.

***Merits:*** This is the simplest and effective method of birth control. There is no need to consult a doctor for using a condom. It also protects against sexually transmitted diseases. Its use can be discontinued when a couple desires a child. It is readily available free of charge from all family planning centres and at a nominal price from chemists, general merchants, grocers and other shops, even in the remotest areas. There is no need for self-restraint.

***Drawbacks:*** In rare cases, an individual may be sensitive to rubber. A few men and women may find the rubber sheath an interference which reduces the sexual sensation.

### Diaphragm and Cervical Caps

The diaphragm is a thin rubber cap which is like a dome with a spring in its ring. It is used by the woman. Before having sexual relations she places it in her vagina so that it covers the opening to the womb (cervix or neck). A diaphragm prevents pregnancy in a very simple way. It blocks the opening of the womb with the result that the sperms cannot find their way towards the womb and no pregnancy can take place. To render it effective, it is better that some contraceptive jelly or spermicidal cream is spread over the diaphragm before use. The cream kills the sperms on contact. It must remain there for about 8 to 10 hours after sexual intercourse and then removed.

***Merits:*** The diaphragm does not interfere with the sex act. It is a reversible and non-invasive method.

***Drawbacks:*** Elaborate preparation is required to insert it before the sex act which may not be possible every time. It has to be removed and washed each time after the sex act. A high standard of hygiene is necessary in storage and use, failing which, it can become a source of infection.

### Intra-Uterine Devices

Intra-uterine means 'inside the uterus', hence, these are devices which are placed in the womb. There are many types of intra-uterine devices (IUDs) but the COPPER-T is most commonly used in India.

### Copper-T (MULTILOAD- 250, ZICOID, ZYLOAD; U-KARE)

Copper-T is also made of plastic but is wrapped with fine copper which enhances its contraceptive effect. Its acceptance is higher than the loop. To secure full contraceptive effect, the Copper-T should be replaced every three years. U-kare is copper containing devise effective for about 5 years after insertion.

***Merits:*** The IUD does not interfere with the sex act. Its presence is not felt. Its insertion does not require hospitalisation. It is a reversible method and can be easily removed when a couple desires their next child. Its failure rate is almost negligible. A plastic thread can be checked by woman herself. If not found she must consult the gynaecologist to ensure that device is in place.

***Drawbacks:*** Side-effects such as heavier bleeding, backache, and abdominal cramps have been reported in some cases. These complaints, however, invariably disappear after a few days or weeks. In case they persist, an alternative method should be adopted. Also, this method is not advised for use in delaying the first pregnancy. Sometimes the device is automatically expelled in about 10% women in the first years; rarely perforation of womb may occur. In 50%-60% cases of pregnancy with Copper-T, miscarriages occur.

## Oral Contraceptives (OC, 'The Pill', and Combined Oral Contraceptives)

The oral contraceptive combines synthetic forms of the hormones, progesterone and estrogen. OCs stop ovulation by interfering with cyclical hormonal changes required for ovulation, render the cervical mucus thick and impenetrable to sperm, and induce endometrial changes. Pills are taken every day for 21 days (7 days off) of 28-day cycles (the last 7 pills are inert or have iron only). A whole cycle must be taken on schedule to work most effectively. When OCs are stopped menstruation occurs.

***Merits:*** Oral contraceptives are highly effective (efficacy is 99.9%) when used properly: they can be easily used and are unrelated to sexual activity.

***Benefits:***

Their use results in:

1. Relief from dysmenorrheal.
2. Less likelihood of ovarian cysts.
3. Regular and painless menstrual periods with decreased blood loss, this may help prevent or help correct anaemia.
4. Decreased risk (50%) of ovarian cancer and uterine cancer by about ½ as compared to non-users of OCs.
5. 50 per cent reduction in risk of certain pelvic (tubes) infections.
6. Protection (1/10 the risk of non-users of contraceptives) against ectopic pregnancy.
7. Protection against benign cystic breast disease.
8. Increased bone mass due to estrogen content.

***Drawbacks:*** The failure rate of the oral contraceptive increases if the pill is not taken regularly. Common minor side-effects include breast tenderness, nausea, headache, vomiting, weight gain, pimples, and spotting between periods or irregular periods for initial few months; these often clear up after two to three months of use. Users of OCs have a greater chance of getting serious cardiovascular diseases, including blood clots, rise in blood pressure, depression, heart attacks, and strokes than non-users. Almost all increased risk occurs among women with conditions predisposing to cardiovascular diseases, especially smoking, age (over 35), and high blood cholesterol. Overall risk of OC-related cardiovascular disease is low, while the risk of death from pregnancy is high. OC users may run a greater risk of having gall-bladder stones and liver tumors (benign) than non-users. There is inconclusive evidence that OCs slightly increase the risk of cervical cancer. Regular *pap smear* test may be requested to exclude such cancer if OC is taken for more than 5 years. Benign liver tumors which may rupture, occur very rarely in women using OCs. They may decrease the quantity of breast milk. Blood clots (particularly in leg veins) occur more frequently in OC user when estrogen dose is high. In a number of women dark patches (melasma) appear around eyes.

**Drug Interactions:** Certain antibiotics (*rifampicin* which is used for tuberculosis, *amoxicillin* and *tetracyclines* for infections) decrease effects of OCs and unwanted pregnancy may occur on continued use of OCs with them. So other method of contraception may be used.

## Selecting the Right OC

Human biological variation is such that no single OC formulation is optimal for every woman. Since major side-effects and most minor symptoms are related to the dose of estrogen, OCs should have less than 50 $\mu g$ estrogen and as little progestin as possible, consistent with a good clinical performance. Some 30 $\mu g$ estrogen-containing formulations perform as well as the 50 microgram preparations, but others less so. There is evidence that switching between formulations causes side-effects, but switching, for example, to a higher-dose formulation is occasionally helpful to help control the intermenstrual bleeding. Various formulations are almost equally effective. If a woman has epilepsy and is taking drugs then a higher-dose estrogen OC may be needed. If cholesterol and sugar levels in blood are marginally high, a low dose estrogen OC is advisable. Over weight women may require high dose OC. A OC pill containing least androgenic (male like effects) progestin such as *desogestril, norgestimate* or *drospirenone* should be used if female has pimples or is hirsuate. A lactating mother may use minipill (as below)

**Oral Contraceptives**

| *Brand Names* | *Hormonal Components* (*Estrogen*) | | *(Progestin)* | |
|---|---|---|---|---|
| **Combined Pills** | | | | |
| DUOLUTON-L OVRAL | Ethinylestradiol | 50 μg | Levonorgestrel | 25 μg |
| OVRAL-G | Ethinylestradiol | 50 μg | Norgestrel | 50 μg |
| OVRAL-L | Ethinylestradiol | 30 μg | Levonorgestrel | 15 μg |
| **Triphasic Pills** | | | | |
| TRIQUILAR | Ethinylestradiol | 5 tab (brown) 30 μg | Levonorgestrel | 50 μg |
| | | 6 tab (white) 30 μg | Levonorgestrel | 75 μg |
| | | 11 tab (ochre) 30 μg | Levonorgestrel | 125 μg |
| **Others** | | | | |
| FEMILON | Ethinylestradiol | 20 μg | Desogestral | 150 μg |
| NOVELON | Ethinylestradiol | 30 μg | Desogestral | 150 μg |

**Warning Signs:** Users of OCs experiencing unusual swelling or pain in the legs; yellowing of the skin or eyes; pain in the abdomen, chest or arms; shortness of breath; severe headache or depression; or eye problems such as blurred or double vision, must seek medical care. OCs are not generally used for longer than 3 to 5 years. It is always good to get a thorough clinical checkup done to exclude the presence of such disease that precludes use of OCs.

***Practical Points:***

1. Fertility returns in 1-2 months of stopping OC. Injectable Ocs may take a longer time.
2. If OC is missed, it is advised take two pills on the next day and use barrier method for 7 days-if intercourse has occurred in past5 days.
3. If pregnancy occurs (failure rate is 0.1% or less), it should be terminated because baby may be malformed.
4. If break through bleeding is troublesome, a high dose pill may be needed.
5. A new *progestin* (DESOGESTRAL-FEMILON TAB.) containing pill may be used if weight gain, acne and rise in cholesterol occurs with usual pills.

***Progestin containing minipill:*** *Norgestrel* or *norethisterone* (AMENOVA, NORGEST 0.35 mg) alone provides protection from pregnancy by effects on womb mainly which becomes hostile to nidation. It is begun on the first day of menses and used like other OCs. It is a choice during lactation because it does not affect milk formation. Cardiac and blood vessel complications are least likely. These are suitable for subjects with sickle cell disease also.

## Emergency Contraceptives

Unprotected sexual intercourse (sexual assault or contraceptive failure in the form of condom rupture, missed contraceptive pills, displaced IUD) may require prevention of pregnancy. For this purpose a common method is called as 'YUZPE METHOD' and involves use of 2 OVRAL tablets (or any other formulation having per Tab. *L-Norgestel* 0.5 mg + *Ethinylestradiol* 50 mg) are taken as soon as possible and 2 tablets 12 hour later within 72 hours of unprotected sex. It prevents 3 out of 4 possible pregnancies. Now a days WHO recommends use of *mifepristone* 200 mg-600 mg (MT PILL, UNWANTED) as a single dose within 72 hours. T-pill contains *mifepristone* (200 mg with *Misoprostol* 0.2 mg). The third drug is *L-Norgestrel.* This agent is marketed as I-PILL, NORLEVE and UNWANTED-72. It can be be taken in two ways: 1. Two tablet to be taken as soon as possible withing 72 hours after unprotected intercourse or 2. One tablet as soon as possible, preferably within 12 hours after unprotected intercourse and second tablet to be taken within 12-24 hours after the first dose. The I-PILL and UNWANTED-72 have double dose of *L-Norgestral* (1.5 mg) so only one pill is needed.

### Injectable Contraceptive and Implants

Trials are going on with depot provera (*medroxy progesterone acetate* 150 mg once in 3 months) but are not freely available. An implantable rod(40mmX2 mm containing 38 mg of longer acting progestin is inserted into arm tissues and provides protection for 3 years. Norplant is in the form of capsule containing long acting form of *L-Norgestral.* Six capsules are implanted under skin of arm and the effect lasts for about 5 years.

### Centchroman (SAHELI)

This is a new type of oral contraceptive developed by the Central Drug Research Institute, Lucknow, which has been approved by the Drug Controller general of India. It makes the environment in the uterus such that the embryo cannot get attached to its wall.

**Who Should *Not* Use Oral Contraceptives?**

Risks associated with OCs increase with age. For women over age 35 who use OCs, smoking increases the risk of heart attack or stroke. Women who have had a heart attack, stroke, angina pectoris, blood clots, cancer of the breast or womb, liver tumor, or impaired liver function should not use OCs.

Consideration should be given to use of an alternative method if any of these conditions are present: irregular periods, unexplained vaginal bleeding, migraine, mental depression, heart or kidney disease, high blood pressure, diabetes, or epilepsy.

Women who had jaundice during pregnancy or a recent fracture of long bones requiring longer period of bedrest should avoid OCs.

It is advisable to seek another method of contraception if cardiovascular risk factors are present. During breast-feeding, intake of OCs can reduce the amount of milk and small amount may also pass into baby through milk so progestin pill may be taken or another method adopted.

***Dosage:*** It is taken twice a week (for 3 months), starting from the 1st day of the bleeding, for example, Sunday and Wednesday. From the 4th month onwards the tablets are taken once a week, e.g. on every Sunday. It is a nonsteroidal and non-hormonal contraceptive, free from the adverse effects of conventional OCs. Failure rate is 1-3%. Some menstrual irregularity may be there during its use.

### Spermicides and Vaginal Preparations

Chemical contraceptives like jelly, creams and foam tablets can help a woman in preventing pregnancies. Spermicides are so called because they kill, on contact, the male sperms deposited in the woman's body during intercourse. The spermicide must be introduced in the vagina only 15 minutes before the intercourse. *Nonoxynol* (TODAY) pessary contains spermicidal agent and is to be inserted into vagina 10-15 minutes before the sexual act.

### Foam Tablet

The foam tablet which a woman inserts in her birth canal, before having sex, produces some foam which provides a protective coating to the whole area. It kills the sperms released from the man's body and thus prevents pregnancy.

### Jelly or Cream

The spermicidal jelly or cream is applied in the vagina with the help of an applicator. It destroys the male sperms on contact in the vaginal canal itself. These creams prove quite effective if used along with a diaphragm or a condom.

***Drawbacks:*** As chemical contraceptives involve intercourse related procedures, some couples find them combersome to apply. They can prove ineffective, if used in insufficient quantity or if they are not of good quality. If, after application of the jelly or cream, more than one hour elapses and sexual intercourse takes place later, there may be a risk of pregnancy.

## Terminal Methods (Permanent Methods)

The methods dealt with earlier offer several choices for those wanting to delay the first pregnancy or to ensure a minimum gap between two children. Once the family is complete, it is useful to consider the terminal methods that put an end to the need for contraceptives.

Sterilization provides permanent protection against pregnancy, allowing a couple to enjoy married life without any further fear of pregnancy whatsoever. Either the husband or the wife can undergo a simple operation for sterilization.

### Vasectomy: Sterilization of the Male

Vasectomy or sterilization of the male is a very simple out-patient procedure which takes hardly 15 to 20 minutes. This involves a small cut equal to the size of the grain of the wheat, above the man's scrotum and a small portion of the vas or the tubes which carry the seeds (sperms) are removed and the cut ends are tied up. The man's sex glands are not touched. He continues to enjoy sex as before. He also continues to ejaculate during sex but now his semen does not contain sperms or those seeds. There is no difference whatsoever in his strength or virility.

Immediately after the operation, the man can return home. However, he should refrain from any strenuous manual labour or cycling for about one week. There is no other inconvenience. He can resume other normal work immediately. Further, it is necessary to use a condom or any other contraceptive for about 15 ejaculations after the operation or abstain for three months. After this the semen should be tested and if no sperms are found, there is no need to use any contraceptive in future.

***Merits:*** Vasectomy is a simple operation, almost one hundred per cent effective, and provides life-long protection against unwanted pregnancies. There are no side-effects or complications. No infection should occur if the minimum requirements of hygiene and cleanliness are observed till the small incisions heal.

***Drawbacks:*** Vasectomy is an irreversible method. Though in some cases surgical recanalisation has been successfully done, the method should be accepted as irreversible.

### Tubectomy: Sterilization of the Female

In sterilization of the female, the doctor removes a small piece from each egg-tube (fallopian tubes) of the woman and ties up the cut ends so as to block the passage of the egg cell. This way, it cannot meet the sperm or the male seed during sexual relations and no pregnancy can take place. Tubectomy is done both by abdominal and vaginal routes. Generally, the woman has to remain in the hospital for 2 or 3 days and need to take a few days' rest.

### Laparoscopic sterilization

Nowadays, female sterilization has been made very simple by the use of a 'laparoscope'. This is an instrument like a telescope which is introduced into the abdomen through a very small opening of hardly one centimeter. The operation requires hospitalisation for a few hours only. Although it is a very quick and easy procedure, it must be handled by a skilled and experienced surgeon.

As stated earlier, sterilization is a permanent method of family limitation and should be undergone only when couples are absolutely certain that they do not want more children.

***Merits:*** Laparoscopy provides a permanent safeguard against unwanted pregnancies. There are no side-effects or complications when it is performed by a competent surgeon.

### Medical Termination of Pregnancy

Medial Termination of Pregnancy (MTP) is not to be taken as a method of family planning. Repeated termination of pregnancies is harmful to women. However, when pregnancy occurs as a result of failure of a contraceptive device and a woman does not want to continue with it, she has the full right to seek its termination before 12 weeks under the Medical Termination of Pregnancy Act, 1971.

Medical Termination of Pregnancy (MTP) or abortion is easy and safe when done within the first 12 weeks of pregnancy by a registered Medical Practitioner registered under the Medical Council Act, 1956, with recognised qualifications as defined in Clause 'H' of section of 2 of the said Act.

MTP should be done as early in pregnancy as possible and only in a place officially permitted to conduct MTP, as well-qualified and trained doctors would be available there. There are usually no complications after MTP and normal routine work can be resumed from the third day onwards. However, occasionally there may be some fever or menstrual disturbance. In all such cases, the woman should immediately report back to the doctor.

It needs to be reiterated that pregnancy should only be terminated through the services of well-qualified and trained doctors as early as possible and before 12 weeks are over. It is important not to fall into the hands of quacks and untrained *dais* in whose hands the procedure can be dangerous. After twelve weeks of pregnancy, the consent of two doctors is necessary before an unwanted pregnancy can be terminated.

### **Mifepristone** (MIFEGEST, MT PILL) + **Misoprostol** (MISOPROST) **for MTP**

This combination has been used by trained doctors for termination of pregnancy of less than 49 days. 600 mg of *mifepristone* are given and then 400 $\mu g$ of *misoprostol* are taken 2 days later. If ectopic pregnancy is suspected, this combination is never used. Intravaginal *Gemeprost* 36 to 48 hours after *mifepristone* is also used by gynecologists.

***Drawbacks:*** Repeated abortions are a health hazard. Abortion is not a substitute for contraceptives and should be the last resort only.

### Emergency Contraception

Emergency contraception is a boon to prevent unwanted pregnancy following unprotected intercourse or expected failure of contraception.The methods used are most effective within the first 72 to 120 hours. Broadly these methods can be of two categories, hormonal and mechanical.

**Hormonal methods:** Combined *estrogen* and *progesterone* pills e.g. Oral (*Ethnyl–estradiol* + *levonorgestrel*) 2 tabs 12 hrs apart.

*Levonorgestrel* pills in a dose of 75 mg. It is more effective, better tolerated, two hourly, with low failure rates.

Mechanical method: ICUD can be used , postcoitally upto 5 days following sexual exposure, with advantage of immediate protection.

*Mifepristone* (RU 486) – 600 mg single dose, efficacy nearly. 100%

Many morning after pills are easily available over the counter.

All these medications have their own side effects, so the failure rates are also present. In case of any side effect or complaints a specialist should always be consulted.

#### When is Medical Termination of Pregnancy (MTP) Permitted?

Under the Medical Termination of Pregnancy Act of 1971, free facilities for MTP are available at all public hospitals under the following conditions:

- ✓ To save the life of the pregnant woman.
- ✓ To prevent grave physical or mental injury to the mother.
- ✓ On humanitarian grounds where pregnancy has been caused by rape.
- ✓ Where there is substantial reason to believe that the child to be born would suffer from such physical or mental abnormalities as to be seriously handicapped.
- ✓ When pregnancy occurs as a result of the failure of a contraceptive device.
- ✓ If there is a fear that the environment or the circumstances of the pregnant woman may cause injury to her health.

# 29

# Drugs Used for Overcoming Sleeplessness

Sleep, like wakefulness, is a natural phenomenon. Both humans and animals sleep. Humans spend almost one-third of their lifetime sleeping. During sleep the activity of the brain is altered, but not completely suppressed. It is an accepted fact that the body needs rest from time to time. Nobody knows why the brain or any other organ should need rest, nor what happens during sleep that is beneficial. Only one thing is certain — that sleep is necessary. If a person is not allowed to sleep for 2 or 3 days (this is often to prisoners to extract secrets), he loses mental co-ordination. Deprivation of sleep increases suggestibility and is, therefore, an effective technique for brain washing.

How much sleep is essential? Children sleep longer than adults. Old people tend to sleep less. Among adults some feel completely rested after 6 hours of sleep; others may need 8 or 9 hours. Mahatma Gandhi used to sleep for only 4 hours, and used to wake up fresh. Stalin needed only a very short sleep and used to receive officials at the odd hour of 3.00 am.

In order to sleep well, some need ideal conditions: a comfortable bed in a noiseless room with controlled temperature. There are others who manage to sleep soundly even on the hard wooden berth of a second class rail compartment. It is really wonderful to be able to sleep well, but there are times when it is not possible to do so due to unavoidable circumstances. Travellers going long distances on jet planes have to readjust their sleeping hours in a new place. Presidents and Prime Ministers take injections of sleep-inducing drugs to overcome travel-induced insomnia and to readjust to new working hours when travelling abroad.

Sleeplessness or insomnia means difficulty in falling or stay asleep, reduced total sleep time or disturbed sleep. Sleeplessness or insomnia may result from various factors such as emotional trauma, fear, apprehension, anguish, drugs, or certain diseases. Loss of sleep for a day or two may not pose any problem, but prolonged insomnia can cause physical and mental fatigue, leading to increase in automobile accidents, alcohol consumption and poor performance and in such cases, medical treatment becomes necessary. A large number of sedatives, hypnotics (causing sleep), and anti-anxiety drugs are available for this, but the greatest difficulty is that all these have varying degree of addiction potential and their withdrawal or discontinuation may pose serious problems. Since they cause addiction, the drug laws prohibit the sale of these drugs without a prescription.

## Treatment and Drugs

The drugs for treatment of insomnia contain a single drug or a combination of two or more drugs causing a similar effect. However, none of the combinations offer any advantage over the single drug. They only add to the cost of treatment. Older drugs like *pentobarbitone* are no longer used for insomnia. *Ticlophos* (PEDICLORYL, TRICLORYL-500 mg/tsf liquid) is some times used for induction of sleep in children when some laboratory test are to be done.

### Benzodiazepine Drugs

***Nitrazepam*** (HYPNOTEX): *Nitrazepam* is effective in initiating and maintaining sleep even when used for a prolonged period. It produces sleep like natural sleep, that is, it does not inhibit REM sleep which is a part of natural sleep. Most people can tolerate this drug. Moreover, it is not addictive. The only problem with this drug is that it has a sustained action, and residual sedative action occurs on the day following its administration. This drug is also unsuitable for patients who develop sudden breathing difficulty and wake up because of it. Its dose of 5 to 10 mg is effective in producing good sleep and is superior to *diazepam* (CALMPOSE) which is frequently used in India for inducing sedation and sleep. The latter drug is used in insomnia due to anxiety.

**Benzodiazepine Family of Drugs for Overcoming Sleeplessness**

| *Drugs* | *Dose/mg* | *Onset of Effect/min* | *Duration of Effect/hrs.* | *Adverse Effects* |
|---|---|---|---|---|
| *Nitrazepam* HYPNOTEX | 5-10 | 30-60 | 6-8 | Daytime drowsiness, dizziness, confusion, visual disturbances |
| *Diazepam* CALMPOSE | 5-10 | 120 | 24 | Drowsiness, fatigue, confusion, nausea depression, visual disturbances, daytime sleepiness, habituation. |
| *Lorazepam* LARPOSE | 1-2 | 30-60 | 8-12 | Lack of appetite, nausea, habituation weakness, dizziness |
| *Chlordiazepoxide* LIBRIUM | 20-40 | 60-120 | 12-24 | Daytime drowsiness, dizziness, forgetfulness, visual disturbances |
| *Alprazolam* (ALPRAX) | 0.5-1 | — | — | Particularly if stress and anxiety leads to insomnia |

### Non-benzadiazepine Hypnotics

A number of new drugs have been developed to induce sleep without disturbing the sleep cycle.

***Melatonin*** (ETERNEX, ZYTONIN 3 mg): It is a hormone of pineal gland. It maintains 'biological clock' which regulates sleep-wake cycle. When sleep is disturbed due to changes in biorythms (jet-lag) *melatonin* can induce sleep in a dose of 3 mg (some preprations like *zytonin* have vitamins $B_6$). It can cause fatigue, headache, itching and confusion. Combinations of melatonin with alprazolam (STRESNIL, MELOPRESS) are also available.

***Zaleplon*** (ZANLOP, ZAPLON, ZASO 5 mg, 10 mg tab.): It rapidly induces sleep but total sleep time is unchanged and therefore daytime hangover is less. It may cause headache, nausea and stomach upset.

***Zolpidem*** (ZOLDEM, SOVE 5 mg 10 mg): This drug induces sleep quickly and increases total sleep time. Dependence potential is less with its use. Its usual dose is 5 to 10 mg at night.

***Zopiclone*** (ZONAP, ZOPICON, ZOLINOX 3.75mg, 7.5 mg): It acts similarly to *zolpidem.*

***Hydroxyzine*** (ATARAX, PRUGO 10 mg,25 mg): It is time honoured medicine for sleep induction when insomnia is due to urticaria (hives) and pruritus (itching).

*Promethazine* (PHENERGAN) and *Diphenhydramine* (BENADRYL cap)are also useful hypnotics.

## Insomnia due to Restless Leg Syndrome (RLS)

RLS is a common sleep disorder in which there is painful creeping-crawling sensations in the legs at night which prevent sleep. The subjects losses in the bed moving legs to alleviate discomfort. Many agents have been tried. Iron is used when anemia is detected. *Gabapentin* (NEURONTIN cap 300 mg) is effective. Other drus are *Pramipexole,* and *Ropinirole* (Antiparkinson's drugs). One must avoid excess of coffee and tee at bed time. One must keep in mind that antihistaminic antiallergics and antidepressants increase the discomfort!

**Choosing a right treatment in elderly:** A common cause of sleeplessness in elderly is age related changes in the sleep cycle. Loss of family support, prostatic enlargement with frequent urination at night, dementia or depression should be looked for and treated. Restriction of excessive fluid intake in elderly, avoiding drugs which cause insomnia and use of short acting hypnotic in smaller doses (because drug disposition is changed in them) initially are some useful measures. Sometimes a glassful of warm milk can be in a good hypnotic. Milk contains "tryptophan" which is needed to make serotonin!! Training in Yoga, meditation can also help in those patients who do not have any discernible cause. There are some drugs which can cause sleeplessness. These are:

**CNS-stimulants:** Caffeine, nicotine, *ephedrine, amphetamine,* appetite, suppressants, nasal-decongestants, *(phenylpropanolamine).*

**Others:** *Chloroquine, ciprofloxacin, metronidazole, levodopa,* some anti-depressants *(Fluoxetine)* and diuretics (if used in evening/at night). Stopping their use or substituting any of them with alternative drugs can treat insomnia.

**Hazards of Overuse**

The drugs described for insomnia are very useful in alleviating human suffering but, when misused, cause serious problems.

Although supposed to be available on a doctor's prescription only, some individuals get these drugs illegally and consume them without medical supervision. Prolonged use leads to remarkable habituation and even addiction, which, at time become difficult to treat. It is the duty of the family members of such persons, not to allow the latter to possess and consume the drugs without medical need and a doctor's prescription. Keeping such drugs in the house in any quantity greater than the amount prescribed for two day's authorized use is risky.

Prolonged and uninterrupted use of most of these drugs may lead to addiction in the form of emotional and physical dependence, causing impairment of mental ability, regression, confusion, emotional instability, and discoordination of movements and reflexes. These should not be used in sleep-apnoea.

These drugs have often been chosen by young persons merely to have a 'good time' and the practice, when not checked, has resulted in loss of valuable time, unsatisfactory performance in examinations, ruining of health, and at times, of brilliant careers.

# 30

# Drugs Used in Sexual Inadequacies

••••••

Sex is a very intimate and important aspect of human life. The problem of sexual inadequacy is very common. About 10% of the world's population suffers from it. Most people do not know where to go and with whom to discuss their sex problems. Sexuality is a large component of one's personality, going far beyond merely the physical organs of the body. The normal sexual act consists of arousal (excitement and erection), orgasm (pleasure) and resolution(relaxation). The common sexual inadequacy is in the form of a defect in arousal and/or orgasm. Not even normal individuals achieve orgasm. It is estimated that 46% of sexually active men have orgasm every time!. The most important causes of sexual inadequacies are ignorance, impotence (erectile dysfunction), orgasmic failure, premature ejaculation, and diminished sexual desire (libido). There has been a major breakthrough in the treatment of erectile dysfunction but far more research is needed to deal successfully with other sexual disorders.

## Erectile Dysfunction (Impotence)

Erectile dysfunction is another name for impotence or the inability to achieve a sexual erection and or orgasm sufficient for a satisfying intercourse.

***Causes:*** It effects one in twenty men at the age of 40-50 years and about 50% males over the age of 65 years. There are four types of disorders associated with impotence. These are: 1. Diseases of blood vessels supplying penis; 2. Diseases of nerves of penis; 3. Use of certain drugs; and 4. Psychological causes (most common).

Narrowing of penile blood vessels occur due to advanced diabetes mellitus and atherosclerosis. Diabetes also damages the nerves. So it is an important known cause of impotence. Certain diseases of backbone, long use of alcohol and stroke can also lead to impotence due to nerve damage. Some drugs such as *thiazides,* antidepressants, *cimetidine,* antipsychotic agents are also known to cause impotence in adults. Low testosterone level is an uncommon cause of impotence. The most common cause is psychological disturbance that is seen frequently in young males. The reasons are many myths and false concepts about sex, feeling of guilt in doing masturbation and excessive anxiety about sexual relationships are some of them.

**Sildenafil** (PENEGRA, ERIX, ANDROZ, 11 PM)

The discovery of *sildenafil* is a major breakthrough in the treatment of erectile dysfunction. The drug's 'potency' enhancing effect was observed by chance in 1990. Before that it was investigated for the treatment of chest pain (angina), it did nothing at all to relieve anginal pain.

**How Does Sildenafil Act?** It acts only on the erectile tissue of the penis. It increases the supply of blood in the organ, causing a hydraulic action. It enhance the physiological response to sexual arousal, causing penile erection. The chemical nitric oxide is released from nerve endings and blood vessels in response to sexual arousal, increases production of another chemical — cyclic guanosine monophosphate (cGMP). This chemical relaxes the smooth muscles of the spongy tissue of the penis, allowing an engorgement due to accumulation of blood. The organ bulges and becomes tight and rigid. The availability of nitric oxide depends on the level of active cGMP. this is normally inactived by an enzyme called phosphodiesterase type-5. *Sildenafil* inhibits this enzyme and allows active cGMP to accumulate in order to sustain the pooling of blood and the erection.

The drug works in 70% men with erectile dysfunction. The outcome may not be as good in drinkers and smokers, and those who eat fatty meals. Eating a fatty meal before taking the drug, hinders its absorption. There are some claims that it increases the blood circulation in the pelvic region, clitoris and may cause sexual arousal in females also. Scientific studies have clearly shown that it does not affect sexual desire (libido). It is effective in men with diabetes, hepatitis, and multiple sclerosis, in spinal injuries, as well as in about 30 to 40% of men whose prostate has been removed.

***Dosage:*** It is available as 25, 50, and 100 mg tablets. The starting dose is 50 mg per day. The maximum recommended dose is 100 mg. If the erection is more than satisfactory, the dose should be reduced to 25 mg. *It must be taken about half to one hour before the act and the effect may last for 4 to 6 hours.*

***Adverse Effects:*** *Sildenafil* lowers the blood pressure only slightly in normal persons but substantially in patients who are taking drugs such as *nitrates* for angina pectoris. Headache, flushing, and dyspepsia are the most common side-effects. Nasal congestion, diarrhoea, dizziness, and rash may occur in rare cases. Transient abnormal vision with a colour tinge (that is, seeing a blue haze), and increased sensitivity to light are uncommon. This adverse effect occurs more frequently with 100 mg than with 50 mg doses. In general, most people do not suffer from any significant adverse effects as the drug is taken infrequently. Moreover the adverse effects have not stopped men from using the drug.

***Precautions:***

1. It should never be taken by patients with coronary heart disease, or those who are taking nitrates or those with blood cancer.
2. Drugs like *erythromycin,* and *ketoconazole* decrease the metabolism and increase its effect. *Rifampicin* increases its metabolism and reduces its effect.
3. A doctor must be consulted by those above the age of 65 years, or have any liver or kidney disorders, or they should start with a smaller dose of 25 mg, and increase it only after consulting the doctor.
4. It should not be taken more than once a day.
5. Alcohol intake may increase drug induced fall in BP.

### Tadalafil (EROTID 10mg, 20mg)

It produces satisfactory erection and has a longer effect. Therefore it can be taken once a day and the sexual performance is successful even upto 24 hours. The adverse effects of *sildenafil* are less often seen with this drug. However some precautions need to be observed.

**Verdenafil** is a newer agent yet to be available in India.

### Direct Injections of Drug into Penis before Sexual Intercourse

Injection of *papaverine* and *phentolamine* (PIPE treatment) into the body of penis by a tuberculin syringe produces erection to permit sexual intercourse. There are problems of longer lasting and painful erection (priapism)and repeated injections cause damage to penis (fibrosis and infections)

### Prostaglandin (ALPROSTADIL)

*Prostaglandin* in the form of urethral suppository can be inserted into urinary passage of penis before sexual intercourse but it may cause irritation and burning sensation.

### Penile Devices

Implants are available which can be placed into penis in such a way that before sexual intercourse they can be inflated (by air) to make penis rigid.

A vacuum constriction device (cylinder) is also available that draws the penis into erected state when suction is applied to create vacuum. When erect, a rubber band is applied over penis-base to keep it in that stage for vaginal introduction. The cylinder is removed before intercourse.

### Surgery Over Penis

If blood vessels are narrowed or blocked, an arterial bypass (akin to heart bypass) surgery is done to allow blood flow into penis. This surgery is rarely undertaken and that too in suitable cases only.

### Herbal Preparations

A number of licensed herbal preparations are available in market. These are recommended for a variety of sexual inadequacies. Examples are HIMCOLIN *gel,* to be applied locally over penis, TENTEX ROYAL, to be taken an hour before sexual intercourse. Their utility is doubtful.

## Premature Ejaculation

This is one of the most common causes of sexual inadequacy in men. Reaching a climax before one wants to, is described as a 'premature ejaculation'. In other words, it is an early orgasmic response. It is mainly a problem of adolescent boys.

***Causes:*** This may be due to anxiety, stressed relationship, fear of pregnancy or fear of lack of self confidence. Some diseases like lower spinal injuries, prostatic inflammation, diabetes are also the causes. The individual looses the ability to exercise control and ejaculation may occur. In some diseases of nerves, there is retrograde (backwards) ejaculation and the person feels dissatisfied as partner complains of 'dry act'.

Some exercises are prescribed to improve orgasmic control. These help an individual to develop control gradually and progressively. A qualified sexologist should be consulted for the programme of exercises. Other measures include:

1. Voluntarily interrupting and restarting the flow of urine repeatedly (to exercise the pubococcygeus muscle).
2. Taking a deep breath and voluntarily contracting the anal sphincter (a ring of muscle surrounding and guarding or closing the anus), holding the contraction for 15 to 20 seconds, and then releasing it. This may be repeated up to 20 times, twice a day.
3. The squeeze technique: voluntarily, the partner squeezes the penis just prior to reaching orgasm.
4. Wearing a condom to decrease sensitivity.

Some local anaesthetics are prescribed to prevent premature ejaculation. They are: *Lignocaine* (XYLOCAINE) 5% ointment, 2% gelly.

*Lignocaine* is generally considered to be effective and safe for use by the public. When applied around the penis, it decrease sensitivity and delays ejaculation. There may be some initial irritation which is followed by a decreased sensation. A small amount is applied 15 to 20 minutes before and may be washed off before sexual act. The vaginal numbness may be complained by partner.

Some antidepressants are found to be effective. *Fluoxetine* (FLUDAC-20 mg/day) is effective in many cases. Other antidepressants have also been tried.

**Adverse Effects:** These anaesthetics may cause allergic reactions such as burning, stinging, and tenderness. In rare cases, there may be very delayed orgasms or even failure of ejaculation due to numbness.

Herbal drugs like CONFIDO and others have uncertain value in premature ejaculation.

## Diminished Sexual Desire (Loss of Libido)

The most common causes are psychological. Many patients are depressed and stressed. In females, frigidity (lack of erotic response) and vaginismus (spasm and pain during penetration) are seen. Psychotherapy and understanding the physiology of sexual act are very helpful. There is a sex centre in the brain which can be stimulated by external stimuli such as sight, odour, touch, and sound A spot (G-spot known after its founder Graefenberg) is found in the anterior part of vagina which when stimulated can arouse a female for erotic response. This may be missing in some females. Several substances, including foods and drugs, have been used to treat impotence or to stimulate sexual desire. These agents are called sex tonics or aphrodisiacs, a name derived from Aphrodite, the Greek goddess of love. An aphrodisiac may work by stimulating the sex centre in the brain or by causing local irritation and increasing the flow of blood in the genital organs.

**Causes:** It occurs in men and women both. It is commonly due to a traumatic experience in past, boredom in relationship (monotony-'midlife crisis'), hormonal decline and use of drugs such as sedatives, antidepressants, *prazosin* and other BP lowering drugs.

While many therapies have been tried to improve sex drive, ultimately counselling and behaviour therapy helps a lot. Various substances which have been used for this purpose are described below:

*Foods:* It is said that a high-protein diet such as eggs, meat, crabs, oysters, and caviar have an aphrodisiac action. The truth of this belief has, so far, not been ascertained though. The psychological aspect appears to be the most important factor in their proposed effect.

*Alcohol:* The effect of alcohol on sexual desire is discussed in detail in the chapter on 'Alcohol'. It causes generalized stimulation by removing the inhibitions which keep a check on behaviour. Alcohol is consumed before intercourse with the idea that it will enhance potency. In his famous drama, *Macbeth*, Shakespeare wrote, 'Alcohol provokes the desire but takes away the performance'. The chronic intake of alcohol may lead to a permanent impairment of sexual functions.

### **Spanish Fly** (CANTHARADIN)

Spanish fly (CANTHARADIN) was originally prepared from a small (Spanish) beetle named *Cantharis vesicatoria*. A few drops of this drug or its synthetic derivative are mixed in a beverage and taken. It passes unchanged into the urine, causing severe irritation and inflammation of the bladder and urethra (urinary tract), and dilating the blood vessels. This stimulates the genitals.

A slightly higher dose may cause severe abdominal pain and painful urination, and destroy the mucous membrane of the urinary bladder and the urethra.

### **Testosterone** (TESTANON, AQUAVIRON)

Testosterone (the male sex hormone) is often used for an aphrodisiac effect. It is rarely effective except in cases where there is a deficiency of this hormone such as in an old age, in the absence of the testes, and in the non-appearance of secondary sexual characteristics in males. In most developed countries, this is not used in the routine treatment of sexual dysfunctions even in ageing males (with andropause!) owing to the risk of adverse effects. Unless one is sure of the decreased level of the hormone, it should not be administered.

An external dose of testosterone may derange the liver functions and lead to jaundice. It may cause enlargement of the prostate gland, causing difficulty in passing urine. Prolonged use may also cause cancer of the liver or the prostate.

**A Genuine Sex Tonic: Does It Exist?**

If you are looking for a real sex tonic, you will be disappointed. A large number of preparations are sold in the market with highly suggestive and tall claims, and you may wonder why people buy them. As it happens, a large number of men are anxious to increase their sexual potency in order to become 'real' men. Manufacturers are aware of this masculine weakness and fully exploit the male ego. And where is the harm if, in this process, they make some money and satisfy some men, though only psychologically? A real biological aphrodisiac has yet to be discovered. The urge for a sex stimulant, it seems, is the same as for a fortune teller, and of the latter, the best tipped are those who predict the most glorious future.

People should, however, realise that there is no sexual magic beyond the natural sex drive itself. The best sex tonic is a harmonious, pleasurable and understanding partnership which excels in a beautiful environment.

## Cannabis

Cannabis is obtained from leaves of *Cannabis indica* or *Cannabis sativa*. (*bhang*); the flowering tops, especially of the female plant, are known as *ganja* (Marijuana); and the resinous exudate as *charas* (hashish).

It causes relaxation, euphoria, increases appetite, and impairs judgement and co-ordination. The overall effect is to remove inhibitions and release more primitive impulses. The assumed aphrodisiac effect of cannabis may be due to an increase in suggestibility or uninhibited behaviour. It has no real aphrodisiac effect.

It causes dryness of the mouth, increases thirst, reddens the eyes, increases the pulse rate, and may even cause fear, panic, and agitation.

## Cocaine

*Cocaine* was once used for sexual stimulation but because of its toxicities its use is not advisable.

## Musk

This is a viscid substance with a pungent odour, found in a sac under the abdomen of the male Asiatic deer. It is believed that if the substance is rubbed on the penis, it will cause an aphrodisiac effect. However, no evidence of the same is available in human beings.

**Drugs for Benign Prostatic Enlargement(BHP)**

| *Drug* | *Formulation* | *Usual dose* | *Adverse effects* |
|---|---|---|---|
| *Finasteride* | FINCAR,FINAST 5 mg | 5 mg once a day | Found in semen, use condom |
| *Dutasteride* | DUPROST 0.5 mg | 0.5 mg once a day | Found in semen, use condom |
| *Prazosin* | PRAZOPRESS XL 2.5, 5 mg | 1 tab at bed time | Fall in BP |
| *Alfuzosin* | ALFUSIN 10 mg | 2.5 to 10 mg once a day | Fall in BP |
| *Doxazosin* | DOXACARD 1, 2 ,4 mg | 1-4 mg at bed time | Fall in BP |
| *Tamsulosin** | Cap CONTIFLO 0.2, 0.4 mg | 1cap at bed time | safer & commonly used |
| *Finasteride* with *dutasteride* | FINAST-T.URIMAX-T | 0.5+0.5 mg | 1 cap at bed time |

BHP is a commom disorder of sex apparatus in elderly males.

# 31

# Sexually Transmitted Diseases and AIDS

There is no disease about which the patient is more secretive than a sexually transmitted disease. He is always worried and even hesitant about discussing it with his personal physician. He does not mind spending a fortune for the treatment. For this reason a large number of quacks who treat such diseases are prosperous and their number is increasing day by day. They advertise on big hoardings at railway stations, street crossings, and commercial areas as clinics for 'restoring youth and happiness' and for treating sexually transmitted diseases.

Sexually transmitted diseases comprise a number of conditions of which AIDS, syphilis, and gonorrhoea are common examples. AIDS has alarmed more than others. These diseases are not transmitted through air, water, food, flies, or casual contacts but through sexual contact. The early signs and symptoms are genital discharges, ulcers, itching, or pain. People experiencing such symptoms should seek immediate medical care.

## AIDS

One of the most talked about and dreaded disease these days is AIDS (Acquired Immune Deficiency Syndrome). This disease is caused by the HIV-1 and HIV-2 (Africa) virus which destroys the defense (immune cells-Lymphocytes-CD4 cells) mechanisms of the body. It makes the patient highly vulnerable to infections. It spreads slowly and there are no symptoms for a few years. These symptom-free persons are carriers of the disease and may spread it to others.

The infection can spread when the blood and/or genital secretions of an infected person come in contact with the blood or mucous membranes of a healthy person. This can happen through sexual intercourse (homo or heterosexual), use of contaminated needles (drug addicts), infected blood transfusion, or by an infected mother to her unborn child. The virus does not spread through everyday social contact such as handshaking, living, playing, or eating together. Food, water, common cups, insects, and toilet seats do not transmit the infection. Its occurrence is increasing in our country and as estimates reveal it is fast becoming an 'epidemic' (prevalence rate is over 1%).

**Regimens for Treatment of**

| Disease/Causative Organism | TREATMENT 1st Choice | Dose |
|---|---|---|
| 1. Gonorrhoea<br>Non-penicillinase producing<br>Penicillinase producing | *Ceftriaxone*<br>*Cefuroxime* | 250 mg IM or<br>250 mg IM, + *Probenecid* 1g orally |
| | *Amoxycillin*<br>*Ampicillin*<br>*Azithromycin*<br>*Procaine Penicillin G* | 3 g orally, or<br>3.5 g orally, or<br>1 mg single dose<br>4.8 million units IM |
| Eye involvement in new born (*ophthalmia neonatorum*) | Eye wash with saline,<br>*Penicillin G Eye drops* | 10,000-20,000 units/ml |
| 2. Syphilis<br>Early (primary, secondary and latent <1 yr.) | *Benzathine Penicillin G*<br>*Procaine Penicillin G* | 2.4 million units IM, 1-3 weekly inj., or<br>1.2 million units IM ×10 days |
| Late (>1 yr) | *Benzathine Penicillin G*<br>*Procaine Penicillin G* | 2.4 million units IM weekly×4 weeks, or<br>1.2 million units IM×20 days |
| Neurosyphilis | *Penicillin G* | 3-4 million units IV 4 hourly for 10-14 days |
| 3. Chlamydia trachomatis<br>Nonspecific urethritis<br>Lymphogranuloma Venereum | *Azithromycin*<br>*Doxycycline* | 1 g orally, single dose or<br>100 mg BD × 7 days orally<br>Same for 2 weeks |
| 4. Calymn. granulomatis<br>Granuloma inguinale/ Donovanosis | *Tetracycline*<br>*Doxycycline* | 500 mg QID × 10 days orally, or<br>100 mg BD ×3 weeks orally |
| 5. Chancroid<br>(*H. ducreyi*) | *Cotrimoxazole*<br>*Erythromycin*<br>*Ceftriaxone* | 960 mg BD × 7 days orally, or<br>500 mg QD × 7 days orally<br>0.25 g IM, single dose |
| 6. Genital Herpes Simplex<br>Early cases | *Acyclovir* | 5% ointment locally 6 times a day 10 days (does not prevent recurrence) |
| Late cases | *Acyclovir* | 200 mg 5 times a day × 10 days orally (in addition to local therapy) |
| Recurrent cases | *Acyclovir* | 200 mg 3 to 5 times a day for 6 months |
| 7. Trichomonas Vaginitis<br>(Treat the male partner also if recurrent) | *Metronidazole*<br>OR<br>*Tinidazole* | 2g single dose or 400 mg TDS for 7 days<br><br>2g single dose or 600 mg OD for 7 days |
| 8. Pubic Lice<br>(P. pubis) | *Permethrin*<br>(PERMITE CREAM RINSE) | 1% cream/rinse single application. Massage hair with about 30 gm, wash hair after 10 minutes |
| | *Lvermectin*<br>(IVERMECTOL 3 mg, 6 mg) | single dose 0.2 mg/kg<br>Wash beddings and clothes. |

## Sexually Transmitted Diseases

*Alternatives (2nd Choice)*

*Cefixime* 400 mg once orally, or
*Doxycyline* 100 mg twice a day × 7 days orally, or
*Erythromycin* 500 mg 4 times a day × 5 days orally, or
*Ciprofloxacin* 250-500 mg orally or
*Pefloxacin* 400 mg orally or
*Ofloxacin* 200-400 mg orally (all once)

*Ceftriaxone* 25 mg/kg (maximum 125 mg) IV/IV

*Doxycycline* 100 mg twice a day × 15 days, or

*Ceftriaxone* 1 g IM × 7 days, or
*Erythromycin* 500 mg 4 times a day × 15 days
*Doxycline* or *Erythromycin* × 30 days, or

*Ceftriaxone* 1 g IM × 15 days
*Proc PnG* 2.4 million units IM daily × 10-14 days
*Probenecid* 500 mg orally 4 times a day or
*Doxycycline* 200 mg twice a day × 21 days

*Erythromycin* 500 mg 4 times a day × 7 days orally, or
*Sulfamethoxazole* 1 g twice a day × 7 days orally
Same for 2 weeks

*Cotrimoxazole* 960 mg twice a day × 2 weeks orally,
*Erythromycin* 500 mg 4 times a day × 3 weeks orally

*Ciprofloxacin* 500 mg twice a day × 3 days orally, or
*Tetracyline* 500 mg twice a day × 7 days orally

*Famcyclovir* (VIROVIR)
125 mg twice a day × 5 days

—

—

*Clotrimazole* (CANESTEN) 100 mg intravaginat
every night 6 to 12 nights

—

*Lindane* (GAMASCAB) 1%
massage hair wash after 10 minutes

(Not to be used in pregnancy
and children

***Common Symptoms:*** There may be unexplained fever, weight loss, diarrhoea, fatigue, night sweats, enlargement of the lymph nodes, muscle weakness, and frequent infections.

Diagnosis is made via a low (<400/mcl) blood counts (CD-4 cell count) and an enzyme-linked immunosorbent assay (ELISA). The confirmation is made by the Western Blot analysis method.

## Treatment

A large number of highly expensive drugs are now made available at an affordable price which can be given alone or in combination. It must be understood that at present drugs only prolong the life and postpone complications, therefore, these are to be used judiciously with regular checkup and blood tests.

| *Drug/Formulation* | *Daily dose* | *Precautions* |
|---|---|---|
| **Nucleoside Reverse Transcriptase Inhibitors(NRTIs)** | | |
| *Zidovudine* (RETROVIR 100 mg Cap) | 300 mg twice with water | Avoid paracetamol,Stavudine |
| *Didanosine* (DDRETRO 250 mg Tab) | 200 mg twice | Use with other drugs |
| *Stavudine* (STAVIR-30 mg) | 20 mg twice | causes neuropathy |
| *Lamivudine* (LAMIVIR-150 mg0 | 150 mg twice | - |
| Hepatitis B-100 mg once | | |
| *Abacavir* (ABAVIR-300 mg) | 300 mg twice | Avoid alcohol |
| **Non- Nucleoside Reverse Transcriptase Inhibitors (NNRTIs)** | | |
| *Nevirapine* (NEVIMUNE-200 mg) | 200 mg once/twice | use in combination |
| *Efavirenz* (EFAVIR-200 mg) | 600 mg once | on empty stoach |
| **<u>Protease Inhibitors(PIs)</u>** | | |
| *Indinavir* (INDIVIR-400 mg cap) | 800 mg | On empty stoach |
| *Nelfinavir* (NELFIR 250 mg) | 750 mg thrice | With meals |
| *Ritonavir* (TITOMAX-100 mg cap) | Usually with other PIs | |
| *Sequinqvir* (SAQUIN- 200 mg) | 1.2 Gm | with meals |
| *Lopinavir* (RITOMAX 400 mg | 400 mg once | with meals |
| **<u>Fusion Inhibitors:</u>** | | |
| *Enfluvirtide* is yet to be available. | | |
| **Some commonly used combinations:** | | |
| COMBIVIR= *Lamivudine* with *Zidovudine* (not available in India) | | |
| LAMIVIR-S= *Lamivudine* with *stavudine* (not available in India) | | |
| TROMUNE = *Lamivudine* + *Zidovudine* + *Efavirenz* (not available in India) | | |

***Preventive Treatment:*** Accidental exposure to needle prick, blood stains and pregnant HIV positive mothers are give onen or two drugs to prevent HIV infection.

Usually *Zidovudine* 300 mg + *Lamivudine* 150 mg are taken twice a day for 4 weeks

In case of higher risk involved then *Indinavir* 800 mg is added as a third drug.

*Zidovudine* 300 mg twice a day from 2ndtrimester onwards and continued throughout post delivery period cuts the chances of infection to new born remarkably. Infected and HIV postive mothers should avoid breast feeding.

Recent developments have established that treatment of HIV positive individuals has become highly specialised and expensive.

**Treatment of Other Infections:** A number of infections (including tuberculosis) flare up in HIV infected individuals due to deficient immunity (ability to resist) against them. These are chronic bacterial, fungal and protozoal infections and require treatment.

**Preventive Measures:** 'Prevention is better than cure', definitely applies to this disease for which there is no cure presently. There is no vaccine against AIDS and it can only be prevented by health education and living responsibly.

The disease can be avoided by having sex with only one faithful partner, use of condoms, avoiding injection or any surgical procedures where sterility of instruments is not ensured. Untested blood should not be used for transfusion. A woman who is an AIDS carrier or suspected to be so, should avoid pregnancy.

## Gonorrhoea

This is an infection caused by the bacteria *Neisseria gonorrhoea*. It infects the private parts, rectum, eyes, and the throat and if not treated, it may involve the bones, skin, pelvic organs and brain.

### Common Symptoms of Acute Gonorrhoea (Urethritis, Vaginitis)

The usual latent or incubation period of its infection is 2 to 7 days. Symptoms include pus like (purulent) discharge, painful and frequent urination, redness of the penile opening in males, vaginal discharge and pain in females. In some women there is involvement of cervix, uterus, tubes and ovaries. This causes pain on intercourse, and abnormal menstrual bleeding in females. In homosexuals, anal and oral infections are common. In infected pregnant women, the infection can spread to newborns. In very severe cases the infection may spread throughout the body (septicemia).

The diagnosis of such a case is confirmed by a microscopic examination of discharge. A cervical, rectal, urethral, or pharynx swab culture may also be done for determining the sensitivity of the organism to antibiotics.

**Condoms: The Sure and Safe Prevention Against AIDS**

An easy, sure, and convenient way of preventing sexually transmitted diseases is the use of latex condoms. In the West these are easily available in grocery shops in fancy packets with nicknames such as 'Yellow rose', and no one knows what is being purchased. These are also available through vending machines located at public toilets in nightclubs, stations, and subways, where a person can buy them just by inserting a coin. In contrast to this, in India though there is wide publicity of condoms through flashy advertisements in magazines, on the TV and radio, their sale is little. The freely distributed condoms at Government hospitals are the non-lubricated ones, which are not liked by the public. In a country where a lady feels shy about asking for sanitary napkins in the presence of another person, the purchase of condoms is out of the question. The distribution system of condoms is very defective, especially for a population which is highly inhibited. There are no outlets available for the purchase of condoms late in the evening. There is an urgent need for a better distribution system (condom vending machines) of good-quality condoms in which the identity of the buyer is not disclosed. This would encourage more men and may be even women to buy more condoms.

See table given earlier for drugs used in the treatment of Gonorrhoea. Disseminated (Systemic) infection requires intravenous drugs such as *Penicillin-G* (10 million units/day x 5 days), *Ceftriaxone* (1 gm/day x 5 days) or, oral drugs such as *Ciprofloxacin* (500 mg twice a day) or *Levofloxacin* (500 mg once a day) for 5 days.

## Syphilis

This is caused by the micro-organism, *Treponema pallidum*. The commonest mode of transmission is through sex. However, it can be transmitted by non-sexual contact such as infection to the baby in the womb by an infected mother or by blood transfusion. The usual incubation period is 3 weeks.

The diagnosis is confirmed by microscopic examination of scrapings of affected areas. Some serologic tests, such as VDRL (Venereal Diseases Research Laboratory), Rapid Plasma Region (RPR) are also performed for reconfirmation.

*Penicillin* injections are the drug of choice for all stages of syphilis. A prolonged treatment lasting for several weeks is required, depending on the severity of infection. In pregnancy, all women should be routinely checked for syphilis. When ever *penicillin* treatment is begun a sensitivity test is a must.

**Follow-Up:** Syphilis patients should be re-examined after every few months as the symptoms may reappear. If the heart and nerves are involved, the patient's case should be followed up for many years. Treatment of other sexually transmitted diseases is given in table.

### Simple Steps to Avoid AIDS

Knowing the facts, one can protect oneself and the society. It is almost always passed on by people who go to bed with different partners or by drug users who share syringes and needles.

**General precautions:**

1. Avoid sharing syringes and needles.
2. Avoid pregnancy if a woman has AIDS.
3. To give and receive blood, sterile disposable needles should be used and blood should be tested for HIV .
4. Universal precautions such as use of gloves. gowns, masks, goggles, specially designed safer needles by health care providers should be observed.

**Sexual precautions:**

1. Avoid multiple and anonymous sex partners (not only for homosexuals but also for heterosexuals).
2. Practices like oral sex, anal sex (receptive) and sex with professional workers could be risky.
3. Use of latex condoms could reduce the risk considerably.
4. Sexual activity leading to exchange of body fluids must be avoided.

# 32

# Drugs for Treatment of Common Skin Disorders

• • • • • •

This skin is as vital as the heart or the brain, and a healthy skin is essential for life. Diseased skin can make life unbearable. Such a person avoids meeting people, and others also like to keep away for the fear of contracting infection. In the last few years, in India like in the west, a multicrore rupee industry has come up to manufacture skin care preparations, so much so that some years ago the Indian Parliament had to amend the Drugs Act of 1940 to the Drugs and Cosmetics Act to include cosmetics in the Act, the use of which has been growing in India at a very rapid rate.

## Scabies

Scabies is a contagious disease caused by a mite (*Sarcoptes scabiei*). This mite lays eggs in the burrows of the skin. The disease spreads through contact with infected individuals, clothing, bedding, or furniture. The commonly affected parts are the finger webs, the palm, wrist, front of the arm, the soles, areas around the nipples, and the groin and inner upper legs causing severe itching (pruritus), specially at night. A person suffering from itching in these areas and not suffering from allergy or pruritus (severe itching of the skin) can be suspected of scabies. This infection may cause small papules and there may be a rash.

The incubation period for the mite is long – about a month – and it can easily be transferred by normal social contact among a group of people living together.

## Treatment and Drugs

All members of the house, whether afflicted or not, should be treated. The clothes, linen, towels, and so on, should be thoroughly washed and ironed.

**Permethrin** (PERLIFE, PERMITE, SCABNIL 5% lotion)

A 5% cream or lotion is considered to be highly effective and safe. It has to be applied once only and if need be repeated after one week. It can be used in children also. It kills lice also. Its toxicity is low and achieves a complete cure usually.

**Gamma Benzene Hexachloride** (EMSCAB, GAMMADERM, GAB, LOREXANE, SCABEX, SCARAB)

It is also called *lindane* and is effective against scabies and lice infestation. In adults single application of its 1% lotion or 2% cream may be necessary to provide a complete cure. If needed it may be repeated after one week.

***Adverse Effects:*** It is an irritant to the eyes and mucosa. It may cause skin irritation if used excessively or for a prolonged period. Such overuse may cause the adverse effect of irritating the brain. Convulsions may occur in rare cases due to its excessive use, as it may be absorbed.

***Precautions:***

1. Do not apply it on the eyes and cuts on the skin as it may cause irritation.
2. Do not apply it repeatedly without consulting a doctor.
3. If skin irritation occurs, which may be due to an allergy, wash it off and don't apply again.
4. Do not apply more than 3 g of the lotion or cream at a time.
5. Wash the body thoroughly after an overnight (8 to 12 hours) application.
6. Avoid its use during pregnancy and in infants. Similarly, if skin is broken due to scratches or ulcers do not apply.

**Crotamiton** (CROTORAX)

It is less effective than *gamma benzene hexachloride (2nd choice)* as it has to be applied for 2 to 4 nights. Its irritant effect is, however, less than *gamma benzene hexachloride*. It is available as 10% cream and lotion. It reduces itching. It is preferred in children.

**Benzyl Benzoate** (SCABALCID, SCABINDON 25%lotion)

Its irritant effect on the skin is more than that of *gamma benzene hexachloride* and may cause a burning or stinging sensation on the area of application. It is applied for 2 days. Itching may continue for a few days. Now a days it is used in difficult cases only.

**Sulphur Ointment**

This is messy, has a bad odour, and stains clothes, but is a very safe and inexpensive remedy. It is preferred in infants, young children, and pregnant women. A 5% sulfur cream (PERSOL FORTE) contains benzoyl peroxide 10%.

**Ivermectin** (IVERMECTOL, SCABITIN, SCABICARE 3 mg, 6 mg tab):

It is the only drug used orally in scabies and lice infestation. Its dose is 0.2 mg/kg (usually 6 mg) once only. Cure rate is very high. It is also available with *albendazole* 100 mg(VERMIN-A, BENDY-Plus) for the single dose therapy of multiple infestations due to worms and scabies.

Some patients have persistent itching and paules after the treatment. This is due to an allegic response to infection and requires local steroid cream (*Clobetasone*-LOBATE or *Triamcinolone acetonide*-KENACORT) for a few days.

## Lice Infestation

This is also called pediculosis as it is caused by common lice – *pediculus capitis* (head louse). Although lice infestation is not injurious to health, it is very annoying due to the itching sensation caused by it. Excessive scratching and excoriation may lead to secondary bacterial infection. The itching is caused by the saliva of the parasite deposited on the skin. If eye lashes are involved, plain vaseline is applied twice a day for about a week and plucking of nits done thereafter.

## Treatment and Drugs

*Permethrin* 1% (MEDILICE lotion) is applied to the scalp and hair with massage and left for 10 minutes before a rinse. Avoid eye contact

### Gamma Benzene Hexachloride (EMSCAB, GAMMADERM, BAG, LOREXANE, SCABEX, SCARAB)

This is described earlier in the chapter. It should be left over the scalp and hair for about 12-24 hours before washing them.. It may be repeated after 7 days only.

*Ivermectin* in the doses stated above is also useful oral drug for lice of body and head.

### Malathion

A 1% lotion is very effective and takes 8 to 12 hours time to kill the lice. However, it has been banned in the USA due to their slow action and toxicity to nerves It is inflammable also. The room should be well ventilated lest vapours may be inhaled.

## Acne (Pimples)

Acne or pimples is a very distressing skin disorder which affects adolescents and young people. As a rule, it is often genetically predisposed. It regresses with time but in some people it may become very severe, disfiguring the face and leaving a permanent scars. It is caused due to an increased sensitivity to the male sex hormones – androgenic steroids. The cells of the hair follicle, which are extremely cohesive, grow faster. The sebum (secretion from the glands of the skin) production increases; which plugs the tubes. This causes growth of *acne bacilli* which form an enzyme (lipase) causing an increase in free fatty acids which are irritant to the skin and cause inflammation. The face, neck, chest, shoulders, and back are most commonly involved. Mild acne is characterized by an oily or greasy skin with closed or open, small sized papules (comedones); in moderate acne, papules or pustules are accompanied by inflammation. In severe form, nodules with inflammatory cysts are formed which leave a scar. Pus-discharging abscesses are rare.

## Types of Treatment

### Non-Drug Therapy

Avoid drugs like *corticosteroids, androgens, iodides, bromides,* and *androgenic progestins* found in some oral contraceptives. If you have to take an oral contraceptive, do not go for the mini pill. Select the one which has a higher ratio of estrogen to progestins. This minimizes the androgenic effect of progestins. Avoid humid environments, occlusive cosmetic oils, and greases.

Diet does not seem to play any role in acne. Minimize the oiliness by washing the area 2 to 3 times daily. Scrubbing with abrasive substances is not advisable as it may damage the delicate opening of the hair follicles through which the sebum flows. Mild soaps are enough. Education of not manipulating comedons due to irritation is a must. This leaves scars causing disfiguration. You should know that at least 4 to 6 weeks time is needed for improvement to occur. Lesions over shoulders, chest and back take longer time than this.

### Drugs

Various measures like reducing the sebum output, action on the follicles, action on *Propionobacterium acnes*, control of infection, are tried. Most of the preparations contain *sulphur*, *resorcinol*, *salicylic acid* or *benzoyl peroxide* alone or in combination, but they do not have any response on acne. The treatment requires regular use of effective medicines under the instructions of a physician.

### Mild Acne

Liquid cleansers, lotions, and creams containing abrasive particles for removing surface debris, for e.g., *aluminium oxide, sodium tetraborate, polyethylene*; drying agents such as *alcohol* or *acetone*; or peeling agents like *sulphur, resorcinol, benzoyl peroxide*, and *salicylic acid* are used for mild acne. Hot compresses may be as effective as some of the agents mentioned above.

## Treatment

### Comedonol Acne

*Tretinoin* (RETINO-A, EUDENA 0.025%-0.05%) very small amount (pea size) of this drug can be applied two times in a week initially at night (to avoid irritation). Then gradually it can be applied every night. Let it be there for about 20 minutes. Then the face can be washed. *Tretinoin* is a vitamin-A derivative and prevents plugging of follicles. Usually it is used for 3 to 4 months.

***Adverse Effects and Precautions:*** It is an irritant drug and should be applied as per instructions. The skin becomes red within 48 hours and begins to peel. It should be applied once at night and the sun should be avoided to reduce irritation. It should not be applied on any part of the skin having eczema. Minimize application on areas near the corners of the mouth, nose, and eyes.

**Benzoyl Peroxide** (PERNOX gel 2.5%, PERSOL FORTE 10%, BENZAC-CC)

It is a water based (without alcohol) formulation so irritation is less. It causes peeling of unwanted skin cells and kills harmful bacteria.

***Adverse Effects and Precautions:*** Due to its peeling effect on the skin, this drug causes local irritation. If it is severe, the dose and frequency of use may be reduced. It is applied for 15 minutes on the first evening. The duration of application is increased by 15 minutes every day until it is tolerated for 2 hours. It may, thereafter, be left on overnight. Allergy may occur with this drug. The chances of allergy may increase if it is applied under occlusive dressings or patches.

### Comedo Extraction

Open comedones (with a black heads) and close ones may be extracted with Comedo extractor by an experienced skin specialist. Recurrence occurs often.

### Acne with Papules and Pustules

Antibiotics are the main form of treatment. There can be given orally or applied locally as lotions.

**For mild acne** local antibiotics are sufficient.

- *Erythromycin* (ACNESOL, ACNEDERM, ERYTOP-LOTION 2%, 3% gel 4%)
- *Clindamycin* (CLINDY 1%)
- *Metronidazole* (METRODERM)
- *Lincomycin* (LYNX gel 2%)
- *Nadifloxacin* (NADIBACT-1% cream)

These can be applied two times a day, *Benzoyl peroxide* may be used alongwith any of the preparations but only in the morning. If required, *Tretinoin* 0.025% may be applied at night.

### Moderate Acne

*Tetracycline* caps (TERRAMYCIN) 500 mg twice a day, *Erythromycin* (ERYTHROCIN) 500 mg twice a day, *Doxycycline* cap (MICRODOX) 100 mg once/twice a day or *minocycline* 50 to 100 mg twice a day are equally effective and are used for about a week. If required topical antibiotics may be used. Some times *spironolactone* (ALDACTONE) 50 to 100mg/day doses act as useful supplementary drug. It acts by opposing androgen effects. Local injections of dilute solutions of *Triamcinolone* (2.5mg/ml) are used by some skin specialists into the papules and small cysts. *Adapalene* (ADAPEN, ACLENE 0.1% gel) is a milder form of vitamin-A derivative used in mild to moderate acne. *Clindamycin* with adapalene (DERIVA-C ) is also available. *Adapalene* is less irritating and has anti-inflammatory effects also.

### Severe Acne

*Isotretinoin* (ISOTROIN, IRET 10mg, 20 mg cap) is a vitamin-A type of drug useful in severe cystic (cavities) acne. It is a potent agent and may cause malformations in new born when taken by pregnant women. Hence an informed consent is to be given by woman of child bearing age. It is given in a dose of 0.5-1 mg/kg in a day for 20 weeks.

***Adverse Effects:*** Increased blood sugar, fats, depression, headache, dry lips, nose-bleed and bone pains are noted. Obviously, it is taken only under regular medical supervision.

### Other Drugs

*Azelaic* acid 10% cream (AZIDERM), *Glycolic* acid 10% (GLYAHA LOTION) are also helpful. AZIDERM reduces grease forming bacteria over skin and decreases melasma and dark circles) also. Tea-tree extract, *Aloe vera* and *allantoin* as cream base are incorporated in a number of OTC cosmetics and soaps. These agents have marginal efficacy only.

One may consider laser dermabrasion by an experienced dermatologist.

### Drugs Aggravating Pimples

If you are suffering from pimples, watch out for drugs like *corticosteroids*, the male sex hormone – *androgen, progestogens, isoniazid, iodides, bromides, phenobarbitone,* and *phenytoin* in any of the preparations you are taking. These aggravate pimples.

## Fungal Infections

Chaya, a young lady, consulted a gynaecologist for a infection in the groin. A corticosteroid ointment (BETNOVATE) was prescribed. She did not get any significant relief and returned to hospital after a week. She was asked to continue the same treatment. However, to her good luck, she met a skin specialist who listened to her carefully and collected a scraping from the affected area for microscopic examination. He confirmed the diagnosis as fungal infection (candida) and prescribed the proper medicine which cured her. Very often we buy an ointment or use one lying at home for skin infection. It would be wiser to consult a skin specialist rather than trying self-medication. Common fungal infections and their treatment are described below :

### Ringworm

Fungal infection, ringworm, and moniliasis, technically called dermatophytosis, may involve any part of the body. In the head it spreads through the barber's instruments, hair brushes, and combs, causing a patchy hair loss. The patient may smell a peculiar odour called a 'mousy' odour. In the skin it starts as a papule which spreads around leaving a central coin-shaped clear area. Another characteristic feature of these fungal infections is an itching sensation.

**Griseofulvin** (GIRFUNGIN-P, GRISOVIN-FP, WALAVIN-FP)

This drug is used for treating ringworm infection. It is available as tablets of 125 mg. The total daily dose is 500 mg. The effect starts slowly and if toes and nails are involved, it takes a few months before significant benefits are seen.

***Adverse Effects:*** It is a relatively safe drug. Some patients may complain of headache and gastric upsets. It is also known to cause photosensitivity reactions (allergy to sunlight).

***Precautions:***

1. Always take this drug with a fatty meal to allow maximum absorption.
2. If you develop photosensitivity, consult the doctor.
3. Avoid alcohol use, as it may cause palpitation and flushing.

**Ketoconazole** (KETOZOLE, PHYTORAL, NIZRAL), **Fluconazole** (SYSCAN)

These have been introduced recently for treatment of fungal disorders. Their spectrum of action is wider, that is, these are effective in rignworm, candida, and other fungal infections. The duration of treatment is short, varying from a few days to weeks.

**Miconazole** (DARKTARIN, ZOLE), **Clotrimazole** (MYCOCID)

These preparations are applied locally in the form of a lotion or ointment and are very effective in controlling most fungal infections. (See Chapters – Antibiotics and Common gynaecological disorders).

**Itraconazole** (ITASPOR,CANDITRAL-100 mg cap)
It is a newer antifungal which has less side effects. (No suppression of steroid formation as done by *ketoconazole*). **Voriconazole** is also likely to be marketed soon.

**Terbinafine** (EXIFINE, TERBEST 250 mgTab): usually given as a single tab daily.

### Duration of Treatment with Oral Antifungal Drugs

It is important. For infection of body skin(ringworm or tinea corporis) usually 3 to 6 week treatment is needed with *griseofulvin, fluconazole* or *ketoconazole*. For ring worm of foot and hard skin 4 to 6week treatment is required, whereas if nails are involved the treatment nust be taken for about a year. *Fluconazole* is usually given once a week.

### Drugs for Dandruff and Seborrhea (excessive sebum formation causing itching and dermatitis)

Dandruff is a common annoying malady of scalp, forehead and upper body surface. It is caused by a yeast called as P. ovale. It requires proper hygiene and care that the infection is eradicated. The drugs used are:

**Ketoconazole** shampoo (KETOZOLE, FUNGIZOLE, KETOVATE 2%), soap (KEYNET) or ointment (PHYTORAL 2%) to be applied once or twice a week over head hair.

**Selenium Sulfide** (SELDAN,SELSUN, 2.5% lotion or shampoo) may also be used. SELDRUFF Plus also contains *Clotrimazole* 1%.

**Zinc Pyrithione** is used as 1% shampoo. It is found in many formulations along with *ketoconazole* 2% (DANCURE, FUNGICIDE, SCALPE NUFORCE Shampoos). DANDRID contains *miconazole* (2%), *tinidazole* (2%) and *zinc sulphate* (2%).

# 33

# Drugs Used in Tuberculosis

There are about 8.8 million cases of tuberculosis (TB) worldwide, more than 40% of these cases are in South East Asia; India has 53.3% of South East Asian burden. About 3 to 5% of cases have Multidrug resistant (MDR)TB. Unless treated, each infectious case can transmit disease to 10 to 15 persons in a year. Globally, one person is infected with tubercular bacilli every second. In India 6 lacs are unaware that they suffer from TB and two persons die in every 3 minutes due to TB. The only treatment available in past, was rest and a protein rich diet, and when possible, the patient was sent to a sanatorium for a change of environment. He would go to any corner of the country to consult the most qualified physicians, the crudest quacks, or priests with assumed healing powers, and was receptive to any available advice. Today, the prospects of a tuberculosis patient have changed entirely. It is no longer considered a dreaded disease but one which can be effectively controlled and cured by drugs.

Tuberculosis, a tissue-destroying (necrotizing) infection, is caused by inhalation of the tubercle bacilli (*Mycobacterium tuberculosis*). The lungs are most commonly affected, but it may spread to the kidneys, bowels, bones, lymph nodes, meninges, or any other part of the body. This infection may cause clinical disease either 1) shortly after inoculation, sometimes called 'primary' tuberculosis; or 2) after months or decades of dormancy which is erroneously referred to as 'reinfection' tuberculosis. Active tuberculosis is potentially fatal and may be transmitted to susceptible individuals. About one-third of the cases are discovered when the patient comes with a low grade fever; another one-third with unrelated complaints; and the remaining are those undergoing routine medical examination. In some cases of HIV infected persons, tuberculosis occurs in the rapidly progressive form poses problems in treatment.

## Diagnosis

A tuberculosis patient may not know about his illness for some time as the symptoms like fever, night sweating, cough, and headache appear slowly and are mild in nature. Sometimes, blood in the sputum (*hemoptysis*), pain in the chest or abdomen and weight loss. The diagnosis is made by a positive tuberculin skin test (Mantoux test), sputum examination for *tubercle bacilli* (acid fast bacilli-the surest test), high ESR (blood test), and X-ray of the lungs and rapid RNA or DNA tests. RNA test is a sensitive test that detects RNA/DNA sequence of TB causing pathogens and is done as polymerase chain reaction (PCR) technique.

## Treatment

The treatment of tuberculosis consists of preventive therapy and curative therapy.

### Preventive Therapy

Preventive therapy of tuberculosis has two major goals: 1) to prevent infection in an individual with a negative tuberculin test but who has had intimate contact with an active case; 2) to prevent active disease in an individual who is infected but does not have any symptoms (significant reaction to tuberculin test but chest X-ray is negative).

In children who come in contact with tuberculosis patients, tuberculin testing should be performed. If the test is negative, BCG vaccination should be given. However, if the test is positive, a chest X-ray is essential. If this is abnormal, a diagnosis of primary tuberculosis is likely and conventional anti-tuberculosis treatment should be given. If the chest X-ray is normal, then *chemoprophylaxis* with *isoniazid* 5 to 10 mg/kg daily for 6 to 12 months is recommended.

Patients receiving corticosteroids or immuno-suppressive treatment, or who develop diabetes, HIV or malignancy should be examined for an old 'inactive' tuberculosis lesion through an X-ray and sputum examination as it may become active in them.

### Curative Therapy

A significant advancement in the treatment of tuberculosis has taken place in recent years. The development of resistance to drugs is prevented by using two or more drugs. The long duration of treatment (1 to 2 years) has been shortened by the introduction of short course chemotherapy. The problem of poor compliance to drugs is minimized by the introduction of intermittent supervised therapy called DOTS (Directly Observed Treatment Short Course) under revised National Tuberculosis Control Programme.

**Short Course Chemotherapy:** A 6 to 9 month regimen consisting of *isoniazid, rifampicin, ethambutol,* and *pyrazinamide* daily for 2 to 3 months, followed by *isoniazid* and *rifampicin* daily for 4 to 6 months, has been found to be satisfactory, provided it is fully supervised. The patient's disease is catagorized depending on the extent of disease (Table-1). The treatment is carried out in two phases. In the initial phase four drugs are to be taken daily or 3 times weekly for 2 months. Then sputum examination is done. If it is positive for TB organisms, drugs are to be taken for one more month. In the second phase or the continuation phase, two or three drugs are to be taken for 6 to 8 months. The details of regimen used are given in the Tables-1 and 2.

**Doses of Drugs for treatment** (Doses mg/kg body weight)

| Alternate Day | Daily |
|---|---|
| H - 10 mg/kg | H - 5 mg/kg |
| R - 10 mg/kg | R - 10 mg/kg |
| Z - 35 mg/kg | Z - 25 mg/kg |
| E - 30 mg/kg | E - 15 mg/kg |
| S - 15 mg/kg | S - 15 mg/kg |

Note: H = Isonizaid, R = Rifampicin, Z = Pyrazinamide, E = Ethambutol, S = Streptomycin

**Treatment of Tuberculosis followed in our Country under Revised National Tuberculosis Control Programme RNTCP (DOTS)**

| *Category* | *Initial Phase* | *Continuation Phase* | *Total Course (in months)* |
|---|---|---|---|
| I | 2 $H_3 R_3 Z_3 E_3$ | 4 $H_3 R_3$ | 6 |
| II | 2 $H_3 R_3 Z_3 E_3 S_3$ + 1 $H_3 R_3 Z_3 E_3$ | 5 $H_3 R_3 Z_3$ | 8 |
| III | 2 $H_3 R_3 Z_3$ | 4 $H_3 R_3$ | 6 |

*Note:* Digits before letters denote months. Digits below letters denote number of doses per week.

## Drugs

The drugs used in the treatment of tuberculosis can be divided into first and second line drugs. Foods such as meat, milk, cereals, legumes, and yeast are rich in vitamin $B_6$. A diet containing these may help in preventing peripheral neuritis.

## First Line Drugs

### Isoniazid (ISONEX)

*Isoniazid* is a first line drug. It is a bactericidal drug and kills both extra cellular and intracellular bacteria. It interferes with the cell wall (mycolic acid) synthesis of the bacteria. It may be administered alone for prophylaxis or in combination with other drugs for chemotherapy of disease. It is almost always required for combination treatment as in DOTS.

***Adverse Effects:*** It increases excretion of vitamin $B_6$ (*pyridoxine*) which may result in numbness pain, tiredness, weakness, pain in the muscles and joints. Patients suffering from diabetes mellitus, malnutrition, or alcoholism should be given 10 mg *pyridoxine* routinely. If there are pre-existing symptoms of peripheral neuritis, a larger dose of *pyridoxine* of 50 to 100 mg may be given daily. Other adverse effects are liver damage, mental disturbance and rarely fits. Liver damage is not common in children but may occur in elderly and alcoholics.

***Precautions:***

1. Get a liver function test (*serum transaminase*) done after a month or two of the treatment. If the *serum transaminase* exceeds 3 times the normal value, the drug should be stopped.
2. A *pyridoxine* supplement is necessary in pregnant women, nursing mothers, and infants as this drug is secreted in milk.
3. The doctor should be consulted if any adverse effects like, allergic reactions, arthritis, or difficulty in vision occur.
5. The drug should be taken regularly as advised by the doctor. Inadequate doses or missing the drug in between causes resistance.
6. Usually, the drug should be taken on empty stomach but if nausea occurs, take it with meals, dividing the dose into two halves, that is, half in the morning and half in the evening.

### Rifampicin (RIMACTANE, RIFAMPIN, RIFA)

It is an antibiotic which kills the bacteria (bactericidal effect). It attacks the nucleus of the bacterial cell (causing disappearance of its ribosome). Bacterial resistance to *rifampicin* can be reduced by combining it with *isoniazid* or other drugs as described hereafter. It increases the activity of oxidizing enzymes of the liver and thus can reduce the effect of various drugs metabolized by these enzymes. It is always included in short course chemotherapy of tuberculosis.

***Adverse Effects:*** Its adverse effects are mild and include abdominal distress and cramps, muscle-aches and cramps in the legs during the first few weeks of therapy. Liver damage (hepatitis) is a dose related adverse effect and is more likely to occur if the liver function is already impaired or when *rifampicin* is combined with *isoniazid* or other drugs which are toxic to the liver. Elevation of the liver enzyme (SGPT/ALT; more than 100 units/ml) occurs in about 4% of the patients treated with *rifampicin* in combination with *isoniazid*, but jaundice is not observed commonly.

Other adverse effects include itching rash (3% incidence), allergic reaction with a flu-like syndrome, and rarely shocks and kidney damage. These are more common when a high dose (900 to 1200 mg) is used intermittently.

*Rifampicin* and its metabolite impart a reddish orange colour to the urine, faeces, saliva, sweat, and tears. However, this is of no consequence but you should know it lest you are alarmed!

***Precautions:***

1. Food reduces absorption of *rifampicin,* therefore always take it on empty stomach, early in the morning.
2. If yellow discolouration of eyes, nails, or skin occurs, inform the doctor.
3. If other drugs like *digoxin, corticosteroids, oral anti-diabetics, quinidine, ketoconazole, dapsone, disopyramide* and *warfarin,* are being taken, consult the doctor for increasing their doses as *rifampicin* increases their metabolism.
4. Urine, stool, saliva, sweat, and tears may become reddish orange. Do not worry about this.
5. Women who are taking oral contraceptives (OCs) may become pregnant if *rifampicin* is also taken. This is because it increases inactivation of OCs so they become less effective! Therefore, they should use alternative contraceptive method!

### Pyrazinamide (PZA, PYRALDINA, PYZINA)

It has become a first line drug in recent years, specially for short course chemotherapy of tuberculosis. It kills (bactericidal) the intracellular tubercle bacilli. Its use with other drugs reduces relapses significantly.

***Adverse Effects:*** It causes dose related hepatotoxicity (liver damage). But this is seen less commonly in our country. The currently used smaller dose of this drug (25 mg/kg daily) rarely causes hepatotoxicity, especially when used for a short period of 2 months. It causes an increase in the uric acid in the blood (hyperuricemia) and may cause gouty joints pains. Sometime the diabetes becomes worse on its use. Skin rash and fever may also occur.Avoid its use during pregnancy and lactation.

### **Ethambutol** (MYAMBUTOL, COMBUTOL, THEMIBUTOL)

*It is a slow acting drug, never used alone.* It is used as an adjunct *isoniazid* and *rifampicin.* Its less frequent adverse effects and good patient acceptance has led to its replacing *aminosalicylic acid* (described later) and is considered to be a substitute for injected *streptomycin.* It prevents development of resistance during treatment.

***Adverse Effects:*** *Ethambutol* causes a dose-related toxic effect on the eyes. After an initial dose of 25 mg/kg daily for 2 months, followed by 15 mg/kg daily for several months, there may be diminution of vision or loss of colour perception in about 1% cases. This adverse effect reverses within a few months of stopping the drug. Other adverse effects include numbness or decreased sensation in the legs, headache, confusion, and increased uric acid levels. Since children (below 6 years) can not report exactly the changes in visual acuity, *ethambutol* is not used for childhood tuberculosis. One should get a complete examination of the eyes done before starting this drug. Do not use if there is optic nerve damage.

### Streptomycin

This was the first drug introduced for the treatment of tuberculosis. It must be given by injection, as it is not absorbed through the intestines. This limits its long-term use.

***Adverse Effects:*** It may cause a derangement of labyrinthine function (organ is for maintaining posture) so postural instability and hearing loss may occur when given in high doses during decreased kidney function or in older patients.

## Second Line Drugs
## (Drugs to be used in Multi Drug Resistant cases)

The safety and efficacy of these drugs are less than first line drugs. They are more expensive and are required in more numbers for treatment of multi drug resistant cases. A brief account is given here :

**Second Line Drugs**

| *Drugs/Brand Names* | *Dose* | *Serious Adverse Effects* | *Precautions* |
|---|---|---|---|
| *Thiacetazone* | 150 mg once a day | Anaemia, Liver damage, Exfoliation of skin, Mouth ulcers | Not to be used in HIV patients<br>Sore throat can be the first sign of bone marrow depression. |
| *Para-aminosalicylate* (PAS-Granules) | 10 to 12 gm in divided doses daily | Loss of appetite, Epigastsic pain Goitre, Fall in blood cell counts | Use with milk |
| *Ethionamide* (MYOBID) | 500 to 750 mg in a day | Liver damage<br>Peripheral neuritis Impotence<br>Mental disturbance | Avoid in psychosis, Diabetics |
| *Cycloserine* (CYCLORINE) | 250 mg twice a day | CNS-toxicity tremor, fits | Short shelf life,do not store |
| *Kanamycin, Amikacin* | 0.75 to 1.0 gm | Ear and kidney toxicity | Avoid in epilepsy and kidney disease |
| *Capreomycin* (CAPOCIN) | Intramuscularly 1g/day | Vertigo, fall in white blood cell count | Avoid in ear/kidney disease. Regularly check liver functions. |

**Newer drugs:** Ciprofloxacin, ofloxacin, sparfloxacin, levofloxacin
These antibacterial drugs have shown good activity against tubercular microbes and at present are used in multidrug resistant [MDR] cases. At present *Moxifloxacin* is being tested in a large number of cases in India.

**Clarithromycin, Azithromycin:** These drugs have been used in a typical mycobacterial infections (affecting lungs and skin) particularly in patients with HIV infection. *Rifabutin* is another drug used in atypical infections.

**Fixed Dose Combinations of Antitubercular Drugs:**

Nowadays FDCs and combikits (containing 2 to 4 tablets in a convenient "daily use strip" are available and increasingly used and some of these are also approved by the WHO. A major advantage is that these simplify use of drugs by patients and rationalize the supply. Following FDCs are available:

| *FDC** | *Form* | *Composition (mg)* | *Dose for adult (wt. 55-70 kg.)* |
|---|---|---|---|
| RHZE | Tablet | *Rifampicin* 150 + *Isoniazid* 75 + *Pyrazinamide* 400 + *Ethambutol* 275 Ethambutol 275 | 4 tablets a day on empty stomach |
| RHZ | Tablet | R-150 + H-75 + Z-400 | 4 tablets a day on empty stomach |
| RHZ | Paediatric tab | R-60 + H-30 + Z-150 | Child (wt 20-24 kg.) 4 tablets |
| RH | Tablet | R-300 + H-150 | 2 Tablets |
| RH | Tablet | R-150 + H-75 | 4 Tablets |
| RH | Paediatric tablet | R-60 + H-30 | Child (20-24 kg.) 4 tablets |
| EH | Tablet | H-150 + E-400 | 3 tablets |

There are large number of formulations (single tablet or combi-pack) available for adults and children. The users are urged to see the contents of the formulation and not change it during treatment.

With the use of drugs, tuberculosis can be controlled very effectively and patient is cured provided regular treatment is taken without break and full course is completed. It is generally observed that almost all patients take treatment regularly for initial 2 to 3 months, however, as they improve, they start ignoring regularity and miss quite a number of doses. It is at this point of time that care is taken to continue treatment even when the person is without symptoms. Supervised treatment as DOTS therapy is available at large number of urban and rural health facilities free of cost.

# 34

# Drugs Used in Worm Infestations

••••••

Over a billion people carry one or other type of parasite in their intestines. Currently this constitutes one of the major public health problems. In tropical countries like India, intestinal infection is largely due to impure water supply and unhealthy environmental factors. Infestation with worms is one of the important cause of anaemia and growth retardation in children. They produce toxins and injure the bowels. Some may migrate to other tissues and obstruct lymph vessels. So worm infestations must be treated. There are a number of worms which infect man, but in this chapter, we shall deal only with those which are more common in India. The drugs used for the treatment of worm infestations are given later in the table, along with their dosage, adverse effects, and precautions.

## Roundworms

*Ascaris lumbricoides* (roundworm) is the commonest worm affecting man. Roundworm disease spreads through handling of contaminated food or soil. In villages or in areas with poor sanitation, children defecate in the area around their homes. In dry climate, the eggs of the *Ascaris* get airborne and are ingested through the mouth. The eggs complete their life cycle in man (partly in the lung and partly in the gut) and lodged in the gut as full adult worms. The disease is prevalent in areas where vegetables are grown on soil fertilized by human excreta. Adult worms may cause no symptoms in light infestation, but severe infestation may lead to abdominal pain, skin rashes, broncho-pneumonia, and even cause obstruction of the intestines. The diagnosis is usually made when ova are found in the stool during a routine examination, or when an adult worm is vomited or passed out in the stools. The adult worm is cylindrical in shape, brown or pinkish brown in colour, 15 to 50 cm in length and 3 to 5 mm in diameter.

### Preventive Measures

1. Children should be trained to use latrines rather than defaecating in the fields. They should not play in dirt and filthy areas.
2. Good sanitation must be observed. The Indian habit of washing hands before eating is extremely useful. This practice should be observed religiously.
3. Wash fruits and vegetables before eating them.

**Drug Treatment:** *Mebendazole, albendazole* or *pyrentel* is the first choice. *Piperazine* or *Levamisole* can also be used. (see table on next page).

## Hookworm

In India, hookworm disease is mainly caused by *Ancylostoma duodenale* and *Necator amaricanus* (hookworm). The ovum (egg) of the parasite grows into larva (baby parasite) in the soil, and usually penetrates the skin of those who walk barefoot. From the skin, the larva reaches the intestines through the blood and there it grows into an adult worm. The female worm lays eggs in the intestines which are excreted in the faeces.

Infected patients may suffer from localized itching or skin rash when the larva enters through the skin. The most serious manifestation produced by the hookworm is anaemia which is due to the sucking of blood by the worm and ulcerations in the intestines. The anaemia may be severe if the infection is heavy and the diet is poor in iron. In children and menstruating woman, it may cause weakness, breathlessness, palpitation, constipation, and headache. The diagnosis is confirmed by examination of the stools for the presence of ova of the worm (see table overleaf for details on drugs).

**Preventive Measures:** The entrance of the worm into the body can be prevented by wearing shoes to avoid direct contact of the skin with the soil.

**Diet:** A diet rich in protein and iron should be taken regularly. The foods most suitable for patients of anaemia caused by hookworm are cereals, spinach, cauliflower, radish, beans, tomato, orange, prune, apricot, almond, walnut, pistachio nut, milk, egg, meat (liver, kidney and heart), fish and poultry.

**Drugs:** *Pyrentel, mebendazole or albendazole* is the first choice. *Levamisole* may be used. (see table)

## Pinworm

Pinworm disease is caused by *Enterobius vermicularis* (pinworm). The eggs of this worm are ingested through contaminated food or drinks. Their life cycle is completed in the gastro-intestinal tract and the fertilized female lays eggs around the anus at night when the patient goes to bed. The movements of the worm in the process of laying eggs, cause intense itching and the patient scratches the affected part. Thus he is reinfested by the direct transfer of eggs by contaminated fingers from the anus to the mouth. This cycle is repeated many times. Children are the usual victims and spread the disease in the family. It is characterized by itching around anus, specially at night. The diagnosis is usually made by stool examination or when the adult worm (0.8 to 1.2 cm in length and 0.3 to 3.5 mm thick, white in colour) is discovered by the patient or by the parents in the case of a child.

**Preventive Measures:** The following preventive measure should be adopted:

1. Fingernails should be regularly trimmed.
2. Underwear should be washed and dried in the sunlight or ironed every day.
3. To control the infection all members of the family should be examined and treated.
4. Hand-washing before meals is a must.

**Drugs Commonly Used**

| *Worm* | *Drugs* | *Dose* |
|---|---|---|
| Roundworm<br>*(Ascaris lumbricoides)* | *Mebendazole*<br>(MEBENDAZOLE, MEBEX, WORMIN) | 100 mg, morning and evening for 3 days; children same dose |
| | *Albendazole*<br>(NOWORM, ALMINTH, ZENTEL) | 400 mg, single dose for adults and children over 2 years |
| | *Pyrantel pamoate*<br>(NEMOCID, EXPENT) | Single oral dose of 11 mg per kg body weight (maximum 1g). |
| | *Piperazine citrate*<br>(ANTEPAR) | 4 g per day, after breakfast, for two successive days. Children — half the adult dose. |
| | *Tetramisole* (LEVAMISOLE)<br>(DEWORMIS) | Single dose of 150 mg; half the adult dose for children. |
| Hookworm<br>*(Ancylostoma duodenale and Necator americanus)* | Pyrantel pamoate<br>(NEMOCID)<br>(equally effective) | As above. |
| | Mebendazole<br>(MEBENDAZOLE, MEBEX, WORMIN) | As above. |
| | Albendazole<br>(NOWORM, ALMINTH, ZENTEL) | As above. |
| Pinworm<br>*(Enterobius vermicularis)* | *Pyrantel pamoate*<br>(NEMOCID, EXPENT) | As above. |
| | *Mebendazole*<br>(MEBENDAZOLE, MEBEX, WORMIN) | 100 mg once only; second dose is repeated after 2 weeks. |
| | *Albendazole*<br>(NOWORM, ALMINTH, ZENTEL) | As above. |
| | *Piperazine citrate*<br>(ANTEPAR) | 65 mg per kg of body weight (maximum 2 g) for 7 days. |
| Whipworm<br>*(Tricharis trichura)* | Mebendazole<br>(MEBENDAZOLE, MEBEX WORMIN) | As above. |
| Filaria<br>*(Wuchereria bancrofti)* | *Diethyl carbamazine*<br>(HETRAZAN) | 2 mg/kg thrice a day (50-100 mg thrice a day) adult for 2-3 weeks |
| | *Ivermectin*<br>(IVERMECTOL) | Single dose of 10-15 mg for adults. Repeat after a year for 5 years |
| Guinea worm<br>*(Dracunculus medinensis)* | *Metronidazole* | 200-400 mg three times a day for 7 days |
| Tape worm<br>*(Taenia solium & Taenia saginata)* | *Praziquentel*<br>(CYSTICIDE) | Single dose of 10 mg/kg |
| | *Albendozole* | As above. |
| | *Praziquentel*<br>(CYSTICIDE) | 50 mg/day in 3 divided doses for 15 days |

**Against Intestinal Worms**

| *Adverse Effects* | *Precautions* |
|---|---|
| It may cause abdominal pain and allergic reactions. | It should not ge given in pregnancy and to children below two years. |
| Mild abdominal discomfort and dizziness | — |
| It may cause abdominal discomfort, headache, and dizziness. | 1. Avoid its use during pregnancy and in children below one year. 2. Do not use *piperazine pyrantel pamoate* together. |
| It may cause abdominal discomfort, allergic reactions, headache, vertigo, tremors, and visual disturbances. | 1. To be avoided in patients of epilepsy. 2. If abdominal pain or diarrhoea is severe, use anti-spasmodic drugs. |
| It may cause mild abdominal discomfort, nausea, vomiting, vertigo, headache, and sleeplessness. | Take after a light meal reduce adverse effects. |
| As above. | As above. |
| As above. | As above. |
| As above. | As above. |
| As above. | As above. |
| As above. | As above. |
| As above. | As above. |
| As above. | As above. |
| As above. | As above. |
| Nausea, vomiting, loss of appetite, dizziness, fever and fall in BP | Some patients may require antihistaminics or steroids for the treatment of adverse effects |
| Itching, dizziness, constipation, abdominal pain | — Should be taken on empty stomach. |
| Nausea, metallic taste headache, dizziness | Avoid alcohol with it. |
| Bitter taste, nausea, dizziness, sedation | Never use in ocular cysticercosis |
| As above. | As above. |
| As above. | As above. |

# 35

# Antibiotics and Antifungal Drugs

Most of us have found it necessary to take antibiotics at some time or other. It is estimated that about one-fourth of prescriptions contains these drugs. Antibiotics are commonly employed in ailments like diarrhoea, respiratory and urinary track infections, and non-specific fevers.

Sulphonamides, the first antibacterials were discovered by Domagk, a German scientist, who was awarded the Nobel Prize for medicine in 1939. Hitler's Nazi regime did not permit Domagk to receive the prize and he had to wait until the downfall of the Nazis to receive this prestigious award, but never received the prize money.

Since then, several antibiotics have been discovered and these are one of the commonest drugs used in many of the developing and developed countries.

**Should Antibiotics Be Used to Prevent Diseases?** Antibiotics are not only useful in an established condition of infection but are also effective as prophylactic agents in a variety of situations. The prophylactic use of antibiotics is advocated to reduce the risk of infection in patients who are more susceptible to infections due to decreased resistance; and to avoid the infection after accidents, injury, dental or general surgery. Penicillin-G is very important to prevent recurrence of rheumatic heart disease. They are also used to prevent infection after delivery, instrumentation (a catheter — rubber tube — inserted into urine-passage) and sexual contact with professional sex workers.

## Problems of Antibiotic Therapy

**Selection of Antibiotics:** Antibiotics are developed for selective action on bacteria without harm to human body. The ideal method of selection is to carry out a bacterial culture sensitivity test before starting the treatment. However, in cases where the infection is severe and the disease is likely to intensify before the sensitivity report is received (it takes at least 24 hours), antibiotic therapy may be started on the basis of doctor's clinical judgement.

**Failure of Response:** The failure of response to antibiotics is frequent and the reasons many. It could be due to a wrong selection, the development of bacterial resistance or inadequate therapy.

The mechanism of the development of drug resistance is quite complex. If a patient has been taking a particular antibiotic frequently, the bacteria in his system are likely to become resistant to it.

**The Patient's Role:** In India, where most of the population is poor, people hesitate to purchase expensive drugs. When a doctor prescribes an antibiotic, the patient thinks twice before he finally makes up his mind to take it, and in the process, loses valuable time. The patient thus postpones the treatment until the infection becomes severe or stops the drugs as soon as the symptoms are relieved, without completing a full course. This leads to the development of bacterial resistance, and the antibiotic becomes ineffective for future treatment of the disease.

In some cases, a patient takes either less than the prescribed dose or decreases the frequency of the intake advised by the physician. If, for example, a correct dose of an antibiotic is 250 mg four times a day (a total of 1g), and the patient takes it only two or three times a day ( total of 500 or 750 mg), this inadequate dose leads to the development of bacterial resistance.

**The Doctor's Role:** Most of the respiratory infections are viral in nature and do not require antibiotics. Therefore, antibiotics should not be prescribed. Depending on the site, duration, associated symptoms and local prevalence of disease, antibiotics are selected. In selection it is ascertained that it should be effective , safe, suitable, and cost-effective. Fevers of long duration, such as in tuberculosis or involvement of the heart (subacute bacterial endocarditis*) require specific drugs.

When a disease is associated with an appreciable quantity of pus, necrotic or dead tissues, and foreign bodies, it is prudent to provide surgical drainage for removal of the pus, dead tissues, or a foreign body and use antibiotics alongwith.

**Adverse Effects:** Almost all antibiotics have two important adverse effects: 1) allergic reactions, and 2) super-infections (added infections) due to other micro-organisms.

Allergic reactions to antibiotics are usually mild, in the form of skin rashes, fever, and joint pain. Serious allergic reactions, such as anaphylactic shock (hypersensitivity to an antigen), are quite rare. A person allergic to one antibiotic is likely to be allergic to other antibiotics of the same group.

Super-infections occur because antibiotics kill one group of micro-organisms, while others keep growing uninhibited. This uninhibited growth of unaffected micro-organisms may occasionally lead to serious consequences, which are most difficult to treat. Specific adverse effects are described with individual agents.

## Anti-Bacterial Drugs

### Sulfonamides

The use of *sulfonamides* is on the decline as bacteria have become resistant to them. Sulphacetamide and silversulfadiazine are two most commonly used *sulphonamides.* A combination of *sulfonamides (SMX)* with *trimethoprim* (which is called *co-trimoxazole) is* described here.

---

* A disease of inner coat of heart and its values.

**Sulfamethoxazole with Co-Trimoxazole** (SEPTRAN, BACTRIM)
This combination has a wider range of efficacy than the two individual drugs. *Trimethoprim(TMP),* like *sulfonamides,* inhibits the formation of metabolites essential for bacterial growth, but by acting at a different site of their synthesis. Thus, these two drugs in combination have more than an additive effect. This combination is very useful in treating infections of the urinary tract, respiratory tract and typhoid fever. This combination has also been used with some success in cholera and acute gastroenteritis.

***Dosage:*** A tablet contains 80 mg of *trimethoprim* and 400 mg of *sulfamethoxazole* (SMX). Its usual dose is two tablets twice a day orally, for 7 to 10 days. Tablets and syrups for children contain 20mgTMP+ 100 mg SMX per tab/tsf.

***Adverse Effects:*** The common adverse effects are nausea, vomiting, loss of appetite, drug fever and skin rashes. Allergic reactions to *sulfonamides* are common and are characterized by skin rashes, inflamed eyes, ulcers in the mouth and intolerance to sunlight. Sometimes a person may suffer from delayed allergy in which fever, joint pain, skin rashes, reddening of eyes, difficulty in breathing and peeling of skin and oral mucosal surface membrane (Stevens Johnson Syndrome) may occur. These medicines may also produce a serious toxic effect known as the which is characterized by severe type of skin rashes and reddening of the eyes

***Precautions:***

1. Always inform the doctor if you are allergic to *sulfonamides* before the prescription is written. There are other drugs which have sulpha-drug structure and these may cause hidden form of *sulfonamide* allergy. Such drugs are *nimesulide, omeprazole, rofecoxib, valdecoxib* (*Etoricoxib* is not a *sulfonamide*), *famotidine, thiazides* and antidiabetic drugs.
2. If skin rashes occur, stop the drug immediately.
3. Avoid these drugs if you have a kidney disease.
4. Drink large quantities of water when you take short-acting *sulfonamides* to prevent their precipitation in the kidneys (crystaluria).

**Sulfacetamide** (ALBUCID, LOCULA 10%.20%, 30%)
This is a highly soluble drug used in eye infections in the form of eye drops. It has been found to be effective in the treatment of trachoma. Allergic reactions due to local use of this drug are quite rare.

**Silversulphadiazine** (SILVEREX, SILVERSHEILD 1% cream)
It is a commonly used preparation to prevent infection in burns.

**Penicillins**

*Penicillin* was discovered by Sir Alexander Fleming in 1928. It was the first antibiotic discovered, yet it is still the most popular in current therapy. Various types of *penicillins* are available in India. *Penicillins* kill the bacteria and for this reason they are the preferred drugs for the treatment of pneumonia, syphilis, gonorrhoea, wound infections, tetanus, gas gangrene (a quick-spreading gangrene of injured tissues infected by a soil bacterium and accompanied by the evolution of gas), brain, liver, lung and abscesses (pus collection). One of the main drawback of most *penicillins* is their inability to inhibit the organisms which produce the enzyme *Penicillinase. Oxacillin* and *cloxacillin* the newer *penicillins* are effective against such organisms.

*Ampicillin,* although structurally related to *penicillin,* has qualities similar to broad-spectrum antibiotics, that is, it is effective against a large variety of micro-organisms. *Amoxycillin* (MOX TORMOXIN) is like *ampicillin* but is absorbed to a greater extent. Some derivatives are very effective against a notorious bug (pseudomonas!). There are *carbenicillin, ticarcillin, mezlocillin* and *piperacillin.* A combination of two drugs may sometimes do wonders in problematic infections. *Clavulanic acid* (stops inactivation of *penicillins* by bacteria), *salbactum* and *tazobactum* are drugs which can be combined with *amoxycillin* or *ampicillin* and empower them to fight against staphylococci, klebsiella and other hospital acquired infective agents.

***Adverse Effects:*** The most serious adverse effects of *penicillin* are allergic reactions. They may uncommonly (0.015%) cause fatal anaphylactic shock (severe hypotension and respiratory arrest) which is more common with injectable preparations than with oral *penicillin.* Other adverse effects, though rare, include brain toxicity (twitching, convulsions) on large doses given intravenously. Procaine element of the *procaine penicillin* can also cause allergic reactions.

With the increased usage of *ampicillin and amoxicillin,* skin rashes are found in 7 to 10% cases. Severe anaphylactic reactions and allergic effects have also been reported. Owing to their structural similarity, patients allergic to other *penicillins* have been reported to be allergic to *ampicillin* and other drugs of this class.

***Precautions:***

1. Inform your doctor of any type of *penicillins* allergy. A sensitivity test by injecting a very small dose of *penicillin,* should always be carried out before injecting a full dose of *penicillin.*
2. Patients allergic to one type of *penicillin* are usually allergic to other *penicillins.*
3. One must avoid the use of *penicillins* locally as ointments or creams

**Some Penicillin Preparations**

| *Drug/Brand Names* | *Route of Administration* | *Doses/day* |
|---|---|---|
| *Penicillin-G* | Injection | 3-6 lac units × 6 hrly IV/IM |
| *Procaine Penicillin-G* | Injection | 5-10 lac units once or twice a day IM |
| *Benzathine Penicillin-G* (PENIDURE) | Injection | 12 lac units once in 3-4 weeks IM |
| *Cloxacillin* (CLOX) | Oral | 0.25-0.5 g × 6 hrly |
| *Ampicillin* (ROSCILIN, BIOCILLIN) | Oral/ Injection | 0.25-0.5 g × 6 hrly |
| *Amoxicillin* (AMOXYVAN) | Oral/ Injection | 0.25-0.5 g × 6 hrly |
| *Carbenecillin* (PYOPEN) | Injection | 1-2 gm × 6 hrly |
| *Phenoxymethyl Penicillin* (CYSTAPEN-V, PENIVORAL) | Oral | 0.25 g × 6 hrly |
| *Piperacillin* (PIPREPEN) | Injection | 1-2 gm × 6 hrly IV/IM |
| *Amoxycillin + Clavulalnic acid* (MOX-CLAV, AUGMENTIN) | Oral/ Injection | 375-625 mg × thrice a day orally 1.2g x 8 hrly IV |
| *Sulbactam + Ampicillin* (SULBACIN) | Oral/Injection | 1-4 gm/day 1 to 5g IV 6 to 8 hrly |
| *Piperacillin* (PIPRACIL) | Injection | 2 gm 8-12 hourly |
| *Piperacillin + Tazobactum* (TAZOBID) | Injection | As above |

NB: A number of antibiotics contain *lactobacilli* or *ambroxol, carbocisteine* and *bromhexine*. Such combinations increase the cost unnecessarily and provide no superiority over antibiotics alone. Combinations of *amoxicillin* with *cloxacillin* (TORMOXIN Plus, SUPRIMOX) may provide additional coverage against resistant staphylocci.

## Broad-Spectrum Antibiotics

Broad-spectrum antibiotics inhibit the growth of the bacteria without destroying them (bacteriostatic action). They are effective against a wider range of bacteria, large viruses, and other organisms like rickettsiae. These drugs are useful in many common disorders in which there is mixed infection caused by more than one group of bacteria. In addition, although broad-spectrum antibiotics are effective in most common infections, they cannot replace *penicillins*, which are both less toxic and more effective in certain cases. Although their use is declining because of development of resistance but some of them are very useful in pimples with infection, chronic bronchitis, resistant malaria, micoplasma pneumonia and Typhus fever.

**Some Broad Sectrum Antibiotics**

| *Drug/Brand Names* | *Doses/day* |
|---|---|
| *Oxytetracyline* (TERRAMYCIN) | 250 mg- 500 mg to be given four times a day |
| *Demeclocycline* (LEDERMYCIN) | 150 mg-300 mg twice a day |
| *Doxycycline* (MICRODOX) | 100-200 mg once a day |
| *Minocycline* (CYANOMYCIN, CNN-50 mg, 100 mg) | 100- 200 mg once a day |

***Adverse Effects of Tetracyclines:*** In about 10% cases *tetracyclines* may cause pain in the abdomen, nausea, and vomiting owing to irritation of the stomach. These drugs may cause diarrhoea owing to disturbance in the intestinal bacterial flora. *Tetracyclines* may cause photosensitive actions in the form of blisters on the exposed parts of the body. This is most common with *demeclocycline* (in about 90% cases). This may also discolour and damage the teeth (cause brown discolouration). All of them may cause kidney damage but *doxycycline* is considered safer. *Minocycline* may cause ear damage and giddiness and unsteadiness.

***Precautions:***

1. *Tetracyclines* should not be taken with milk or antacids as their combination makes insoluble complexes which cannot be absorbed.
2. The use of *tetracyclines* should be avoided during pregnancy (cause liver damage) and in children up to 12 years of age owing to the adverse effects on teeth and bones (bone growth is retarded)
3. They should not be given to patients with a pre-existing kidney disease.

## Macrolide (Bulky molecules) antibiotics

**Erythromycin** (EMYCIN, ALTHROCIN)

This is a valuable drug for infections of throat, tonsils and airways, particularly in those patients who are allergic to *penicillins*. It is very effective in whooping cough and atypical pneumonia. Usually it is given in a dose of 250 to 500 mg four times a day in adults and 30 mg/ kg body weight dose in children as syrup of 100 mg/ 5 ml.

***Adverse Effects of Erythromycin:*** *Erythromycin* usually affects the gastro-intestinal tract causing nausea, vomiting, and diarrhoea. *Erythromycin estolate* (not others) is reported to be toxic to the liver. Recent reports indicate that it may cause spasms and narrowing of the gastric passage in newborns. *Erythromycin* inhibits inactivation of *theophyline, terfenadine, cisapride, carbamazepine* and *valproate*. Therefore, dose adjustments or change in drug may be required.

***Precautions:***

1. This drug should be withdrawn if it induces diarrhoea.
2. Never use it with *terfenadine, astemizole ,ketoconazole or cisapride.*

**Azithromycin** (AZITHRAL,AZIWOK, AZIFAST 250 mg 500 mg Tab; 50 mg/tsf), **Clarithromycin** (CLARIBID) and **Roxithromycin** (ROXITHRO, ROXID)

These are newer type of drugs which have broader activity against many infections on which *erythromycin* is not effective. Another advantage is that these are used in two divided doses in a day. They are concentrated in the infected (inflamed) tissues (tonsils, pharynx and soft tissues). *Clarithromycin* and *Azithromycin* are effective in tuberculosis and peptic ulcer causing organism H.pylori. Usual doses are:

| *Drugs* | *Dose* |
|---|---|
| *Roxithromycin* | 150 mg twice a day in adults; 2.5-5 mg/ kg (two doses) in children (dispersible tab 50 mg) |
| *Clarithromycin* (CLARIBID, CLARIMAC 125 mg, 250 mg) | 250 mg twice a day in adults. |
| *Azithromycin* | 250 mg twice a day for 3 days in adults; 10 mg/ kg in one or two divided doses in children. |
| *Spiramycin* (ROVAMYCIN forte 3MIU tab) | It has effects against protozoa and cryptosporiodosi. |
| *Bacitracin* (NEBASULF-ointment, powder) | is commonly used for skin infections, eye ulcers. |

## Aminoglycosides

*Streptomycin, Gentamicin, Kanamycin, Netilmicin, Amikacin* and *Tobramycin* are *aminoglycosides*. All of them are injectables and not effective orally. *Streptomycin* is used in tuberculosis only. *Framycetin* (SOFRAMYCIN 0.5%, SOFRA-TULLE dressing 1%) is commonly used in skin infections and boils. Other drugs have special uses.

*Gentamicin* is commonly used for infections. It is a valuable drug for prevention and treatment of lung infection in hospitals and to treat resistant infections of kidney and urinary passages, meningitis and heart infections. It is available as injection (20 mg/ml) and eye/ear drops 0.1%.

***Adverse Effects of Gentamicin (and other Aminoglycosides):*** The most important adverse effects of *gentamicin* are felt on the ears, muscles and the kidneys. It causes hearing defects and frequently damages the nerves to the vestibular apparatus (an apparatus in the ear responsible for maintaining the equilibrium of the body). Skeletal muscle weakness may be there in high doses.

***Precautions***

1. Due to its toxic nature it should be taken only when other antibiotics are ineffective.
2. It should be taken in correct doses, as low doses may cause bacterial resistance and high doses may cause kidney damage.
3. It should not be taken during pregnancy.
4. It should be used cautiously along with drugs potentially toxic to the kidneys, such as *cephalosporins, polymyxins, ethacrynic acid,* or *furosemide.*

## Cephalosporins

*Cephalosporins* are antibiotics which act like *penicillins* and kill an array of harmful bacteria. They are considerably safe for use. They are divided into four major groups or generations; depending mainly on their microbiological spectrum of activity.

### First-Generation Cephalosporins

These have a narrow spectrum of activity and include:

**Cefadroxil** (DROXYL, ODOXIL, LYDOXYL, KEFLOXIN-250mg, 500 mg, 125 mg/tsf syp), **Cefazolin** (LYZOLIN, REFLIN-500 mg), **Cephalexin** (SPORIDEX, BLUCEF 250 mg, 500 mg cap).

The first-generation *cephalosporins* have a broad spectrum of activity and are relatively non-toxic. Oral drugs may be used for the treatment of urinary tract infections, for minor staphylococcal lesions, or for minor poly-microbial infections such as cellulitis or soft tissue abscesses. However, oral *cephalosporins* should not be relied upon in serious systemic infections. Some of these are available along with *lactobacilli* and *ambroxol.* These only increase the cost without increasing clinical efficacy.

### Second-Generation Cephalosporins

These have an intermediate spectrum of action and include the following drugs:

**Cefaclor** (KEFLOR), **Cefuroxime** (CEFOGEN, SUPACEF), **Cefprozil** (3-CEF 250 mg tab)

Due to its activity against *beta-lactamase*-producing *H influenza* or *Branhamella cartarrhalis cefaclor* is used to treat sinusitis and otitis media (inflammation of the middle ear) when patients have not responded to *ampicillin* or *amoxicillin. Cefuroxime* is the only second-generation drug that crosses the blood-brain barrier well enough to be used for the treatment of meningitis, especially H influenzae meningitis, and sepsis.

*Cefuroxime Axetil* (CEFTUM) is orally effective in resistant infections. Single dose is effective in gonorrhoea. It is commonly used in roadside injuries when mixed infections are usual.

### Third-Generation Cephalosporins

These have a broad spectrum of activity and include the following drugs:

**Cefotaxine** (BIOTAX, CLAFORAN, OMNATAX), **Ceftazidime** (FORTUM), **Cefoperazone** (MAGNAMYCIN), **Ceftizoxime** (CEFIZOX), **Ceftriaxone** (CEFAXONE, MONOCEF), **Cefixime** (BIOTAX, OMNATAX-O, TOPCEF 50 mg Dt,100mg, 200 mg Tab), **Cefdinir** (ADCEF-300 mg cap), **Cefpodoxime** (CEPODEM, PODOCEF 200 mg), **Cefetamet pivoxil** (ALTACEF 250 mg) and **Ceftibuten** (PROCADAX, 200 mg) - last five are effective orally.

Due to their ability to penetrate the central nervous system, third-generation *cephalosporins* — except *cefoperazone* and *cefixime* —are used to treat meningitis, including meningitis caused by pneumococci, meningococci, *H influenzae* and *P. aeruginosa.* Other potential indications include sepsis of unknown causes in the immunocompetent patient and susceptible infections in which *cephalosporins* are the least toxic drugs available. In neutropenic, febrile immunocompromised patients, third-generation *cephalosporins* can be effective if used in combination with an *aminoglycoside.* Intravenous *cefalosporins* may enhance bleeding tendencies and alchol intolerance is also noted. Patients should avoid alcohol beverages with these drugs.They are commonly used in hospital settings in patients with serious systemic infections. Oral drugs are expensive but more effective and thus are used as follow-up drugs after intravenous *cephalosporins* used to cure hospital acquired infections. *Cefixime, cefdinir, cefpodoxime, cefetamet pivoxil* and *ceftibuten* are effective orally.

### Fourth-Generation Cephalosporins

*Cefepime* (MAXICEF, NOVAPIME inj. 250 mg, 500 mg, 1g) can be used in resistant infections due to gram negative rods and staphylococci causing septicemia. *Cefpirome* (BACIROM, CEFROM inj. 250 mg, 500 mg, 1g) has same utility as *cefepime.* These are very expensive.

***Adverse Effects of Cephalosporins:*** Allergy: *Cephalosporins* are sensitizing and may cause a variety of hypersensitivity reactions, including anaphylaxis, fever, skin rashes, nephritis, granulocytopenia, and hemolytic anaemia. The chemical nucleus of *cephalosporins* is sufficiently different from that of *penicillins,* enabling some individuals with a history of *penicillin* allergy to tolerate *cephalosporins.* However, patients with a history of anaphylaxis to *penicillins* should never receive *cephalosporins.*

Toxicity: Local irritation can produce severe pain after intramuscular injection and thrombophlebitis after intravenous injection. Renal toxicity, including interstitial nephritis and even tubular necrosis, has been demonstrated and has caused the abandonment of *cephaloridine.*

### Super-Infection

Many second and particularly third generation *cephalosporins* are ineffective against gram-positive organisms, especially *stayphylococci* and *enterococci.* During treatment with such drugs, these resistant organisms, as well as fungi, often proliferaite and may induce super-infection.

### Linezolid (LIZOLID, LINOX-600 mg)

It is effective in multidrug resistant pneumococci, staphylococci and enteric organisms induced infections in a dose of 600 mg twice a day. It may cause suppression of bone marrow and interacts with decongestant drugs whose dose should be reduced.

## Fluoroquinolones

In 1990 fluoroquinolones were introduced to tackle ever increasing menace of resistance in gram negative rods. Since then many more drugs have been developed which have effects against both gram positive and negative bacteria, anaerobes and tuberculosis organisms. These drugs destroy the DNA of bacteria. Unfortunately due to overuse, resistance is becoming the problem again.

### Ciprofloxacin (CIPLOX, CIFRAN,QUINTOR-500 mg)

Presently a drug of choice for typhoid fever, (*chloramphenicol* is no longer used) gonorrhoea, abdominal (bowel) pelvic infections and diarrhoea, soft tissue and bone infections. It can be used by mouth 500 mg twice a day or intravenously in serious cases.

***Adverse Effects:*** Some adverse effects are loss of appetite, nausea and bowel upset, dizziness, restlessness, loss of sleep, poor concentration and tremulousness (avoid driving). Drug allergy may cause skin eruptions. A potentially serious problem is that it may cause cartilage damage as based on animal studies so should be used sparingly in children (although it is best to avoid it). Tendon (Tendo Achilles-heal tendon) rupture has been reported. *Theophylline, caffeine, warfarin* show toxicity when taken with *ciprofloxacin* and require staggering or reduction in dose. Pain relievers may cause more CNS adverse effects of *ciprofloxacin.* Antacids, milk and iron salts reduce absorption, do not take with milk or after meals.

**Norfloxacin** (NORFLOX, UROFLOX 200 mg) is less potent to *ciprofloxacin* but is effective in the treatment of urinary tract infecting diarrhoea (usual dose 400 mg twice a day in adult).

**Pefloxacin** (PEFLOSYN, PFLOX-200mg) is a good drug for meningeal infections and typhoid fever. A single dose of 400 mg cures gonorrhoea. No dose adjustment is required in mild to moderate renal disease.

**Ofloxacin** (OFLOMAC, ZANOCIN 200 mg, 400 mg, ZANOCIN-OD 400 mg) is effective in urethritis, cervicitis and atypical pneumonia. It is useful in tuberculosis also (never given alone). Food does not reduce its absorption. It is a commonly used drug in enteric fever also.

**Sparfloxacin** (SPARFLOX-200 mg) has greater activity to treat pneumonia, sinus infection, and ear infections. It is longer acting so it is given in a dose of 200-400 mg once a day. It may cause disturbed heart beats particularly when other drugs are given along with it (drugs for depression and *cisapride*).

**Gatifloxacin** is like *sparfloxacin* in action, it is associated with unwanted effects in diabetics and heart disease so is withdrawn in many countries. We discourage its use.

**Levofloxacin** (LEVOMAX, LOXOF, LEVODAY 500 mg) is completely absorbed orally and does not interact with drugs (unlike *ciprofloxacin* and others). High cure rates are achieved in pneumonia, sinusitis, acute kidney infections and soft tissue infections. It is used in a dose of 500 mg once a day. Diabetics may experience low sugar episodes so caution should be exercised.

**Moxifloxacin** (MOXIF, MOXICIP 400 mg) has greater effects on pneumonia organisms. It is likely to cause heart rhythm disturbance. At present it is being evaluated as an alternative drug for MDR tuberculosis.

**Gemifloxacin** (GEMEF, GEMIF, GEMBAX 320 mg) is the most potent weapon against pneumonia causing bacteria. Its dose is 320mg once a day for 10 to 14 days and can be given with or without meals. No adverse effects are observed given with other drugs.

**Nadifloxacin** (NADIBACT 1% Cream) is the *fluoroquinolone* available astoical agent for the treatment of skin infections.

**Nalidixic acid** (GRAMONEG 500 mg) is a *quinolone* effective in chronic and recurrent urinary infections and sometimes in the treatment of bacterial diarrhoea.

## Other Antibiotics

**Clindamycin**(DALCIN 150 mg, 300 mg) is a special antibiotic used in the treatment of anerobic infections of bones, lungs and abdominal lower organs. It is very toxic and causes severe infection with C.difficile.

**Vancomycin** is used in staphylococcal heart valve infections.

**Mupirocin** (T-BACT 2% cream) and **Fusidic acid** (FUSIDIN 2%) are used for skin infections

**Nirofurantoin** (FURADANTIN with LIQUORICE 200 mg tab)) is a urinary antiseptic and has a preventive value in cathereised patients. It should not be used for more than 2 weeks because of its toxic effects on nerves. It causes nausea and vomiting.

## Anti fungal drugs

There are two types of anti-fungal drugs: agents which are used as creams, ointments, lotions, and pessaries for local effects and; drugs which are used by mouth or by injections for the treatment of systemic fungal infections.

### **Griseofulvin** (GROSOVIN- FP)

This antifungal antibiotic used by mouth for the treatment of skin fungal disease such as *Tinea corpris* (ring worm), *Tinea capitis* and fungal disease affecting toes and nails. Usual dose is 125 to 250 mg twice a day with food. Usual duration of treatment is 3 weeks for skin infection and 12 months for toes/ nails infection.

***Adverse Effects:*** It is well tolerated but alcohol should not be taken during medication. It may cause headache and bowel upset.

### **Fluconazole** (ZOCON, SYSCAN)

It is very commonly used for the treatment of systemic fungal infection and moniliasis (*candida* — a mould). Its usual dose is 150 mg capsule once a day for 2 weeks. In light skin infection it is advised to be taken once in a week because it stays longer in body. Eye drops are used for fungal infection of cornea (front visible part).

***Adverse Effects and Precautions:*** It may cause bowel upsets, pain in abdomen and headache. In some cases liver may be affected. It is not given in pregnancy and during breast feeding. When *phenytoin, cisapride, warfarin* and *antidiabetics* are taken with it some changes in doses are required.

### **Itraconazole** (ITOSPOR)

It has broader activity than *fluconazole* and effective against Aspergillus fungal infections. Its usual dose is 200 mg once a day. It may cause stomach upset, dizziness, fall in blood potassium, unsteadiness and loss of sexual desire. Adverse effects and precautions are same as for *fluconazole*.

### **Voriconazole** (VFEND tab. 50 mg, 200 mg; inj. 200 mg)

It is a newer drug considered to be more effective against candila and aspergillus fungi. It is better absorbed orally than fluconazole. Its usual dose is 200 to 400 mg daily.

### **Ketoconazole**

It has been used for quite sometimes but it causes a number of adverse effects such as loss of appetite, vomiting, loss of hair, headache and numbness, hormonal disturbance (decreased male hormones) such as enlargement of male breast, loss of desire and fall in spasm-counts. In females it may cause irregular menstrual cycle. It may cause mild degree of liver damage also.

The most dreaded problem with *Ketoconozole* is occurrence of heart rhythm disturbance with concurrent use of *cisapride, terfenadine* or *astemizole.* It raises blood levels of other drugs such as *Rifampicin, Phenytoin, Warfarin* and antidiabetic drugs. Because of these reasons and availability of safer drugs *Ketoconazole* is less preferred nowadays. Topical *ketoconazole* as shampoo or lotion is commonly used in dandruff (see chapter on drugs for common skin diseases).

**Other Antifungal Drugs**

| *Drug/Brand Names* | *Form* | *Uses* |
|---|---|---|
| *Nystatin* (MYCOSTATIN) | Oral tablet-5 lac* units, vaginal tablet- 1 lac units, eye ointment 1 lac/g | For candida infections and oral thrush |
| *Hamycin* (IMPRIMA) | Suspension 2 lac units/ ml, Ointment 1 lac/ g | Oral thrush and vaginal moniliasis |
| *Clotrimazole* (SURFAZ) | Lotion 1%, Cream 1%, Vaginal tablet 100 mg/ tab, Powder | Oral thrush Vaginal moniliasis (fungal vaginitis) |
| *Miconazole* (DAKTARIN) | Gel 2%, Solution 1%, Ear drops 1%, | Highly effective in fungal vaginitis and ear infections |
| GYNODAKTARIN) | Vaginal tab 100 mg/ tab | |
| *Ketoconazole* (FUNGICIDE) (KETOVATE) | Ointment 2%, Shampoo 2% Cream 2% | Dandruff and skin lesion |
| *Econazole* (ECODERM) | Ointment 2%, Cream 2% | Oral thrush and ear infection |
| *Tolnaftate* (TOLNADERM, TINADERM) | Lotion 1%, Cream 1% | Pityriasis vorsicolor (Superficial skin infection of chest and back) |
| *Ciclopirox olamine* (OLAMIN) | Cream 1% Lotion 1% | Pityriasis vorsicolor (Superficial skin infection of chest and back) |
| *Undecylenic acid* (TINEAFAX) | Ointment | Nappy rash and skin fungal infection |
| *Benzoicacid* (WITH SALICYCLIC ACID) | Ointment | Fungal infection of thick skin, corns, warts |
| *Sodium Thiosulfate* (KARPIN) | Lotion 20% | Pityriasis vorsicolor |
| *Oxiconazole* (OXICON) | 1% Cream, Lotion | Skin ringworm |
| *Terbinafine* (TERBIDERM) | 1% Cream | Pvorsicolor & ringworm |
| *Butenafen* (BUTOP, FINTOP) | 1% Cream | As above |

* 1 Lac = 1/10th million.

# 36

# Antioxidants and Phytonutrients

••••••

A number of oxygen-radicals are formed in our body during process of metabolism of nutrients in body cells. These oxygen-radicals (by virtue of having free electrons) are highly reactive (oxidants) and can damage DNA molecules, proteins and cholesterol rich LDL molecules. In defence, body produces substances to prevent damage caused by oxidants or free radicals. These endogenous antioxidants may be inadequate when there is excessive formation of oxidants. This results in disease processes. Numerous studies have shown that oxidative stress plays role in causation of atherosclerosis, Parkinson's disease, stroke, Alzheimer's disease, cancer, diabetes, smoking induced lung damage and cataract formation. It is also believed that normal ageing process is hastened by oxidative stress and free radical induced cell damage and death. Antioxidants are powerful agent to quench (scavenge) free radicals in body.

## Role in Disease Prevention

It is obvious that when body's defenses are weakened and production of antioxidants such as superoxide dismuthate and metal binding proteins are reduced it is helpful to supplement antioxidants in the form of antioxidant-foods and dietary supplements called Nutraceuticals. Thousands of clinical trials have been done to investigate the effects of such supplementation on the risks of cancer, and heart diseases. A diet, rich in antioxidants, is associated with lower risk of development of common cancers and may prevent cancer recurrence. The risk of heart disease may be reduced by the use of antioxidants. The eye is yet another organ affected by oxidant-injury. High doses of antioxidants may prove to be useful in prevention of degeneration of the retina (where visual images are formed) and cataract. Thus useful vision can be preserved.

**Foods High in Antioxidants:** Anti-oxidant rich fresh fruits and vegetables use may prevent aging of skin and wrinkle formation. Antioxidants are abundant in fruits and vegetables, nuts, grains and some meats, poultry and fish.

- Beta-carotene is found in many foods that are orange in colour, including sweet potatoes, carrots, cantaloupe, pumpkin, and mangoes. Green leafy vegetables including collard greens, spinach, and kale are also rich in beta-carotene.

- Lutein, best known for its association with healthy eyes, is abundant in green, leafy vegetables such as collard greens, spinach, and kale.
- Lycopene is a potent antioxidant found in tomatoes, watermelon, guava, papaya, pink grapefruit and other foods.

| ORAC* Units per 100 g | |
|---|---|
| Dark Chocolate | 13,120 |
| Milk Chocolate | 6,740 |
| Prunes | 5,770 |
| Raisins | 2,830 |
| Strawberries | 1,540 |
| Spinach | 1,260 |
| Raspberries | 1,220 |
| Brussel Sprouts | 980 |
| Plums | 949 |
| Alfalfa Sprouts | 930 |
| Broccoli Florets | 890 |
| Oranges | 750 |
| Red Grapes | 739 |
| Red Bell Pepper | 710 |
| Cherries | 670 |
| Onion | 450 |
| Corn | 400 |
| Eggplant | 390 |

Tomatoes, broccoli, green tea (and its extract containing catechins) and cauliflower are excellent source of natural antioxidants. Fruits and vegetables which have rich hue of colours are also rich sources of antioxidants. Clinical studies show that phytonutrients, present in the skin of these fruits and vegetables, enhance body's defense system (immunity) and can prevent cancer. Therefore, next time when you stroll through vegetable market, don't forget to buy red onion instead of white variety, and, crisp and fresh green leafy vegetables. The thumb rule is the deeper and richer the colour of fruits and vegetables, the more phytonutrients are present in them. Organically grown plants are richer in polyphenols which are strong antioxidants. Celery juice has anticancer nutrients such as phthalates and polyacetylene antioxidants and potassium which reduces BP. Soya beans contain isoflavones which are helpful in cholesterol control, improving cognition and cancer prevention.

**Alternatives to Antioxidant Foods:** When you don't have regular access to organic fruits and vegetables, you may consider addition of food supplements or nutraceuticals and phytonutrient-supplements. These have extra nutrients without excess of sugar and calories. It must be remembered that pills containing antioxidants are prescribes and sold in the market a great deal, but these are nowhere as effective as the antoxidants from 'natural foods' which remain the best source. Overdose of these pills may enhance free radical induced tissue injury, hence should best be avoided. Many of them have not stood the test of time in well controlled studies. The various antioxidants available, contain one or more than one of the followings.

1. Natural Carotenoids: There are various carotenoids in plants.

*Lycopene:* It is a carotenoid which gives tomatoes a red colour. It is very much effective in attacking oxygen-radicals in body and acts as a cell protector. Lyco-Red is the market preparation which is claimed to be effective in male infertility, pregnancy associated high BP, post menopausal syndrome and pregnancy with a history of bad outcome previously. It prevents premature delivery and foetal growth retardation.

*ß-Carotene:* Synthetic ß-Carotene is also a quencher of free radicals and prevents *peroxidation* of fats. Both natural carotenoids and synthetic ß-Carotene are present in a number of formulations.

* ORAC (Oxygen Radical Absorbance Capacity) is a measure of the ability of the foods to subdue harmful oxygen free radicals that can damage our bodies.

*Lutein and Zeaxanthin:* They are found in corn and green leafy vegetables and prevent the process of cataract formation.

2. Vitamin-E (A-TOCOFEROL): It is fat soluble vitamin and it works as a membrane bound antioxidant. It is found to preserve membrane functions and prevents lipid oxidation. Interestingly, it prevents oxidation of vitamin A in the intestines so more vitamin A is absorbed. Vitamin E also preserves activity of immune cells. It has been tried in prevention of oxidative injury in diabetes, heart disease, inflammation, cataract and infections.

3. Alpha Lipoic acid (EBIZA-L): It is a powerful antioxidant which is found to be useful in diabetes mellitus. In diabetes, uncontrolled high sugar itself favours formation of injurious oxidants. Alpha lipoic acid increases glucose uptake in cells and quenches free radicals which play a role in causing diabetic neuropathy (nerve damage). In Germany it is licensed for the treatment of diabetic neuropathy for over 20 years and is also available in India. It is also found to be protective against development of eye and kidney complications in diabetics.

4. Selenium: It is an antioxidant mineral, needed for making natural anitoxidants in our body. It is given along with other antioxidant supplements.

*Vitamin C (Ascorbic acid):* It is a strong reducing agent and is given along with vitamin E for its antioxidant effects.

5. Ginseng (REVITAL): It is known to increase body defense mechanism. Asian Ginseng helps to rebuild damage nerve cells and is available in combinations with multivitamin preparations.

6. Flavonoids (ISOFLAV-CR-60 mg cap): Bioflavonoids have antioxidant properties as they quench free radicals. They have role in prevention of Cardiovascular disease, improve memory in ageing and Alzhiemer disease and in cancer prevention.

7. Co-enzyme Q 10 or Ubiquinone (ZYME- Q 10): As an antioxidant it is useful in Parkinson's disease and strokes.

8. Curcumin (TURMIX tab 300 mg): It is given in a usual dose of 300 mg in a day. It is a cardio-protective antioxidant. If used for long period it may cause nausea, vomiting and anemia.

9. Others: Immunocal is a natural protein and raises blood glutathione levels. It has powerful antioxidant properties and detoxifies liver. Immunocal contains albumen, lact-albumen and lactoberrin, ZMC, Copper and Manganese are also used for their antioxidant properties.

**Points to Ponder**

- Eating 6 servings of fruits and vegetables per day ( per1000 calories) can reduce the risk of head and neck cancer by 29%.
- Isoflvones were associated with a mean 9.3% reduction of total cholesterol,12.9% reduction in LDL-C and 10.5% reduction in triglycerides. These reduce the activation of *tau* brain protein which is associated with Alzheimer's disease.
- In well controlled trials Vitamin-E failed to show benefit in Heart Protection study (HOPE-Study). It may actually hinder the beneficial effects of statins!

**Common Market Preparations with Antioxidant Activity**

| *Brand Names* | *Antioxidants* |
|---|---|
| ANTOXID | ß-carotene, Zinc sulfate, Selenium, Manganese, Copper |
| ANTOXID-HC | Cis & Trans- ß-carotenes, Selenium, Manganese, Copper |
| CARDIVIT | Vitamin A, $B_6$, $B_{12}$, Folic acid, Vit C, Selenium, Vit E |
| EBIZA-L | Alpha lipoic acid, Chromium, Vit E, Folic acid, Vit $B_6$, $B_{12}$, Selenium |
| GYNACEA | Soy-isoflavones, Calcium, Phosphorus, Vitamin $D_6$ |
| IMMUNOSE | Natural cortenoids, L- carnitine, Vitamins, Cystine |
| OCUGOLD | Luetin, Zeaxantin, ß-carotene, Vit E, Vit C, E,P |
| LYCOGOLD | Lycopene, Selenium, Vit-C, mixed carotinoids, Zn, Wheat germ oil, B12 |
| OXYACE | ß-carotene, Copper, Zinc, Selenium, Manganese, Vit C, and E |
| OXYVIT | Vits A, C, E, Zinc, Selenium, Manganese, ß-carotene |
| RECHARGE | Co-enzyme Q 10, Vit E |
| VITOXID- OD | Vits A, E, C, $B_3$, Zinc, Selenium |
| ZYME | Coenzyme-Q10 |
| LYCOVIT | Lycopene |
| WINOFIT | Omega-3 fatty acids, Chromium, Vits A,C,E |
| MENOEASE | Soy Isoflavones, Vits B complex and antioxidants |
| I-VIT | Vit-A,E,C,Zn,Cu,Selenium |
| CAVIT-PM | Isoflavones, Calcium, Vit D3, Mg |
| MULTIZAC | Lutein, ß-carotene, Vits $B_1$,$B_2$,$B_{12}$, folic acid, Vit-C,Vit-E,Selenium, Niacin, L-lysine, L-cysteine |
| XEELO | ß-carotene, Lycopene, Vits-B,C,E.$B_2$, $B_6$, Zn, Folic acid, selenium |
| BENFAGE FORTE | Benfotiamine, $B_6$, Alpha linolic acid, Vit-$B_{12}$, inositol |

# 37

# Commonly Used Ayurvedic and Unani Drugs

Sometimes ago an executive at the French consulate, Pondicherry had an excruciating backache. It was so severe that she could not even sit on a chair. The specialist at the hospital took a series of X-rays but could not find any abnormality. He prescribed her pain-relieving tablets, which she refused to take as perceived that these provide only temporary relief and produce harmful effects. She consulted the *Ayurvedic* physician at the Aurobindo Ashram and we were surprised to see her dancing after a couple of days. The miraculous relief from her pain is a mystery for us. Whether the *Ayurvedic* medicines provided the relief or the major cause of her illness was psychological and she got relief due to faith in *Ayurvedic* medicine is a question that intrigues us.

There is greater recognition for non-allopathic schools of medicine in the West now than ever before. Ayurvedic concepts and herbal medicine are attracting attention. There is also more scientific research conducted in India, on herbal remedies. There are some diseases for which Ayurvedic treatment can claim superiority over other systems. The physicians of these traditional medicines claim that to be effective all the ingredients (which range from 3 to 30) should be mixed in a specific way and then administered. Patients often use these traditional medicines in some of the ailments such as arthritis, diseases of the lungs, heart, liver, nervous system etc., for which effective medicines are not available in allopathic system. The information on use of these medicines is given below.

### AIDS

*Bhallataka, Guddoochi, Chitraka* and some time-tested mercurial compounds are used in the treatment of AIDS. Extensive research is now on about the use of Ayurveda and Siddha medicines in the treatment of AIDS as the allopathic treatment is expensive and beyond means of most of the patients and the patients tend to switch to comparatively cheaper alternatives of Ayurveda.

### Arthritis

There are several *Ayurvedic* and *Unani* preparations in the Indian market with claims of effectiveness in arthritis. Various arthritic conditions can also be treated by internal and external remedies. For external application oils such as *Pinda Tailam, Vishamusti Tailam* and *Amavatha Tailam* are commonly used. *Guggulu* (resinous extract of the bark of *commifera mukul*) and other herbo-mineral compounds are taken internally.

Most popular among them are RUMALAYA, R-COMPOUND, SALLAKI., RUMAYOG, RUMAYOG-GOLD and MYOSTAL. RUMALAYA tablets contain 16 herbo-mineral ingredients including *commiphora mukul (Guggul)* and calcined conch *(shankh bhasma)*. Besides, a RUMALAYA cream (containing herbal extracts, oils, camphor, and bee wax) is also available for topical use. Many studies (sponsored by the manufacturing companies and published in their own house journal) have been made on the effects of RUMALAYA tablets and cream on rheumatoid arthritis, ankylosing spondylitis, and osteoarthritis, with encouraging results. One such study on 50 patients reported a slow onset of recovery with no side effects during the clinical trial. The anti-inflammatory effects of the chief ingredient *commiphora mukul* are well documented in the scientific journals. R-COMPOUND is a herbo-mineral preparation. It contains *commiphora mukul (Guggul),* calcined gold *(swarna bhasma),* and *maharasndi quoth* processed in *curcuma longa rhizome (haldi)* powder. SALLAKI is a single-ingredient preparation containing a standardized extract of *boswellia serrata.* The anti-inflammatory and pain relieving properties of most of the ingredients are well documented. Although not systematically investigated, these are claimed to be non toxic.

### Cancer

CANCER GAJ KESRI, a preparation containing gold and diamond *bhasma* is used in the treatment of cancer. It is an extremely expensive preparation.

### Diabetes

NISHA *(Curcuma longa and Manjal* in Tamil) AMALAKI CHURNAM, TARAKESHWARA RASA as bhasma, *Shilajit (Bituman), gudoochi satvam* (starchy portion of the guduchi stem) are used in diabetic treatment. Other preparations are GULDIBIT, NISHA AMLIKI, HYPONID and TRIBANG SHILA.

### Heart Diseases

*Guggulipid* (containing 4 g, Z and E *guggulsterones* per 100 g) from *Commiphora mukul* has a cholesterol lowering property. Scientific data (pharmacognostic, phytochemical, pharmacological, toxicological, and clinical) based on experimental and clinical studies show that *guggulipid* is a safe and effective lipid-lowering agent, comparable to *clofibrate,* with better patient compliance and lesser side-effects. The recommended dose is 500 mg (one tablet) three times a day. Due to paucity of data, it is not recommended for use in children . Other products used are ARJUNA powder and ARJUNA RISHTHA as cardiotonic medicines.

**Ayurveda: The Ancient Science of Healthy Living**

Ayurveda, the ancient Indian 'Science of Living', traces its etymology to *Ayush,* meaning 'life', and *Veda,* which originates from *vid* or knowledge. Ayurveda helps the human body keep fit while providing cure of illnesses through use of plant materials, animal products, and minerals.

The main body of text of Ayurveda is found in the fourth *Veda* — the *Atharva Veda.* However, even though Ayurveda is part of the *Atharva Veda,* it is also recognized as an *upa* or supplementary Veda in its own right. Ayurveda maintains that there is a definite relationship between illness and the metaphysical state of an individual. Its approach to medical treatment focuses on the individual rather than the disease.

KHAMIRA ABRESHAM ARSHADWALA is a reputed cardiotonic paste used in *Unani Tibb.* It has 22 ingredients, the chief ingredient is the cocoons of the silkworm. Pharmacological studies have revealed antihypertensive, antiarrhythmic, and cholesterol lowering effects. However, data on systematic clinical trials is not available.

*Amritkalash* is claimed to be effective in the prevention and treatment of cardiovascular diseases. It is reported to possess anti-oxidant, fibrinolytic, and immuno-enhancer properties and prevent free radical damage, clot formation, degenerative diseases, and premature ageing. It is available as paste and tablets. It contains 41 herbal ingredients. The major constituents of it are, *Emblica officinalis (amla), terminalua chebula (haritaki), withania somnifera (ashwagandha), glycyrrhiza glabra (mulehti)*. The data supplied by the company gives sufficient justification for carrying out systematic clinical trials with this formulation.

## Hypertension

Sarpagandha (*Rauwolfia Serpentina*) is considered effective. The warning here is that the same prescriptions or dosage are not viable for all patients, as individual constitutions differ. A good physician who has analyzed the patient's nature will be in a position to prescribe the medicine required.

*Allium sativum (lahsun)* is used in heart disease and hypertension for its hypolipidemic activity. It also has anti-microbial, hypoglycaemic, and anti-inflammatory properties. Pharmacological and clinical studies on garlic oil have been extensively carried out at many centres in India. Garlic oil is now being commercially marketed in the form of capsules. The most popular among these is GARLIC PEARLS and capsules. SUMANTA tablets are used in cases of hypertension associated with anxiety and depression.

## Liver Disease

More than 100 herbal formulations are available in the Indian market for use in liver ailments. About 81 medicinal plants have been used in such formulations. Herbs like *pippali (Piper Longum)*, *bhoomiamla (philanthus niruri)*, *bringaraj (eclipta alba)*, and *maricham (piper nigrum)* are effective in the treatment of liver disorders. The most popular and widely used preparations among these are LIV-52, LIVOMYN, LIVOTRIT, VIMLIV and TEFROLI. These preparations contain 20 to 25 plant ingredients.

Pharmacological and toxicity data on most of these plants is available. The formulation LIV-52 seems to have been extensively investigated from pharmacological, toxicological, and clinical aspects with very encouraging results. It is claimed to have protective and regenerative effects on hepatic parenchyma with anabolic, diuretic, chloretic, and appetite-improving properties. It is used in cases of anorexia, childhood cirrhosis, infective hepatitis, chronic active hepatitis, adult cirrhosis, and jaundice. Though the manufacturers claim it to be useful in cancer, diabetes, dermatological disorders, burns, digestive problems, degenerative and debilitating diseases, as an adjunct to prolonged antibiotic therapy, and for alleviating fatigue and stress in athletes, scientific evidence on these aspects is insufficient and equivocal.

The preparations (available in the form of tablets and syrup) have, however, made a significant impact in the treatment of liver diseases, which do not respond favourably to allopathic medicine.

## Respiratory Diseases

Two traditional preparations, namely *Chyavanprasha* from *Ayurveda* and *Joshanda* from *Unani Tibb* are widely used for the prevention and treatment of common cold.

*Chyavanprasha* is claimed to increase immunity of the body and strengthen defense to fight infections. The formula is taken from an ancient *Ayurvedic* text *Bhaishajyaratnavali* and contains about 40 ingredients. *Emblica officinalis (amla)* fruits form the chief ingredient of this formulation. This fruit is rich in vitamin C in natural form believed to be a resistance-building agent in respiratory diseases. The contents in fruits, pulp, and juice are about 600, 720, and 920 mg/100 g respectively. Comparative data on bio-availability from synthetic and natural sources of vitamin C is not available. Some manufacturers add saffron, calcined mica, *Siddha makardhwaja* (an *Ayurvedic* mercury preparation), and silver foil to the formulation and call it SPECIAL CHYAVANPRASHA with enhanced activity but such claims have not yet been substantiated. *Chyavanprasha* is also used as an adjunct tonic in cases of asthma and tuberculosis. It is claimed to prevent aging. Well planned, double blind multi-centric clinical trials on this ancient recipe are warranted to establish its real worth.

*Joshanda* is a Persian word derived from *joshanidan* (boiling) and *andah* (prepared by) meaning 'prepared by boiling'. This formulation, available in packets containing 6 to 8 crude dried drugs in a particular proportion, are meant to be used in the form of a freshly prepared decoction to which sugar can be added for palatability. A pack contains *althea officinalis* seeds *(khatmi), cordia latifolia* fruits *(sapistan), glycyrrhiza glabra rhizomes (mulehti), malva rotundifulia* seeds *(khubbazi), onosma bracteatum* leaves *(gaozaban), viola odorata* stems, leaves, and flowers *(banafsha),* and *zizyphus jujuba* fruits *(unnab).* These days a concentrate of crude ingredients of *Joshanda* is available under the name JOSHINA for convenience and instant use. A spoon full of it is mixed in hot water and sipped like tea. While the formulations used are very popular and claimed to be highly efficacious, no scientific reports are available.

Literature reveals that the ingredients of *Joshanda* have anti-microbial, broncho-dilatory, anti-allergic, cough suppressing, spasm relieving, anti-inflammatory, mucus stimulating and liquefying *(expectorant)*, and respiratory stimulant properties. Fomentation of the palate and throat by the hot decoction might be responsible for some of its effects and feeling of well being. The soothing effect of sugar, the aroma, the hot beverage-type of administration, and interplay of psychic factors may also be contributing towards its beneficial effects. Experimental studies in recent years have confirmed the expectorant, decongestant, anti-allergic, and anti-cough effects of *Joshanda.*

## Skin Diseases

*Manjishta (Indian maddar), neem (azadiracta indica), saribha (hemidismus indicus)* and the barks and varieties of the family of Ficusaceae are used in treating skin ailments. NEEM capsules, HERBOLINE ointment are available for these disorders. Oil 777 is used in psoriasis.

**The Unani Tibb System of Medicine**

Unani Tibb is based on the ancient Greek and Indian theories of four humours (phlegm, blood, yellow bile, black bile). The imbalance in the humours is responsible for ill health. Faulty digestion is the cause of the imbalance.

Diagnosis entails 'touching' of the skin and examination of general characteristics of the patient to identify his inherent type of temperament and compare it with his current diseased state. Treatment aims at restoring the balance in the body's self-preservation power by correcting the diet and lifestyle and prescribing appropriate drugs.

### Tooth and Gum Paints

GUM TONE reduces inflammation of gums and relieves dental pain. It arrests bleeding and tightens the gums after scaling. This in turn reduces any dental pockets that have formed. It inhibits the growth of salivary bacteria and prevents the formation of cavities in the mouth.

### Anti-anxiety and antidepressants

Tablet, SUMENTA and tablet and syrup BRENTO are used for treatment of anxiety, mental depression and insomnia.

### Memory-Improving Drugs

Popular medicines include VIDYARTHI AMRIT, DIMAGHEEN SYRUP. SHANKHPUSHPI, and DIMAG POUSHTAK RASAYANA. These contain 4 to 12 herbal ingredients, two medicinal plants, *Centella asiatica (brahmi)* and *convolvulus pluricaulis (shankhpushpi)* appear to be common to all the formulations. There is considerable amount of evidence for their CNS effects and facilitation of learning process in the animals. However studies on human beings about the efficacy and safety on individual ingredients or the formulations are scanty.

A widely practised system, Unani Tibb can be used successfully for many day-to-day problems and some chronic ailments.

### Nerves Tonics

Paralysis, neurosthenia, dystrophy and atrophy are treated using *ashwagandha (withania somnifera) bala, dasha moolas* etc. oils (tailas) that are used for external applications are *Dhanwantara Taila, Karpastatyadi Taila, Visha Musti Taila, Mahanarayana Taila, Mahamasha Taila* etc.

### Miscellaneous

The concept of blood purification is unique to *Ayurveda* and *Unani Tibb.* Two popular blood purifiers sold in Indian markets are SURAKTA and SAAFI. The claimed efficacy of these preparations for clearing the complexion and in dermatological diseases is largely uninvestigated.

A large number of digestive and gas-relieving *churans* and tablets are being marketed by various companies. These have not been included in this review. *Ayurvedic* and *Unani* manufacturers, physicians, and self-styled sex-specialists are doing flourishing business by selling aphrodisiacs and sex tonics to gullible patients. There is no true aphrodisiac in any system of medicine. Scientific studies on these are conspicuous by their absence. This aspect is, therefore, left untouched

***Note:*** The herbal medicines are invariably cheaper and available locally. The general belief that herbal drugs are without any side effects is not true. Recently there has been a resurgence of interest in herbal medicines for treatment of various ailments chiefly because of prohibitive cost of allopathic drugs, unavailability in remote areas. Unfortunately, no accurate information about the rational use of these products is available.

Some of the ayurvedic preparations exported from India to Canada and the USA were found to be containing metals in toxic concentrations and have resulted in the banning of these drugs in Canada. The Drug Controller General of India has since made stricter control on the manufacture and analysis of such products.

# 38

# Corticosteroids And Anabolic Agents

••••••

Cortisone was isolated from the adrenal cortex by Kendall in 1939, and he was later awarded the Nobel Prize for this discovery. This discovery was followed by the successful use, not only of *cortisone,* but of several synthetic derivatives of this naturally-occurring substance in the body which are collectively known as *corticosteroids.* During the initial years of their use in the 1950s, these were regarded as miracle drugs because they provided dramatic relief in a variety of disorders related to inflammation and allergy. For this reason, they were more indiscriminately used than any other group of drugs known in medical history. In almost all conditions, except in the case of decreased activity of the adrenal gland, their use is empirical. These drugs do not cure the disease, but only provide symptomatic relief, giving a false sense of well being. In spite of this drawback, these drugs are very useful in certain conditions and their relevance cannot be disputed.

***Functions:*** The function of these hormones is to maintain the internal environment (homeostasis) of the body and to protect against stress (in a stressful situation there is increased secretion of cortisol). These hormones have powerful anti-inflammatory and anti-allergic actions and modify the metabolic functions involving carbohydrates, proteins, fats, minerals, and fluids. They may raise blood sugar and produce a condition similar to diabetes, or may even precipitate diabetes in some individuals. The breakdown of protein is enhanced, whereas, the synthesis is showed down, resulting in weakness and wasting of the muscles. There is increased excretion of *calcium,* causing thinning of the bones. There is loss of potassium and retention of sodium in the body. Along with sodium, water is also retained causing edema (tissue swelling under the skin). In children linear growth retardation is due to early cessation of growing activity in long bones.

## Drugs

The prominent trade names and doses of important *corticosteroids* are given in the table below:

**Some Commonly Used Corticosteroids**

| *Corticosteroid* | *Trade Name(s)* | *Dose Range/mg* |
|---|---|---|
| *Hydrocortisone* (Hemi succinate) | EFCORLIN Soluble | 100-300 mg/day (IV) |
| *Hydrocortisone* (acetate) | WYCORT (TOPICAL) | 25-50 mg intra articular injection |
| Prednisolone | DELTACORIL, WYSOLONE | 10-80 mg |
| Methyl Prednisolone | SOLUMEDROL, LUPUS | 500-1000 mg IV/IM |
| *Triamcinolone* (acetonide) | LEDERCORT, KENACORT | 4-40 mg intra articular |
| Dexamethasone | DECADRON, DEXONA | 4-20 mg/ day IV0.5-5 mg/day Oral |
| Betamethasone | BETNELAN, BETNESOL | 0.5-5; 0.5-5 mg/day Oral |
| Fludrocortisone | FLURICORT | 100 micrograms |
| Desoxycorticosterone acetate | DOCA | 10 mg IM |
| Deflazacort* | DEFZA | 3-18 mg |

* less likey to cause osteoporosis and worsen diabetes.

### Uses

Due to their wide and varied adverse effects on the body metabolism and organ systems, there are no real therapeutic uses of *corticosteroids,* except in substitution therapy for adrenal insufficiency. However, in certain acute inflammatory and allergic conditions associated with severe illness, when other drugs fail, these may be life-saving. Their use is empirical (without any sound basis) and palliative (relieving the symptoms without curing the disease). It must be remembered that if at all necessary, these should be used for as short a duration as possible.

**Substitution Therapy:** *Corticosteroids* are given in conditions associated with the decreased functioning of the adrenal or pituitary glands (e.g. Addison's Disease). In these conditions the level of natural cortisol in the body falls below normal and needs to be substituted till the organ regains normal activity. In this condition small dose is required (*Hydrocortisone* 20 mg morning and 10 mg in the evening) for very long period may be required for lifetime..

## Uses In Large Doses

**In Arthritis:** In rheumatoid arthritis and other kind of arthritides (diseases of the bones and joints) *corticosteroids* should be used only if the disease is progressing in spite of the treatment with other drugs. It must be remembered that once this treatment is begun it has to be continued for several years. If there are periodic attacks of acute inflammation in one or two joints, characterized by reddening, swelling and pain in the joints, *corticosteroids* can be directly injected into the joint cavity. But this should not be done frequently as there may be chances of painless destruction of the joint (Charcot's arthropathy).

**In Rheumatic Heart Disease:** Some physicians prefer *corticosteroids* to *salicylates* for the treatment of acute rheumatic carditis. *Corticosteroids* are more potent anti-inflammatory agents but are more likely to cause rebound inflammation when stopped. Therefore, aspirin cover is provided.

**In Allergic Diseases:** In very severe type of allergic reactions such as anaphylactic shock due to *penicillin,* intravenous *dexamethasone* (8 to 12 mg) may be helpful but it takes more time to act than *adrenaline.* In minor forms of allergic reactions, an antihistaminic drug should be tried before resorting to these drugs (see chapter on 'Drugs Used in Allergy'). In allegic rhinitis, *flunisolide* (SYNTARIS nasal inhaler 25g per puff).

**In Bronchial Asthma:** *Corticosteroids* are used in cases of uncontrollable acute severe asthma. Intravenous soluble steroids are needed in addition to bronchodilating drugs. Inhaled steroids (BECLOMETHASONE DIPROPIONATE 50-100 $\mu$g BECLATE INHALER), *Budesonide* 200-400 $\mu$g (PULMICORT inhaler), *ciclasonide* (CICLOHALE 80-160 $\mu$g) or FLUTICASONE 100-250 $\mu$g (FLOHALE INHALER) are commonly used for maintenance therapy). In chronic bronchial asthma, *corticosteroid* therapy may be considered when all other measures have failed. In such cases the aim of the therapy is to give *corticosteroids* on alternate days or to keep the dosage low enough to reduce the symptoms partially. The patient is encouraged to take the usual medicines along with *corticosteroids* in order to keep the doses of the latter at the minimum level. For this reason a short-acting *corticosteroid* such as *prednisolone* is preferred to the long-acting *betamethasone* or *dexamethasone* (see chapter on 'Bronchial Asthma'). Currently, inhaled drugs are preferred in this situation.

**In Disease of the Eye:** *Corticosteroids* ointment or drops reduce pain, redness, and secretions of the eye caused by the inflammatory condition and provide remarkable relief. These should never be used in bacterial, fungal, or viral infections of the eye as the symptoms of the progression of the disease may be masked until sight is lost. C*orticosteroids* also increase the pressure of the fluids in the eye (intraocular pressure) in some cases and if the pressure is already higher, a painful and disabling condition called Glaucoma may be precipitated. Soft steroids are being developed to reduce the ocular complications.

It is quite depressing to note that a large number of eye drops and ointments available in India contain a combination of these drugs with antibiotics for the treatment of inflammatory conditions of the eye. It is advisable to use an antibiotic separately in case of bacterial infection and *corticosteroid* alone for inflammation. When given in combination, these prolong the infective state. Oral or ocular injections are needed in the treatment of opticneuritis to save eye-sight.

**In Skin Diseases:** Preparations of *corticosteroids,* like ointments, creams, and pastes, are often used for various skin disorders. These do provide dramatic relief, but unfortunately the effect does not last too long. An important use of *corticosteroids* is in eczema in which *hydrocortisone* ointment is usually applied. Pemphigus* is another very important conditions in which it is life-saving is where large doses of *prednisolone,* ranging from 40 to 120 mg per day, are required to be given orally.

**In Shocks:** *Corticosteroids* are often administered in septicemic shock as a desperate attempt to save life. There are many other conditions in which steroids have role to play as palliative drugs. In brain oedema due to tuberculosis and infections, intravenous *dexamethasone* is some times life-saving. Similarly, in injury of backbone large doses prevent paralysis. Steroids are essential component of combined chemotherapy of blood cancers (acute leukaemia) and lymphomas. They are also useful in breast carcinoma and also prevent rise in blood calcium levels in advanced cancers. High doses are given to prevent graft rejection (skin and kidney) in organ

---

*Pemphigus — A distinctive skin disease marked by successive outbreaks of blisters.

transplantation. Steroid enema is useful in ulcerative colitis. They prevent lung damage in aspiration pneumonia and occurrence of respiratory distress in premature newborn. For this purpose they are given to mother in late pregnancy.

***Adverse Effects:*** *Corticosteroids* are known to cause a number of adverse effects, depending upon the dosage and the duration of treatment. A short-term treatment may not pose any problem but when used for a longer time (more than 2 to 3 weeks) three types of problems are known to occur:

1. Adverse effects of *glucocorticoids*
2. Suppression of pituitary control on adrenal gland and
3. Adverse effects due to sudden stoppage of them.

***Adverse Effects of Glucocorticoids:***

1. Fat deposition on face (moon face), shoulders (buffalo hump) and abdomen (pot belly)
2. Skin striation and Fragility
3. A high blood sugar precipitation of diabetes
4. Muscle weakness and thin legs
5. Proneness to infections and delayed healing of wounds
6. Epigastric pain, activation and silent perforation of peptic ulcer
7. Water accumulation in body; weight gain and rise in BP
8. Mental irritability and psychosis
9. Loss of calcium and weakness of bones-flat bones can break easily
10. Rise in tension in eye (glaucoma) and cataract formation
11. Growth retarded (stunted) in children
12. Fetal damage (when used by pregnant mothers)

Alternate day treatment with *prednisolone* reduces these complications

***Adverse Effects Due to Sudden Stoppage After Long-term Use:*** When the steroids are taken for a longer period, normal pituitary control on adrenal is markedly suppressed and adrenal gland shrinks in size. On sudden withdrawal of external steroids, these small adrenals are unable to cope up to increased needs so there are symptoms like generalized body muscles and joint pain and falling blood pressure. This is called adrenal crisis and needs to be avoided by gradual withdrawal of steroids under doctor's supervision. A similar situation may occur in surgical stress because adrenals can not cope up for extra need so additional doses are needed. Any patient who take more than 20 mg hydrocortisone in the last one year may require steroid protection during stress (infection or surgery).

***Precautions:***

1. Newer take corticosteroids on an empty stomach. Patients of hyperacidity or peptic ulcer, should take an antacid tablet or at least milk, along with the medication.
2. A diet rich in proteins should be taken to minimize muscle wasting.
3. Patients of diabetes, should get their blood sugar checked repeatedly and, if necessary, dosages of *insulin* may be increased.

4. Patients of high blood pressure need to get blood pressure checked at frequent intervals and adjust the dosages of the anti-hypertensive drugs if required. It may be necessary to supplement potassium chloride and restrict sodium intake. Hypertensive drugs (oral diuretics) and *corticosteroids* cause loss of potassium from the body.
5. Intensive antibiotic therapy must be instituted without stopping steroids, if there is any kind of infection.
6. Extra calcium and vitamin D should be taken to prevent osteoporosis.
7. Never stop *corticosteroids* abruptly. Sudden withdrawal may cause unpleasant symptoms such as fever, headaches, nausea, vomiting, restlessness, and muscle and joint pains. The best way to withdraw is by supplementing them with other conventional drugs and reducing the doses of *corticosteroids* gradually over a period of time.

### Mineralocorticoids

A *mineralocorticoid* differs from the *glucocorticoids* in that it retains the sodium in the body longer than normal. *Deoxycorticosterone* is one such preparation used as a replacement therapy in chronic primary adrenocortical insufficiency. It is available in a combination with anabolic steroid (DOCABOLIN).

### Anabolic Steroids

These are testosterone (an androgen or male sex hormone derivatives) which are useful in certain conditions with muscle wasting.Some agents which are available and uses are:

**Androgens:** *Testosterone* (Inj AQUAVIRON) 25 mg twice a week.
*Testosterone propionate* and *enanthate* (Inj SUSTANON 100 and 250) once in 3 to 4 weeks.
*Dihydrotestosterone gel* (ANDRACTIM 25 mg/10 Gm ) once daily.

**Anabolics:** *Methandienone* (ANABOLEX 2mg,4 mg) tab
*Stanozolol* (NEURABOL 2mg)
*Oxymetholone* (ADROYD- 5 mg) tab
*Nandrolone phenypropionate* (DURABOLIN 25mg, 50 mg) Inj IM once in a week
*Nandrolone Decanoate* 25mg, 50 mg (DECADURABOLIN) inj IM once in 3 weeks

### Uses

These agents are used in severe muscle wasting in critically ill patients, testicular failure with infertility and hereditary angioneurotic edema(rare). Anabolics are helpful in bone marrow failure (Referactory Anemia), osteoporosis and chronic renal failure.

Unfortunately, these are misused by athletes to increase their performance, but identified in 'Dope tests' leading to disqualification. Actual benefit is also doubtful.

# 39

# General Tonics

••••••

Tonics are popular all over the world. Men take them to increase their vigour and potency. Women take them to overcome weakness and children are advised to take them for better health. Tonics are not new to us. If you trace their history you will find that the *nawabs* and *maharajas* of days gone by patronized *hakims and vaidyas* who fed them expensive tonics to prolong their youth, vigour, and life. These *hakims* and vaidyas were not only treated as VIPs but given exalted titles in addition to gold, silver, and jewels. *Hakims* and *vaidyas* have been replaced by big pharmaceutical companies and the practice of taking tonics has been extended from the rich to the common man.

The manufacture and sale of tonics is a big business today. At one time, only a few pharmaceutical houses in the country made them but during the last few years, companies, new and old, have vied with each other to bring out new brands of their own Many international pharmaceutical houses do not make these tonics for consumption in their own countries, but only for use in India and other developing countries.

## Vitamins and Their Role

Vitamins are naturally occurring 'vital amines', either biosynthesized in the body or made available from foodstuffs like meat, fish, eggs, vegetables, and fruits. These are required for their metabolic role in nutrition and in deficiency diseases. An average Indian diet contains a sufficient amount of vitamins for average daily requirements. The general belief that a slight deficiency of vitamins causes weakness or lowers body resistance, is not correct. On the contrary, excess vitamins may do much harm (discussed later). However, vitamins are required to be given in certain specific situations where the diet is inadequate in quality and quantity such as in alcoholism, to the elderly, debilitated persons, or those on a slimming diet, but it must be remembered that vitamins are no substitute for rich food. Vitamins may also be needed in certain illnesses like prolonged diarrhoea, dysentery or vomiting, infections and worm infestations, or any other prolonged disease. There are other situations in which the requirement is increased, as at the time of pregnancy and lactation. In these cases vitamins are needed in higher quantities than normally required. Besides these, there are certain specific vitamin deficiency diseases in which large doses of a specific vitamin are required in preference to other constituents of the tonic. Same is true for protein and amino acid containing tonics which are available in various flavours along with vitamins. They are no substitute for a balanced diet.

The highly publicized tall claims that a particular tonic increases vitality and zest, muscle strength and memory, or height, are false and misleading. Vitamins do increase metabolic activity and promote growth but this happens only when there is a deficiency. The general belief that if 100 units of a vitamin do good, 1,000 units would do better, is unfounded and erroneous. Most of the popular preparations contain huge quantities, several times more than the daily requirement, plus the extra vitamins added (up to 100%) to cover the loss in storage. A look at the table on 'Important Constituents of Some Popular Tonic Preparations' will indicate the excess of vitamins found in the preparations marketed by some of the most reputed pharmaceutical companies. This is not only an economic waste for an individual but for the entire nation as many of these vitamins or their raw materials are imported by India.

## Methylcobalamin

It is an active form of vitamin B12 and is needed for proper nerve function (Neurotropic factor). Many formulations contain it along with other vitamin B forms, some have Alpha Lipoic acid or ALA (needed for membrane function in nerves) and gabapentin (for diabetic neuritis). Vitamin B12 is stored in our body and if deficiency develops it means all the stored amount is exhausted. Pure vegetarians, chronic alcoholics, those who take too much coffee and those on crash diets develop its deficiency. Executives on the move and taking imbalanced diet are susceptible to its deficiency. Usually deficiency of iron and folic acid coexists and needs to be corrected. Therefore many iron capsules and tablets have all of them together. Some common preparations are:

| | |
|---|---|
| Tab MCBM, METHYCOBAL, MECONEURON | 500µg and Inj MCBM 500µg IM |
| Capsule NEUROKIND-OD, METHYNEURON-OD | 1500µg to be used once a day |
| Capsule MECOLIFE Plus, NERVE-UP Forte, NEUROKIND | Plus have methylcobalamin with ALA and other vit-B factors. |
| Tab PREGAB-M, MAHAGABA-M has Pregabalin | 75mg with methycobalamin 750µg |

Benfotiamine (BENFAG tab 100 mg, 200 mg): It is a modified form of vitamin B1 and is widely used for diabetic and alcoholic neuropathy. It may cause allergic reactions.

### Vitamins : Hazards of Excessive Use

Previously it was believed that the water soluble vitamins like B complex and C are retained in the body up to a certain limit and whatever extra we take are passed out in the urine and unlikely to cause any adverse effects. However, today a number of reports on the adverse effects of large doses of these vitamins are available. The use of these vitamins in large doses, specially by injections, which are completely absorbed, must be avoided. The situation in case of Fat-Soluble vitamins like A and D is still worse. The extra amount taken is deposited in the body to produce a number of adverse effects.

It is not an uncommon observation that patient buys only tonic, instead of antibiotic or other drugs, prescribed by the physician in the hope of curing his weakness. The weakness may in fact be due to infection which requires antibiotic rather than a tonic! So poor man's precious little is lost in vain!

## Iron and treatment of Anaemia

Iron deficiney anaemia is very commonly seen in communities. Females are more affected than males. Iron is required for formation of hemoglobin found in red blood cells.

## Dietary Sources

Liver, dry beans, wheatgerm, yeast, meat, chicken, fresh spinach, banana, apple are good sources. Average daily diet contains 10 to 20 mg of elemental iron.

## A Few Facts about Iron

1. Absorption is better with haem-iron (animal) than others.
2. If food has too much of phytate (maize, wheat) iron is poorly absorbed.
3. Antacids retard absorption.
4. Iron is largely conserved in body. Only negligible amount is lost in urine.
5. We always talk of elemental iron. Various salts available for use have varying amount of elemental iron ferrous sulphate has about 20%, ferrous gluconate about 12% ferrous fumarate 33% and colloidal ferric hydroxide has 50% iron. Iron hydroxy polymaltose is better absorbed.
6. Many preparations have multivitamins also.
7. Among the vitamins, folic acid and vitamin $B_{12}$ are required for formation of hemoglobin. Others may not be needed.
8. It is not true that if higher dose is taken then absorption and effect will be more. In fact there is 'shut-valve' mechanism in the intestinal lining to block absorption of iron if body does not need it.
9. Iron taken by mouth or injections raises hemoglobin by 0.5gm to 1.0gm in a week.
10. Even when the iron deficiency anaemia is fully corrected the treatment is continued further for 2 to 3 months to replete the stores.

## Preparation and Doses

About 200 mg of elemental iron is required per day to be taken by mouth in 3 divided doses. There are only a few products available in market which provide such quantities (See page 234). In selecting a particular preparation, one should consider the amount of elemental iron in it, rather than the quantity of iron-salts in the formula.Carbony iron and iron polymaltose complex are better tolerated and absorbed.

| Daily Requirement of Iron | |
|---|---|
| Male (adult) | 0.5-1.0 mg/day |
| Female (adult) | 1.0-2.0 mg/day |
| Pregnant women | 3.0-5.0 mg/day |
| Children | 25 μg/kg (body weight) |
| Infants | 60 μg/kg (body weight) |

***Adverse Effects:*** Oral iron may not be tolerated equally by all individuals. Epigastric pain, heart burn, nausea, staining of teeth, metallic taste, constipation occur frequently. A smaller dose in between meals initially may improve acceptability. Injectable iron (intramuscular IMFERRON or JECTOFER) may cause joint pains, local pain and pigmentation at the site of injection, fever, headache and allergic reaction with a fall in BP may also occur. Acute iron poisoing may occur due to ingestion

**Some Common Vitamins**

| *Vitamin* | *Normal Daily Requirement* | *Food Sources* |
|---|---|---|
| Vitamin A | 3,000 to 4,000 IU | Liver, fish liver oils, *ghee*, butter, egg, fish, spinach, carrots, green vegetables (carotenoids) |
| Vitamin D* | 400 IU | Fish, egg, butter, milk, exposure of the body to sunlight, yeast |
| Vitamin E | 10 mg | Vegetable oil, leafy vegetables, legumes, egg-yolk, wheat germ oil. |
| Vitamin B Complex | | |
| a. *Thiamine* or Vitamin $B_1$ | 1.5 mg | Unmilled cereals and pulses, meat, dairy products, vegetables, nuts, fruits |
| b. *Riboflavin* or Vitamin $B_2$ | 2 mg | Found in most foods |
| c. *Nicotinamide or Niacin* | 20 mg | Liver, meat, fish, whole cereals, pulses, and groundnuts |
| d. *Pyridoxine* or Vitamin $B_6$ | 2 mg | Liver, meat, fish, whole cereals, pulses, yeast, soybean |
| e. *Folic acid* | 0.2 mg in pregnancy, 0.8mg | Liver, eggs, leafy vegetables, milk |
| f. *Cyanocobalamine* and *Hydroxy cobalomin* Vitamin $B_{12}$ | 1-3 microgram | Liver, fish, eggs, milk, cheese, pulses (legumes) |
| *Ascorbic acid* | 50 mg | Citrus fruits, guava, green leafy vegetables, germinated pulses, tomatoes, potatoes |
| Vitamin K | 50 microgram | Green leafy vegetables, liver, cheese |

*Note:* If you think you really need to take multivitamins, choose the one containing not more than the daily recommended requirement. This will not only save you from its adverse effects but prove to be extremely economical.

* 1 g = 1,000,000 mcg: Initial dose is high 100-200 μg by injections.

**and their Characteristics**

| *Deficiency Diseases* | *Requirement in Deficiency Diseases* | *Adverse Effects of Excessive Intake* |
|---|---|---|
| Diminished vision, rough and dry skin, decreased growth and resistance, corneal softening/opacities, night blindness, sterility | 50,000 to 1,00,000 IU for 3 days | Headache, body aches, irritability, nausea, vomiting, loss of appetite, itching skin, loss of body hair, bone pains, liver disease. |
| Decreased bone growth in children (rickets), thinning of bone in adults (osteomalacia), muscle spasm Deficiency of vitamin-K | 1,000 to 5,000 IU or 3-6 lac IM once in 3-6 months (It is found to cut cancer risk also) | Loss of appetite, nausea, vomiting, diarrhoea, deposition of calcium in tissues, kidney failure, increased thirst. |
| Rupture of red cells, degeneration of nerves, muscles and heart, anaemia | 100 mg or more | Abdominal cramps, delayed wound healing, lethargy. |
| Weakness and tingling sensation in the hands and feet, nervousness, wrist and foot drop, palpitation, heart failure | 100 mg | |
| Ulcers in the mouth, burning sensation in the eyes, scaliness of the skin, loss of hair | 5 to 10 mg | Not much known yet. |
| Diarrhoea, mental symptoms, dementia, ulcers in the mouth, headache, insomnia, skin cracks peels and turns black, anaemia | 200 to 500 mg in divided doses | |
| Ulcers in mouth, nerve damage, convulsions, anaemia, growth retardation | 10-50 mg (10mg with *isoniazid*) 50mg with oral contraceptives | Convulsions, appearance pimples, skin rashes, sensory neuropathy with high dose (2g) |
| Anaemia (large red cells), soreness of tongue, general weakness, loose motions, sterility, weight loss | 5 mg | — |
| Anaemia, sterility, nerve damage, numbness tingling sensation, poor memory, weakness, mood changes | 5 to 10 mcg* (Upto 1500 leg/day in diabetic neuropathy) | Not much known yet. |
| Weakness, anaemia, swelling & bleeding of gums, loose teeth decreased resistance | 500 to 600 mg | Diarrhoea, stone formation in kidneys. |
| Excessive bleeding below skin, blood in urine, nose bleed | 5 to 10 mg | Rupture of red cells in G-6PD deficiency, jaundice in new born. |

* Vitamin D exists in many forms — Cholecalciferol ($D_3$), Calciferol ($D_2$), Calcitriol (potent and active forms), Alphacalcidol.

## Appetite Stimulants

| Brand Names | Vitamins (mg) | | | | | | | |
|---|---|---|---|---|---|---|---|---|
| | $B_1$ | $B_2$ | $B_3$ | $B_6$ | $B_{12}$ | A(IU) | C | D(IU) |
| BAYER'S TONIC LIQUID | — | — | — | — | — | — | — | — |
| BIO VITAL CAP | 10 | 10 | 75 | 2 | 7.5 | — | 150 | — |
| CYP-L LIQUID | — | — | — | — | — | — | — | — |
| NEOGADINE LIQUID | 0.5 | — | — | — | — | 2000 | 15 | 200 |
| SANTEVINI PLUS LIQUID | 0.6 | 0.9 | 10 | 1 | 1 | — | — | — |
| BESTOZYME LIQUID | — | — | — | — | — | — | — | — |
| MERIZYME SYRUP | — | — | 25 | — | — | — | — | — |
| UNIENZYME MPS SYP. | — | — | 25 | — | — | — | — | — |
| UNIENZYME TAB. | — | — | — | — | — | — | — | — |
| VITAZYME | — | — | — | — | — | — | — | — |
| NERVITONE | — | — | — | — | — | — | — | — |

## Mineral-Tonics

| Brand Name | A (IU) | D (IU) | E (mg) | $B_1$ (mg) | $B_2$ (mg) | $B_3$ (mg) | $B_6$ (mg) |
|---|---|---|---|---|---|---|---|
| BECOZINC CAP | — | — | — | 10 | 10 | 50 | 3 |
| BECADEX TAB | 2500 | 200 | — | 2 | 2 | 25 | — |
| DIANUTRIN TAB | 10 | — | 10 | 1 | 1.5 | — | 1 |
| NUTRISAN CAP | 3000 | 300 | 7.5 | 2.5 | 2.5 | 25 | 0.75 |
| POLYZEE CAP | — | — | — | 10 | 10 | 50 | 3 |
| REVITAL (GINSENG) CAP | 2500 | 200 | 10 | 2 | 3 | 20 | 1 |
| SUPRADYN TAB | 10000 | 100 | 25 | 10 | 10 | 100 | 3 |
| Z&B CAP | — | — | 20 | 10 | 10 | 50 | 3 |
| NEUROBION FORTE TAB | — | — | — | 100 | 5 | 45 | 3 |
| COBADEX FORTE CAP | — | — | — | 10 | — | 100 | — |

## and Digestive Syrups

| *Enzymes* | *Proteins* | *Liver Extracts* | *Yeast Extract (mg)* | *Alcohol /15ml* | *Others* |
|---|---|---|---|---|---|
| — | — | 12 | 178.5 | 1.65 | — |
| — | — | — | — | — | Zinc Ginseng extract |
| — Citrate 275 mg | Tricholine | — | — | — | *Cyproheptadine* 2 mg *sorbitol*, tricholine |
| — | — | — | 100 | — | Cyproheptadine 2 mg |
| — | Iodised Peptone 29 mg | — | — | 0.95 ml | Calcium, Magnesium., phosphoric acid, vanadium |
| — | Peptone 300 mg | — | — | — | Calcium, Magnesium., Lysin 100 mg |
| Amylase, papain | Lysine 100 mg<br>Papain | —<br>— | —<br>— | —<br>— | Caraway oil, arise oil |
| Fungal diastage | Papain | — | — | — | Wood charcoal *dimethicone* |
| " " | Papain | — | — | — | Charcoal |
| " " | Papain | — | — | — | *Simethicone* |
| " " | — | — | — | — | Caraway, Cinnamon, Cardamom |
| — | 75 mg | — | 400 mg | 1.75 ml | Calcium, Magnesium, Mineral |

## and Multivitamin Preparations

| *Pentothenic (mg)* | *Biotin (mg)* | *Folic acid (mg)* | *$B_{12}$ (mg)* | *C (mg)* | *Zinc (mg)* | *Calcium (mg)* | *Selenium (mg)* |
|---|---|---|---|---|---|---|---|
| 12.5 | — | 1mg | 15 | — | 54.93 | — | — |
| — | — | — | — | 30 | — | 250 | — |
| — | — | — | | 50 | 15 | 162 | 7.5 |
| — | — | 0.5 | 2.5 | 40 | 20 | 150 | — |
| 25 | — | — | 15 | 150 | 22.5 | — | — |
| 5 | — | 03 | 1 | 50 | — | 75 | — |
| 16.3 | 0.25 | — | 15 | 150 | 2.2 | 129 | — |
| 12.5 | — | 1 | 15 | 150 | 27.5 | — | Chromium |
| 50 | — | — | 15 | — | — | — | — |
| 50 | — | 0.15 | 15 | 150 | — | — | — |

## Iron Preparations*

| Name | Iron Compound | Other Ingredients |
|---|---|---|
| CONVIRON-TR Cap | Fe. Sulfate (dried) 60mg | $B_{12}$ 15µg, folic acid 1.5mg, $B_6$ 1.5mg, vit. C75mg |
| FESOVIT-SPANSULE Cap | Fe. Sulfate (dried) 150mg | $B_{12}$ µg, folic acid 1mg, nicotinamide 50mg, $B_6$ 2mg |
| FEFOL SPANSULE Cap | Fe. Sulfate 150mg | Folic acid 0.5mg |
| HEMGLOB Syrup (15ml) | Fe. gluconate 300mg | $B_{12}$ 15µg, $B_1$ 5mg, $B_2$ mg, $B_6$ 1.5mg, niacinamide 45mg |
| AUTRIN Cap | Fe. fumarate 350mg | $B_{12}$ 15 µg, folic acid 1.5mg, vit. C 150mg |
| DUMASULES Cap | Fe. fumarate 300mg | $B_{12}$ 7.5µg, folic acid 0.75mg, B. 5mg, niacinamide 50mg, vit. C 75mg, $B_6$ 1.5mg |
| HEMSYNERAL Cap, FIFA Tab | Fe. fumarate 200mg | $B_{12}$ 15µg, folic acid 1.5mg |
| HEMATRINE Cap | Fe. succinate 100mg | $B_{12}$ 2.5µg, folic acid 0.5mg, vit. C 25mg, niacinamide 15mg |
| POLYRON Tab, BIOFER Tab | Iron hydroxy, polymaltose | Folic acid 0.35mg |
| POLYFER chewable Tab | Iron 100mg | |
| TONOFERON Syrup (5ml) | Colloidal ferric hydroxide 500 mg (iron 250 mg) | Folic acid 0.5mg, $B_{12}$ 5µg |
| Drops (1 ml) | - do – 50 mg (Iron 25 mg) | folic aid 0.2 mg, $B_{12}$ 5 µg |
| FERROCHELATE Syrup (5ml) | Ferric ammon, cit. (Iron 60 mg) | $B_{12}$ 5 µg, folic acid 1 mg |
| Drops (1 ml) | - do – (Iron 20 mg) | $B_{12}$ 4 µg, folic acid 0.2 mg |
| HAEM UP Liquid (15 ml) | Ferric ammon. cit. 100 mg | Cu $SO_4$ 30 µg, Mn $SO_4$ 30 µg, Zn $SO_4$ 30 µg |
| HAEM UP Gems | Ferric ammon. cit. 100 mg + Haemoglobin 0.65 µg | Cu $SO_4$ 2.5 µg, Mn $SO_4$ 2.5 µg, Zn $SO_4$ 4.5 µg |
| RARICAP Tab | Iron cal. complex (Iron 25 mg) | folic acid 0.3 mg |
| Syrup (5 ml) | - do-(5% iron) 500 mg | Vit. A 200 i.u., $B_1$ 1.5 mg, $B_2$ 2 mg, nicotinamide 20 mg, Vit $D_3$ 150 IU |
| PROBOFEX Cap | Fe. aminoate 600 mg | $B_{12}$ 15 µg, folic acid 1.5 mg, $B_6$ 3 mg |
| Syrup (15 ml) | - do-(10% iron) 300 mg | $B_{12}$ 15 µg, folic acid 1.5 mg, $B_6$ 3 mg |
| DEXORANGE Cap | Ferric ammon. cit. 160 mg | $B_{12}$ 7.5 µg, folic acid 0.5 mg |
| HEMFER Cap | Ferrous glycine (50 mg iron) | $B_{12}$ 7.5 µg, folic acid 0.5 mg, Vit. C 75 mg, Zinc 5 mg |
| FEROX Cap | Carbonyl iron 60 mg | $B_{12}$ 5 µg, folic acid 1 mg, Vit. E 15 IU selenium 60 µg, |
| FEROMALT, FERRIUM Tab | Iron (III) Hydroxide polymaltose complex 100 mg | folic acid 0.3 mg |
| DUMASULES-Z Cap | Ferrous fumerate 100 mg | $B_{12}$ 1 µg, Folic acid 0.3 mg, Vit. C 50 mg, Zinc 41.4 mg |
| DEXORANGE Cap | Ferric amm. citrate 160 mg | $B_{12}$ 7.5 g, Folic acid 0.5 mg, Zinc sulphate 20.0 mg |
| GLOBAC-XT Tab | Ferrous bisglycinate 60 mg | Folic acid 1 mg, Methylcobalamin 0.5 mg, Zinc 15 mg |
| FERISAN Tab | Sod Ferredate 700 mg | Folic acid 1.5 mg, B12 15µg, zinc 61.4 mg |
| AXIFER, IREX Tab (33 mg) | Feredate sodium | |
| ALOHA-XT (100 mg) | Ferrous ascorbate | |

*Many preperations have multivitamins also.

of large quantities of liquid iron preparation by children the anti dale is *desferrioxamine* (5 to 10 gm) milk and egg yolk may be given as first aid, after inducing vomiting by tickling of fauces.

## Other Minerals

Copper, cobalt, selenium, zinc, manganese, molybdenum, selenium and magnesium are required in very small quantities (trace amounts). All of them are needed for activation of certain enzymes. Zinc deficiency may cause growth retardation in children, copper deficiency leads to anemia in under nourished children. A number of multi vitamin and iron preparations contain varying amounts of these trace elements. The use of these in normal persons can not be recommended.

**Choosing a right vitamin preparation**

If we are eating a balanced diet there is no need for extra vitamins. In persons older than 35 years, eating out frequently and on pure vegetarian diet, some vitamins may be needed. A multivitamin preparation which contains RDA of vitamins is ideal. Since it is to be used regularly it should not be costly. We feel, if used for limited period, Tab SUPRADYN (it has fat soluble vitamins so avoid overuse), BECOZYM C FORTE, BEPLEX FORTE TAB, POLYZEE, COBADEX FORTE, BECOSULE, NUTRISAN and alike are suitable for use ( We do not endorse any of these brands of course!). Addition of extra frills such as ginseng, green tea extract, gingko, brahmi primrose oil just are flavours (have unproven efficacy) and increase cost unnecessarily.

One must avoid overdoses of fat soluble vitamins(A,D,E,K), vitamin C and others. Excess of vitamin D reduces vitamin K and calcium absorption, iron in large amount reduces absorption of zinc, copper and calcium. Excess of folic acid reduces zinc absorption.

# 40

# Slimming Drugs

We are becoming one among the top obese nations. Half of the Indian workforce is considered overweight and about 3% of all females are obese. Our country would incur an accumulated loss of over $ 20 billion by 2015 due to unhealthy life style. Indian men are more prone to develop truncal (belly) obesity-a risk factor for heart disease. A study shows that 17% of Indian youth aged 14 to 18 years are overweight or obese. Your child should be considered obese if the BMI is in excess of 21.5 (boys) and 21.6 (girls) at the age of 14 years, 22.7 (boys) and 23.7 (girls) at the age of 16 years and 23.2 (boys) and 23.9 (girls) at the age of 18 years.

The measure of overweightness is called as Body-Mass-Index (BMI) and is obtained by dividing weight (kg) with square of height in metres. Table-1 shows the BMI values.

## Do Obesity and Inactivity Run Parallel?

Some highly obese individuals have been men of eminence and action. Napoleon heads this category. Winston Churchill was highly obese and so was Mussolini. Khwaja Nazimuddin, the former Chief Minister of undivided Bengal, who later became the Prime Minister of Pakistan, was really fat. In our own country, the 'Nightingale of India', Sarojini Naidu, who had won millions of hearts and delighted us not only with her captivating poetry but also by her beautiful prose for more than half a century, was highly obese.

**How to Calculate Your Body Mass Index (BMI)**

A good way of determining whether you are overweight or not is to look at your Body Mass Index. Body Mass Index factors both your height and weight in determining excess weight.

$$\text{Body Mass Index} = \frac{\text{Weight in kg}}{(\text{Height in metres})^2}$$

The result is compared with the table below:

| | *Underweight* | *Ideal* | *Overweight* | *Obese* | *Externaly obese* |
|---|---|---|---|---|---|
| BMI for Men | <18.4 | 18.5-24.9 | 24-29.9 | 30-34.9 | > 35 |
| BMI for Women | 33700 more | — | — | 30000 more | 82000 more |

This does not mean that obesity is not a disadvantage. These individuals have been exceptions rather than the rule. Who knows, they may have done better and even more work than they did, but for their obesity. Generally, a fat man carries a psychological burden of rejection by his colleagues, relatives, peers, employers, and even by his physician. The life expectancy is reduced as the body weight increases (See table). Recent studies have clearly shown that persons overweight by 8 kg or more have a much higher probability of getting a heart attack than individuals in the normal weight range.

The cut off for action to be initiated is waistline over 72 cms in Indian men (as against international level of 80 cms).

***Causes:*** Excessive intake of calories (fats) results in fat deposition particularly when physical activity is limited. There are various causes of obesity such as hormonal changes during pregnancy, genetic or familial obesity and hormonal diseases such as hypothyroidism, alcoholism, and stress. Emotional disturbance and stress may result in abnormal eating patterns such as night-time over-eating and binge eating. Research shows that fat cells are larger and more in number in obese persons and this could be a developmental factor. Some drugs like antipsychotics, antidepressants, corticosteroids and oral contraceptives may also cause a gain in weight. Change in lifestyle and domestic invasion of electronic gadgets leads to obesity. The risk of obesity rises 65% when one takes a cola drink daily.

The fat truths about children are poor eating habits such as eating while watching TV, not taking tiffin in school and taking excess of junk-food-pizzas, burgers etc and lack of physical activity are responsible for childhood obesity. Women who resort to 'fasting as a religious ritual' and take 'fasting food' should be alarmed at the calories they are taking as be the 'junk food' gulpers (Table-). It is observed that many working women starve in the day and guzzle calories at night! Drunkrexia — not taking day meals to have enough drinks at a night party — should be discouraged.

| *Ready-Food* | *Calories (Kcal)* | *How to burn them* |
|---|---|---|
| 1 slice pizza | 250 | 1.5 hour cycling |
| 1 Cheese burger | 330 | Swimming 1 hour |
| 1 medium French fries | 300 | Jogging 30 mins |
| 1 Pastry | 500 | Tennis 1.5 hours |
| 1 samosa | 150 | Dancing 30 mins |
| 1 Cola (200 ml) | 110 | Skipping 15 mins |
| *Fasting Indian food* | | |
| Dry Fruit Khoya Barfi | 350/2 pieces | — |
| Sabudana Namkeen | 250/100 Gm | — |
| Potato-pakoda | 250/2 pieces | — |
| Kuttu-atta Puri | 100 per puri | — |

***Why is it Necessary to Treat Obesity?*** The successful treatment of fatness or obesity can be highly gratifying both to the patient and to the physician. Based on statistics, there is enough evidence to show that obesity may lead to diabetes, thyroid dysfunction, infertility and poor sperm quality, respiratory distress, and various other diseases. Obese people get tired soon, develop sleep apnoea (moments of cessation of breathing at night) have frequent low backaches and, knee pains, swelling of feet (oedema) and sweat more often on exertion. Fat accumulates in the abdomen in males and in thighs and buttocks in females. Abdominal obesity is a risk factor for coronary heart disease (Syndrome-X is a constellation of abdominal obesity, high blood pressure, high cholesterol, heart disease and resistance to insulin impaired glucose tolerance).

***What Measures Are Necessary to Correct or Avoid Obesity?*** The imbalance between energy needed and consumed can be corrected in two ways: by reducing the food intake and by physical exercise. It is said that the best principle of dieting is to eat when you feel like it and eat only to inhibit your hunger but not to fill the belly. The diet should be low in calories. Cakes, pastries, nuts, *samosas, kachoris,* pizzas, chocolate, ice-creams, sweets, and fried foodstuffs should be avoided. Fruits and vegetables have relatively fewer calories and should be eaten in abundance. *If a rich man eats the poor man's diet and the latter eats the rich one's, it will be good for both.*

Vigorous exercise such as jogging or skipping can be helpful in reducing weight at a faster rate. Although it is easy to suggest ways of losing excess weight, in practice it is difficult and requires considerable effort, determination, and will-power. In one extensive survey it was found that only about 25% of the grossly obese cases were able to reduce as much as 10 kg, and only 5% as much as 20 kg or more. The follow-up study indicated that the majority of them returned to their former weight after the strict regimen was withdrawn. It is, therefore, important that once the weight loss is achieved, the patient should maintain it. He must make it a routine to do every activity at a swifter rate. He should walk briskly, climb the stairs faster, make every movement quicker. It has been estimated that by walking briskly for a particular distance, person consumes about 4 times the amount of calories than while walking slowly.

***Can Drugs Really Help?*** It is common knowledge that fat persons often have a liking for foods *jalebis* or *halwa, and* fried potatoes which are rich in calories and comparatively poor in proteins. When they start eating they seldom stop. They appear to suffer from some kind of a psychological disorder of compulsive eating. So, are appetite-inhibiting pills the answer? Drugs help as long as you take them, but even these may fail if you are not determined to eat less. Drugs can achieve about 10% reduction in body weight when taken for about 3 to 6 months. The effect lasts only as long as the drug is taken.

## Drugs

For reducing weight two types of drugs are used: 1) those which form a bulk in the stomach and give the feeling of fullness, and 2) those which act on the feeding centre of the brain to inhibit the appetite.

### Drugs that Make You Feel Full

**Methyl Cellulose** (METHYL CELLULOSE GRANULES, LIMICAL BISCUITS, BRAN)
In an attempt to reduce the caloric value, while providing a feeling of fullness, *methylcellulose,* a non-digestible substance, is available in the form of granules or biscuits (3 to 4 gm/day). It is taken with water before meals and swells in the stomach. It does fill the stomach and may help some obese patients to overcome the feeling of emptiness and decrease the intake of other foods, but is no more effective than the high-residue, low-calorie diet. This is of very little value as a

slimming aid. However, it has no CNS stimulant effect and is thus free of the side-effects associated with the drugs described later. Abdominal bloating and faecal impaction may occur.

*Medislim* and similar powders (low calorie, low fat nutraceuticals) are promoted for obesity. These are costly substitutes to a strong will-power!

## Drugs Acting on the Feeding Centre of the Brain

**Sibutramine** (OBESTAT, SIBUTREX 5 mg, 10 mg)
It is a commonly used drug for obesity. It suppresses appetite and increases heat production from fat by activating Beta-3 receptors of fat cells. It can reduce weight by 3 to 9 kg in 5 to 6 months. Its adverse effects are constipation, dry mouth, anxiety, loss of sleep and some rise in blood pressure and may pose problems in diabetics. It has also caused cardiac problems and at present it is being evaluated further.

**Orlistat** (ORLICA, LIPOPHAGE , ZEROFAT 60 mg, 120 mg cap)
This is a new anti-obesity drug which inhibits the absorption of fats in the diet. As a result 30% of the dietary fat remains unabsorbed and is excreted in the faeces. One of the adverse effects of this drug is oily spotting from the rectum and faecal incontinence. This drug is to be taken in a dose of 120 mg during or before every main meal. Fat soluble vitamins supplementation should be taken with it. If 5% weight reduction is not achieved in 12 weeks then it should be discontinued.

**Olestra** is a sucrose polyester which can be used as substitute for cooking oil. It is not utilized by the body and is eliminated in stools.

**Rimonoband** (RIMOSLIM, RIOMONT 20 mg tab):
This is an interesting drug which controls weight and is most suitable for diabetics with Syndrome-X. In diabetics it controls metabolic (fats) disturbances. Its actions are on brain hunger-centers which are activated by special receptors (CB1 receptors), blocked by this drug. Its usual dose is 20 mg a day. Unforunately it causes depression and suicidal tendencies. Hence, should never be used in depressive illness. Presently it is withdrawn from market in India and many other countries.

*Metformin* (GLYCIPHAGE-500 mg), a drug for diabetes is also found to reduce weight in nondiabetic obese individuals. Females with polycystic ovarian disease and obesity benefit most from this agent.

**Note:** A word of caution! Slimming is good only within limits. Don't overdo it. Excessive slimming, with or without drugs, cannot make every woman look like a model. It may even end up making her look like a starved! The average middle-class Indian woman has much less flesh and more fat in her body than her Western counterpart. She cannot afford to lose too much of the fat or she will look like a skeleton. Someone has said aptly that a little fat makes a woman look enviable; if it is more, she is called pleasantly plump, but if it is too much, she can only be pitied.

# 41

# Drug Abuse

Any drug when used for a non-medical purpose, is said to be misused or abused. During the last few decades, drug abuse has become a serious problem for the individual and society. Besides adversely affecting the well being, progress, and the health of the user, it is a cause of tragedy to the family life of these persons. Amongst those who handle drugs, that is, the doctor, the nurse, the pharmacist, and the patient, the maximum responsibility for the proper distribution of drugs is that of the pharmacist. Under the laws of India drugs, which can be abused, are dispensed by the pharmacist, only under a doctor's prescription and are controlled by the legal provisions of the Drugs and Cosmetics Act. Non-compliance of this Act by the pharmacist can promote the misuse of drugs and thus bring misery to the user.

To understand the phenomenon of drug abuse it is important to know a few terms which are commonly used in this context and the classification of drugs of abuse.

**Drug Dependence:** This is a biological phenomenon which consists of psychic dependence and physical dependence. Psychic dependence is seen in the form of compulsive and repeated drug-taking for personal satisfaction. Heavy cigarette smoking is an example. Physical dependence which is present when withdrawal of a drug produces symptoms that are opposite to those sought by the user. Alcohol withdrawal syndrome is a common example. The term 'addiction' is also used sometimes in place of dependence and includes both psychic and physical dependence.

**Drug Tolerance:** After repeated use of a drug, a larger dose is needed to produce the same effect, indicating the tolerance is supposed to have developed in the individual for that drug. Tolerance is closely associated with the phenomenon of physical dependence and in almost all such cases, the person needs a larger dose of the drug for the same effect. For example, persons who are dependent on *morphine* may, at times, need 200 times the usual dose for its euphoric effects.

**Drugs as Reinforcers:** A number of psychoactive drugs serve as reinforcers to initiate a self-administration habit, and when the drug is repeatedly used, it can cause compulsive drug abuse behaviour. In humans, reinforcement is in the form of a feeling of pleasure, relief of pain, discomfort, or an altered perception. Reinforcement behaviour has been extensively studied in rats, monkeys, and baboons and shows certain patterns of self-administration of drugs. In humans, it may act as a reinforcer even in the absence of physical dependence or any pre-existing psychopathological conditions.

### Drugs in Beverages and Tobacco

1. *Caffeine* in tea, coffee, cold drinks: A cup of tea may carry 30 to 45 mg, coffee, 80 to 100 mg; and cola drinks, about 30 mg of *caffeine.* No serious harm is done by repeated consumption. Non-availability of these drinks can lead to a mild headache and bodyache.
2. *Ethyl alcohol:* If used habitually, it may cause dependence or addiction and tolerance, and may thus end up causing physical and economic ruin to the user and associated misery to the family. If alcohol is taken in high doses, it causes behavioural changes, mental confusion, incoordination, and coma. Diagnosis of alcohol toxicity can be extremely difficult if a sick or injured person happens to have taken alcohol as well. Alcohol enhances the sedative properties of antihistaminics and of tranquillizers, and thus causes unwanted side-effects. In these situations its use is contraindicated. Ethyl alcohol, if adulterated with or substituted by methyl alcohol, can cause severe poisoning, leading to acidosis unconsciousness and blindness.
3. *Nicotine:* it is taken in a number of forms of tobacco, in bidies, cigarettes, in *paan,* or as snuff (intranasal administration). While tobacco consumption does not benefit the user, it has been clearly established that it is the cause of many chronic ailments and it can decrease longevity which is evident from the adjacent graph:

**Adverse Effects of Smoking:** Men smoke more often than women in India but the incidence of smoking in villager women is very high. One of the common ill-effects of smoking is lung cancer. Giving up smoking reduces the risk of premature death, and after 10 years, the risk approximates to that of a lifelong non-smoker. The risk of developing cancer of the mouth and throat is 5 to 10 times more in smokers than in non-smokers. Under the age of 65, smokers are about twice as likely to die of coronary heart disease as are non-smokers, and heavy-smokers, about 3.5 times as likely. The narrowing of the smallest coronary arteries is enormously increased in heavy and even moderate smokers. Other problems faced by smokers are chronic bronchitis and chronic lung disease leading to congestive heart failure. Women who smoke are more likely to be infertile or take longer to conceive than women who do not smoke. They also run the risk of spontaneous abortion.

**How Smoking Increases the Risk of Death Before 65 Years of Age**

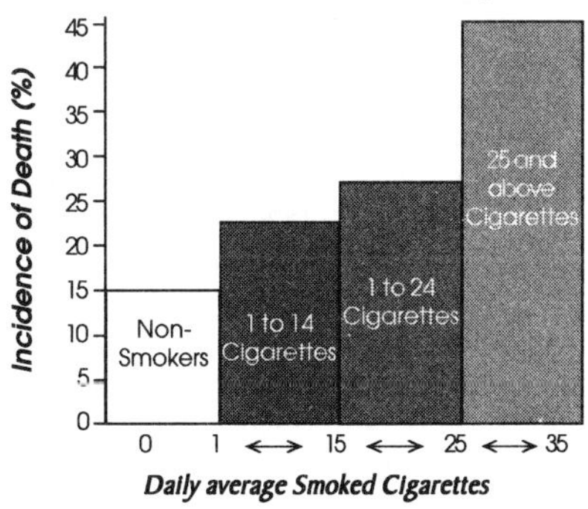


**Smoking Cessation Techniques:** There are many smokers who wish to quit, but peer pressure and withdrawal effects reinduct them back to smoking. They are often heard saying 'Smoking is easy to quit, I have done it many times'! Proper education and behavioural interventions help them. Some drugs also help. Nicotine replacement therapy and role of *Bupropion* is discussed in the chapter on 'Smoking and effects of drugs'.

## Prescribed Drugs

Drugs like *morphine, meperidine (pethidine),* barbiturates, tranquillizers, and *amphetamine* are to be used only on a doctor's prescription but those who have easy reach to these drugs tend to misuse them and thus develop drug depend.

Tolerance to these drugs is not as severe as that to alcohol and *morphine.* Only a psychological dependence is perceived. A physician, pharmacist or a nurse should not hesitate to familiarize patients with their harmful effects and the risks involved therein.

The patterns of addiction development and types of behavioural symptoms of drug dependence vary from drug to drug and the socio-cultural background. It is, therefore, difficult to prescribe any one uniform treatment for various forms of drug abuse. The management of drug addiction should be carefully worked out for each drug but psychotherapy and later, social rehabilitation programmes, help considerably in bringing back the addicted person to a normal life.

For long-term management of opiate dependence, two pharmacological methods are basically employed: opiate maintenance and use of opiate antagonists. *Methadone* maintenance aims to achieve a stabilisation on the drug, gradually increasing the dose until a high degree of cross tolerance develops, so much so that the euphoric feeling even from high doses of other opioids is not experienced (narcotic blockade). In this program the patient is given a daily oral

**Banned Drugs**

1. *Heroin* is the most dangerous drug because of its addiction liability which includes both psychological and physical dependence components, both of a very severe type. It is for this reason that the manufacture, sale, and distribution of this drug is banned. It is a synthetic derivative of *morphine* and is available through clandestine sources. Anyone dealing with *heroin* is severely dealt with by law enforcement authorities. *Codeine* is a milder drug present in a number of cough syrups. These liquid preparations have been misused by those who find difficulty in procuring *heroin* and *morphine.*
2. *Cocaine* is obtained from plant sources and is also highly addicting. It is used intravenously and also intranasally. It can produce severe toxicity, sometimes unexpectedly, even under a doctor's supervision. It became popular in the 1930s and in the 1980s, it came back with a bang and has done considerable harm to the population.
3. *Cannabis (charas, ganja), marijuana,* and other hallucinogens like *lysergic acid diethylamide* (LSD) are not used medically but used by individuals for the strange feelings and experiences provided by them. These drugs cause changes in thought, perceptions, mood and behaviour. Of these LSD is the most potent. *Ganja* and *charas* are more potent than *bhang* and unlike *bhang* which is taken orally, these are mostly smoked. The active principle present in these substances is *tetrahydrocannabinol* which is absorbed in the blood from the lungs and, therefore, brings about an effect as immediate as seen by intravenous administration. It leads to an increased heart rate and reddening of the conjunctiva. The blood pressure may fall and the appetite is increased. Heavy smokers of *marijuana* suffer from chronic bronchitis and tracheal obstruction. Their driving ability may be adversely affected.
4. A combination of *methaqualone* and *diphenhydramine (MANDRAX)* originally introduced as a hypnotic agent, went into extensive abuse, particularly by the student community, and is now a banned preparation. However, off and on, this preparation is found in the clandestine market.

dose of *methadone* that does not cause sedation, constipation or other effects but is high enough to prevent the craving for the opiate. The *methadone* dose is gradually tapered down to zero in the course of the next 4 to 6 weeks. When the patient does not get the desirable euphoric effect, he may stop craving for the drug and may soon discontinue it. *Naltrexone*, an opiate antagonist effective by mouth, is given to post-addicts to reduce craving. The patient should be opiate free for 7 to 10 days, then 25 mg *Naltrexone* (NALTIMA) is given initially then dose increased to 50 mg once a day.

### Misuse of Antianxiety and Sleep-inducing Drugs

Now a days *benzodiaozepines (Diazepam)* are increasingly used for inducing sleep and to allay anxiety. When used for more than two weeks some degree of physical and psychic dependence develops. Persons may have poor muscular coordination (driving may be erratic) and reduced alertness. Judgement errors and lack of concentration may affect studies. There may be sleep disturbance.

If stopped all of sudden, then a state of drunkenness and excitation may occur. These features may resemble acute alcohol intoxication. The *benzodiazepines* may have to be given again in smaller doses to avoid serious consequences and then gradual reduction is done over several days.

# 42

# Alcohol

Any discourse on medicines will be incomplete unless it includes alcohol. Alcohol has been more misused than any other substance in history, billions of rupees worth of alcohol is being consumed daily. Only a small fraction of it is employed for its medicinal properties. Nevertheless, this does not decrease its value as an effective and basically useful medicinal substance. If used discreetly, it can serve as a very useful therapeutic tool, while its indiscriminate consumption results misery and the ultimate ruin of many families.

**Where Does Alcohol Go in the Body?** Alcohol is one of the very few substances which goes into the bloodstream directly from the stomach. Most of the other foods and drugs travel right up the intestines before passing into the blood. After reaching the blood it goes to other parts of the body, but the liver is where it is primarily metabolized (broken down) to carbon dioxide and water.

**Is it a Food?** Yes, it is, but incomplete and expensive! It provides energy more quickly than any other food. It is rich in calories and carries 7 calories per gram, while carbohydrates and fats provide 4 and 9 calories per gram, respectively. A bottle of beer (650 ml) contains 250 calories, while 100 ml of whisky carries 400 calories. Since it does not require any digestion, it can serve as a ready source of energy. However, due to its quick metabolism, the energy cannot be stored and are called empty calories. A normal person metabolizes about 10 g of alcohol (a small peg of whisky) in 1 hour, and if the intake is limited to one peg per hour, one may never get drunk and the blood concentration will not rise beyond 0.1%.

**Beverages and their Alcoholic Content**

| *Beverage* | *Source* | *Alcohol %* |
|---|---|---|
| Beer | Cereals | 4-8 |
| Wine | Grape Juice | 10-22 |
| Champagne | Grape Juice | 12-13 |
| Cider | Apple Juice | 8-12 |
| Whisky | Cereals | 51-59 |
| Brandy | Wine/ Fermented Fruit Juice | 43-57 |
| Rum | Molasses | 51-59 |
| Gin | Cereals | 51-59 |
| Rectified Spirit | Cereals | 95 |

**Does it Make You Fat?** Since alcohol provides readily available energy, it spares carbohydrates, proteins, and fats from their breakdown for the supply of energy, and even if you eat the normal diet along with it, you will get fat. Ordinarily one tends to eat more after consuming alcohol and if this becomes a regular habit, it soon makes one excessively obese.

**Is it a Stimulant?** It is generally believed that alcohol is a stimulant but this belief is only a myth. It is not a stimulant of the nervous system; rather, it has a definite depressant action. In adequate doses it promotes sleep and in very high doses, it may depress most of the areas in the brain and cause respiratory arrest and even death. This is a common method of death due to ingestion of large quantities of alcohol.

The general impression that alcohol is an excitant, is due to the fact that it also depresses the areas of the brain responsible for playing an inhibitory role. We all have our inhibitions which guide our conduct and behaviour, which vary according to the circumstances and environment. Our behaviour, choice of words, and responses vary considerably when we are in the presence of our teachers and parents on the one hand, and our friends and colleagues on the other. Under the effect of alcohol, the inhibitions which keep our true behaviour masked in the presence of seniors, are suppressed and our true self emerges. This aberration of cultivated social behaviour or, more truly speaking, the exposure of our true self, if generally mistaken as the result of the stimulant action of alcohol. However, all available scientific evidence indicates that it has a depressant action.

**Does Alcohol Benefit Heart?** Yes and no? Yes, because regular intake of small amount (one drink) raises heart-protective cholesterol fraction (HDL-C) and decreases activation of LDL-C (which is harmful). This may be the cause of lower (15 to 30%) rate of occurrence of heart attacks. This protective effect is lost if intake is over 3 drinks per day. Moderate intake also raises blood pressure and directly weakens the heart muscles. Heart rhythm irregularities are common in chronic alcoholics. Wines (red wine) have antioxidants and are considered to provide better protection than other preparations.

**Does It Affect Acquired Skills?** Most habitual consumers of alcohol boast that their performance of skilled tasks is not adversely affected by alcohol, but this is not true. In vehicle driving, the judgement is impaired, the reaction time increases, and alcohol is the major cause of road accidents. The same is true for typing or marksmanship, where the speed may increase but inaccuracies multiply.

**Does It Affect Behaviour?** The behavioural pattern of the individual is dependent on the blood concentration of alcohol, which, in its turn, is primarily dependent on the quantity ingested and the frequency of intake. If the blood concentration of alcohol is within 0.1%, the behaviour of the person is apparently normal, self-confidence increases, shyness disappears, after-dinner speeches come easy, and he is altogether delightful company. In higher concentration, up to 0.3 %, he becomes emotionally unstable and his thoughts get disoriented. There is motor incoordination, loss of all self-control; the speech gets slurred and the gait (walking) is affected. Higher concentrations may result in unconsciousness, coma, and eventually death.

**Is Alcohol A Sexual Stimulant?** Such is the general impression. It is true that a large number of sex offences are related to the influence of alcohol but it does not necessarily mean that alcohol is a sexual stimulant. Alcohol, by dulling inhibitions, removes shyness and promotes sexual advances (which would not otherwise be made) but the sex act, if it takes place at all, suffers. Shakespeare writes in *Macbeth* (Act 2, Scene 3): 'It provokes the desire but takes away the performance'. This is a fact.

**How to Manage Alcohol Intoxication?** Quite often one faces a situation when someone has taken too much alcohol and his condition is bad. If a doctor is not available, some simple measures can be taken. The first thing to do is to remove unabsorbed alcohol from the stomach. If the patient is conscious, he should be encouraged to vomit it out by putting two fingers on the back part of the tongue and pressing it. This should be followed by giving him a preparation containing about 100 mg of caffeine. Alternatively, one or two cups of strong tea or coffee may be given. If he has vomited, he should be given plenty of fluids to make up the fluid loss.

## Chronic Alcoholism

Habitual indulgence in alcohol in excess is easily understandable when one considers that it is taken not only for its local effects on the organs of taste and on the mucous membrane of the mouth and stomach, but for its action on the brain in dulling the consciousness of unhappiness. This weakening of the higher sensibilities by alcohol, is generally the objective sought by a drunkard. He finds that under the influence of alcohol, his habitual depression disappears; he loses the sense of degradation and remorse which possesses him when sober; he attains false courage and is inspired with a sense of adequacy which he normally lacks otherwise. As has been so aptly expressed by Samuel Johnson; 'In the bottle, discontent seeks for comfort, cowardice for courage, and shyness for confidence'. The depression and senses of frustration and inadequacy return in exaggerated form after the effects of alcohol have worn off, and though they can be removed again by the same means, the habit is formed, each successive dose being rendered necessary by the depression produced by its predecessor. This descent into chronic drunkenness is facilitated by the lessening of self-control owing to the action of alcohol on the brain. The victim may form the best of resolutions, but his impaired will-power and self-control prevent him from carrying them out.

Excessive and prolonged use of alcohol (chronic alcoholism) may cause weakening of the mucous membranes of the throat, stomach, and intestines. There are frequent attacks of sore throat (chronic catarrh) and poor absorption of nutrients from the intestines. Other organs affected are the liver and heart. In these organs degeneration of tissues occurs with the deposition of fat (fatty degeneration). The liver appears to be more susceptible. In the advanced stage, cirrhosis of the liver may occur with a fatal outcome. The chemical 'aldehyde' formed in the liver and loss of protective materials (gluthathione) in the presence of deficiency of nutrients is the cause of liver fibrosis. However, in Scotland, where the consumption of whisky is very high, cirrhosis is very rare. It may have something to do with the nutrition as chronic alcoholism is associated with the poor absorption of nutrients.

## Treatment

It is not easy to treat an alcoholic. Generally, his craving for alcohol is stronger than any reasoning. It would be a great mistake to suddenly stop him from taking alcohol. Such a step may precipitate many other serious health problems which may worsen his condition. He may, however, be encouraged to reduce the consumption. *Diazepam* like drugs may be given to reduce his agitation and to promote sleep. Simultaneously, psychotherapy and intensive nutritional therapy including vitamins (particularly vitamin $B_1$) are given. After the treatment, his environment should be changed, otherwise he is likely to fall prey again.

Some drugs like *disulfiram* (ANTABUSE) create a distaste for alcohol, but their effects are short and do not necessarily prevent the alcoholic from taking alcohol in the future. These are, therefore, of limited value for those who will fully want to quit.

If alcohol had not been discovered at all, the world would in no way be a poorer place to live in. But now that we have it, it is best to know its proper use. Some call alcohol the 'devil'. In fact, the devil in not in alcohol; it's in the person who drinks. Everyone who tastes it does not turn alcoholic. We believe that those who become alcoholics have a weak character, poor self-control, and are generally cowards. People with will-power do not fall prey to it; rather they make the best use of it. If taken discreetly, sparingly, and only occasionally, one can get more out of alcohol than it can get out of us.

The following guidelines may be followed usefully:

1. Alcohol should never be taken on an empty stomach. It is best to drink after or along with some snacks to prevent its quick absorption, which would lead to a high blood concentration.
2. It is wrong to gulp it quickly. Besides being bad etiquette, it may 'hit you in the head' and spoil your evening.
3. Its occasional consumption does not harm but if it becomes a habit, it does no good.
4. It should not be consumed to kill boredom due to lack of company. Rather it is best used to make company livelier. Those who drink alone, are more likely to end up as alcoholics than others.
5. Alcohol should never be taken by those who suffer from a liver or kidney disease or a peptic ulcer.
6. Use of alcohol with anti-allergics, hypnotics, sedatives, tranquillizers and many other drugs can produce dangerous sedation, leading to respiratory depression.

## Useful Applications of Alcohol

1. As a skin antiseptic, 70% alcohol is very useful. Quite often people use rectified spirit (which is 95% alcohol) for this purpose, which is not right. This high concentration of alcohol does not penetrate and is a poor antiseptic. Three parts of rectified spirit should be diluted with one part of water to make it 70%, before application.
2. Alcohol in a concentration of 50%, if rubbed, prevents development of bed sores in bed-ridden patients.
3. A drink or two, prior to dinner, can be useful to stimulate appetite and improve digestion. A glass of beer is recommended for those who wish to put on weight.
4. Those who consume moderate amounts of alcohol 3 or 4 times a week are known to live longer.
5. It is a good preservative. Alcohol in 5% concentration is used to preserve other drugs in solution form.

6. It can be rubbed over the skin sprains and joint pains.
7. Doctors inject alcohol around the nerves in trigeminal neuralgia.

## Methyl Alcohol Poisoning

Every now and then we read in the newspapers about death due to hooch consumption. The number of people who become blind or disabled is huge. These tragedies occur due to consumption of illicit liquor containing poisonous methanol liquids (methyl alcohol), or ethylene or propylene glycol (antifreeze used in cars). These liquids are indistinguishable from alcohol as their smell, taste, and effects are similar to it. The only difference is of fatal toxic effects on the eyes and vital organs of the body. Since there is no excise duty on these agents, they are cheaper and mixed in illicit beverages by unscrupulous elements.

### Treatment

The treatment of poisoning due to the intake of any form of illicit liquor is similar. In order to save a life or prevent a disability, it is important to know what measures can be taken in case there is any delay in consulting a doctor. There are two areas of treatment: to precipitate the excretion of the poison and to prevent acidosis. An amount of 60 to 120 ml of alcohol, in the form of ordinary whisky, gin, or rum can be given every 6 to 8 hours for a week or so to accelerate excretion of the poison. A teaspoon of soda bicarbonate given every 2 to 4 hours neutralizes the increased acids in the body. It can be mixed with juice or a sweet drink to make it palatable. However, it is imperative that a doctor should be consulted at the earliest.

# 43

# Drugs and Your Child

A child suffering from mild diarrhoea was once taken to a well known specialist. After attentively recording the history and a careful physical examination, the specialist asked the mother about the diet of the child. She replied, 'A little milk with sugar.'

'Ah , ha! That is it. Sugar! Just avoid it and he will be all right,' said the doctor.

A few minutes later another woman came with her child who was suffering from a similar condition. After the examination, the doctor posed the same question about the diet. The mother replied that she fed her baby unsweetened milk.

'No sugar in the milk? Add a bit of sugar, he will be all right.'

Can you guess the logic of a doctor recommending two different diets to cure the same ailment? He believes that many of the aliments in children are self-limiting and require time and patience rather than drugs. What this doctor did was to free the mother from anxiety, and yet did

**Immunization Schedule: Infants and Children**

| *Age* | *Vaccines* |
|---|---|
| *At Birth* | BCG, $OPV_0$, Hepatitis-$B_1$ |
| *6 weeks* | $DTPw_1$/$DTPa_1$, $OPV_1$, Hepatitis $B_2$, $Hib_1$ |
| *10 weeks* | $DTPw_2$/$DTPa_2$, $OPV_2$, $Hib_2$ |
| *14 weeks* | $DTPw_3$/$DTPa_3$, $OPV_3$, Hepatitis $B_3$ *, $Hib_3$ |
| *9 months* | Measles |
| *15-18 months* | $DTP_w$ $B_1$/DTPa $B_1$, $OPV_4$, Hib $B_1$, MMR |
| *2 years* | Typhoid+ |
| *5 years* | DTPw $B_2$/DTPa $B_2$, $OPV_5$ |
| *10 years* | Td#/TT |
| *16 years* | Td#/TT |

Pregnant Women 2 doses of Td#/TT.
$3^{rd}$ dose of Hepatitis B can be given at 6 months of age
+Revaccination every 3-4 years
#Td preferred over TT

* Chapter contributed by Dr Deepak Shivpuri, Sr. Consultant and HOD Pediatrics and Neonatology, Fortis Escorts Hospital, Jaipur.

**Vaccines that can be given after discussion with the parents**

| Age | Vaccines |
|---|---|
| > 15 months of age | Varicella Vaccine# |
| > 18 months of age | Hepatitis A Vaccine+ |
| > 6 weeks | Pneumococcal Conjugate Vaccine* |

#<13 years of age: 1 dose; > 13 years of age: 2 doses at 4-8 weeks interval +2 doses at 6-12 months interval.
*3 primary doses at 6, 10 & 14 weeks followed by a booster dose at 15 months.

not prescribe drugs. From the history of frequency and quantity of feeds, the colour and consistency of the stool, he found that the diarrhoea was due to indigestion rather than infection. On physical examination, he noticed that it was not severe enough to cause dehydration. He knew that in such cases, once the intestines were emptied, their normal activity would start and the diarrhoea would be automatically controlled.

In contrast to this, most other doctors would have prescribed an anti-diarrhoeal antibiotic and possibly, also a vitamin preparation. Even if the doctor does not do so, patients often demand a drug for each and every symptom i.e. 'pill for every ill'. They erroneously believe that drugs switch the activity of the body on or off. *Drugs should be used only when absolutely necessary.* No doubt they do good, but they also cause adverse effects which may become apparent only after some time. In today's world of evidence based medicine a drug should only be prescribed/used when evidence suggests that it will do more good than harm. It is advisable that parents have patience in simple and short-lasting ailments of their children like coughs, colds, mild diarrhoea, headache, or mild fever in which frequent, unnecessary, and indiscriminate use of drugs may, at times, cause permanent harm to vital organs like the liver, ears, bone marrow, and kidneys, The child's growth may also be retarded in some cases. Since the child's health is extremely important for his future growth and development great discretion is advised while giving drugs.

Drugs to neonates and infants can be administered orally, through the rectum or by injection. The rectal route is more unpredictable than the oral route but is useful in children who are vomiting persistently, are unconscious or having convulsions. Rectal suppositories are available for *diazepam, paracetamol* and *antiemetics.*

**Drugs Commonly Used in Diseases of Children**

1. **Anti-bacterial Agents**
   *Ampicillin, Amoxycillin*
   *Cephalexin, Cefadroxil*
   *Amikacin, Azithromycin*
   *Cotrimoxazole, Nalidixic acid*
2. **Fever and Pain Relievers**
   *Paracetamo, Ibuprofen*
3. **Vitamins and Minerals**
   Iron Preparations
   Vitamin A, Vitamin D
4. **Deworming Agents**
   *Albendazole*
5. **Antimalarials**
   *Chloroquine*
   *Quinine*
6. **Antivomiting Agents**
   *Domperidone, Ondansetron*

In neonates, these drugs should be given on the advice of the doctor, as even a slight overdose may lead to serious side-effects. The drug metabolizing and drug excretory systems (liver and kidneys) of neonates are underdeveloped to deal with drugs. In addition, in neonates, the blood protein binding capacity of a drug is low and a large amount of the drug remains in the free form, and is responsible for both excessive effects and adverse effects. These deficiencies are further enhanced in the prematurely born, who are, therefore, more likely to be harmed by drugs.

The side effects can be minimized to an extent by giving the correct dose of the drug. Dispersible tablets and liquid preparations are commonly used. It is best not to administer liquid medicines in teaspoon doses as teaspoons vary greatly in size. A standard 5ml or 10ml measure should always be used.

When two or more drugs are administered to the same patient at a time they may interact resulting in unpredictable effects or toxic responses.

Almost all drugs administered to lactating woman are secreted to some extent into their milk and may be ingested by the nursing infant. Although drug use should be as minimal as possible during pregnancy and lactation, it is not possible or desirable for lactating women to stop taking medication which are necessary.

**Drugs to be Used with Caution in Children**

| *Drugs* | *Adverse Effects* |
|---|---|
| *Chloramphenicol* (PARAXIN, CHLOROMYCETIN) | May cause bone marrow depression |
| *Betamethasone* (BETNELAN, BETACORTIL) | Stunted growth, lowered body resistance |
| *Dexamethasone* (DECADRON, DEXONA) | Prolonged use may cause steroid effects |
| *Prednisolone* (WYSOLONE, OMNACORTIL) | Stunted growth, lowered body resistance |
| *Diphenoxylate* (LOMOTIL), *Loperamide* (RIDOL) | Margin of safety in children is low |
| *Aspirin* (DISPRIN, ECOSPRIN) | May cause Reye's encephalopathy |
| *Metoclopramide* (PERINORM, REGLAN) | May cause extrapyramidal symptoms |
| *Combination antidiarrhoeals* (NORBEX-M, NORFLOX-TZ) | Offer no benefit over single drug formulations, add to side effects |
| *Combination antipyretics* (FLEXON, COMBIFLAM) | No advantage over *paracetamol* |
| *Tetracyclines* (ACHROMYCIN, TERRAMYCIN) | Gets deposited in teeth and growing bones. Not recommended for children below 8 years. |

# 44

# Drug Treatment in the Elderly

Every type of machinery functions normally for some years but starts giving problems with age. This is true for a bicycle, a car, a railway engine, or an aeroplane. The body functions also, do not remain as efficient in old age as in youth or middle age. Besides physiological changes associated with ageing, other factors such as the multiple disease processes, nutritional deficiencies, inability to adhere to drug-schedules, and the decline of financial resources multiply problems in old age. Besides these, in those who are not aware, lack of proper physical exercise and the ability to modify the diet suitably are also responsible for causing undesirable responses to drugs. The doctor who treats the elderly has to be more knowledgeable, more careful. As individuals age, they are more likely to have disability and side effects of drugs.

Before 1947, the average age of an Indian was 37 years, but now it has reached as high as 67. This means that the percentage of older people in this country has increased considerably. In many ways, our situation is coming close to that of the more developed countries of the west where the average age is as high as 77 or 78 years. These countries have learnt to overcome the problems of old age, including those of altered drug response.

This chapter discusses the mechanism of altered clinical responses of drugs in the elderly and outlines a preferable approach to therapeutic management with examples of disease entities.

**Altered Organ Functions Result In Changes In Drug Effects And Disposal:** Ageing affects many a physiological function of the body. The functional capacity of most of the major organs like the kidneys, heart, liver and lungs shows a continuous decline after the age of 45 years. Thus kidney functions which are usually cent per cent till the age of 45 are reduced to 80% by the age of 60 years and 70% by the age of 80 years. The cardiac functions are affected even earlier, and are reduced to 80% at the age of 50, 70% at 60, and 65% at 80 years. Similarly, the maximal breathing capacity comes down to 85% at the age of 50, 60% around the age of 60, and 40% around the age of 80 years. Besides this, the elderly have a reduced lean body mass (as % of body weight), reduced body water (as % of body weight), and increased body fat (as % of body mass). The impact of all these changes, coupled with a progressive decline in functional capacities, results in an altered handling of the drug by the aged body in terms of its absorption, distribution, metabolism, and excretion.

***Metabolism of Drugs in the Elderly:*** The capacity of the liver to metabolise drugs does not appear to decline with age. Yet, for some drugs, a decreased metabolism is noted in the elderly. In addition, certain extra hepatic diseases like congestive heart failure may dramatically reduce the ability of the liver to metabolise drugs.

## Drug Therapy in Elderly

With altered organ-functions, the effects and efficient removal of drugs is affected in elderly. Elderly people are more likely to experience adverse effects of drugs. They may not be able to tolerate full doses of drugs (adult doses). Medicines may exhibit abnormal responses in elderly people. For example, *Diazepam* (a sedating drug) may cause prolonged sleep and behavioural problems in elderly.

There is decline in kidney and liver functions. Liver blood flow is also decreased. Elderly have low total body water so drug distribution is affected. Serum albumen levels (which allows binding of drug) decrease and total body fat increases with age. Distribution of fat is on abdomen and there is thinning of legs and arms. These changes result in altered drug metabolism. Generally metabolism of drugs and excretion by kidneys is reduced due to age dependent reductions in their function and hence dose adjustments are needed for several drugs.

Finally elderly people suffer from a number of diseases at a time and hence they take many drugs which interact (adversely) with each other. Older patients are likely to cause dosage errors due to forgetfulness, poor vision and hearing problems. These aspects need to be addressed by a conscientious prescriber.

***Note:*** It is important to understand that a healthy old person is different from diseased old person. Drug related changes are minimal in the former group.

***Precautions:***

1. Always try non-drug methods for trivial ailments.
2. Treatment should be started with lower than adult doses. Dose increments should also be gradual.
3. As far as possible number of medicines be kept minimal. This improves compliance.
4. A family member should be asked to bring all medications at each visit and instructions are taken again for efficient management.
5. Errors in taking correct/exact doses of drugs may be due to physical disability such as tremor, limited joint movements and visual problems. Liquid drugs to be taken as 1 to 2 teaspoonful may not be taken correctly by elderly because of above reasons.
6. Cataract formation may diminish vision and thus labels should be large enough for patients to see instructions clearly. It is important to understand that a healthy old person is different from diseased old person. Drug related changes are minimal in the former group.
7. Extreme care and caution is needed in the use of following drug-groups.
   a *Anticoagulants:* If dose is not regulated, formation of blood collections (haematoma) on slight fall may be there.
   b *Antiglaucoma drugs:* TIMOLD eye drops can be absorbed and cause slowing of pulse and fall in BP. Loss of appetite and weight is noted with the use of *Acetazolamide.*

c *Meperidine* (PETHIDINE) may cause excitation and confusion in elderly. *Paracetamol* is safe. Other anti-inflammatory analgesics may worsen kidney function. *D-propoxyphene* may cause drowsiness.

d *Cough and cold remedies:* They cause dryness, hesitancy of urination, constipation, fall or rise in BP and confusion.

e *Antivomiting drugs: Prochlorperazine* and *metoclopramide* may induce abnormal movements (dyskinesia).

f *Antipsychotics* and *antidepressants* may cause unacceptable adverse effects like dryness of the mouth.

g Antihypertensive drugs such as calcium channel blockers may cause swelling of feet and *diuretics (thiazides)* may not be useful in this case. Low dose *thiazide* alone have excellent BP reducing effect because of gradual fall in BP over days. *Propranolol* like drugs may be more hazardous in older patients with lung problems (particularly when they are smokers or ex-smokers). Alpha blockers *(Prazosin)* are useful in high BP and prostatic problems but postural fall on standing (at night) may be hazardous as falls, stroke or fractures may occur. This is particularly true when *thiazides* are also given.

h Once a drug is initiated a close watch is kept on drug induced adverse effects which may be subtle and evade detection.

Doses of certain antibiotics require alterations or alternative drug may be preferred in certain diseases in elderly. A few examples are given in Table below.

| Group | Drugs and expected changes | Preferred drug of that group |
|---|---|---|
| Sleep-Aids | *Diazepam* / longer duration of sleep, confusion | *Oxazepam, Alprazolam, Zolpidem, Zopiclone* (low doses) |
| Antipsychotics | *Chlorpromazine* / more fall in BP, sedation and abnormal movements | *Thioridazine, pimozide* |
| Antidepressants | Imipramine, Doxepin, Amoxapine/ Dryness of mouth, constipation, urinary retention. | *Nortriptyline, Desipramine Fluoxetine, Trazonil* |
| Drugs for Heart and BP | *Digoxin* / less excretion, more heart irregularities | Reduced doses |
| | *Propranalol* / cold limbs, longer effects, sedation | *Atenolol* |
| | *Nifedipine* / palpitation, edema | Longer acting form preferred |
| Antibiotics | *Penicillins* / longer duration of action | dose adjustments if poor kidney function |
| | *Cephalosporins* / longer duration of action | dose adjustments if poor kidney function *Ceftriaxone* dose same; |
| | *Aminoglycosides (gentamicin, Amikacin)* Reduced removal in elderly | Dose adjustment for *aminoglycosides* |
| | Fluoroquinolones / reduced excretion | Pefloxacin preferred |
| | Tetracyclines / reduced excretion | *Doxycycline* preferred |
| Antidiabetic Drugs | *Chlorpropamide* / prolonged lowering of blood sugar | Avoided, prefer Tolbutamide |
| | *Glibenclamicle* | preferred in low doses |
| | *Metformin* | used in overweight patients only |
| Drugs for Constipation | Castor oil, liquid paraffin, magnesium sulphate Avoided | *Bran, Isabgol, Bisacodyl* preferred |
| Drugs for Peptic ulcer | Cimetidine - avoid | Omeprazole preferred |
| | Antacids | Avoid long-term use |

# 45

# Drugs to be Avoided During Pregnancy and Breast-Feeding

Pregnancy is a normal physiological phenomenon in women. It is accompanied by changes in the body giving rise to certain abnormal symptoms like nausea, vomiting, and discomfort. These symptoms are collectively called 'morning sickness' because of their greater frequency during morning hours. In pregnancy, except for certain vitamins (which are adequate in a good nutritious diet), no other drugs should be ordinarily given. However, if the symptoms of morning sickness become unbearable or there is some associated disease, drugs may become necessary. In recent years, information about possible adverse effects of drugs on a pregnant women and her unborn baby (embryo or foetus) has been causing serious concern.

Till the early and 1960s, there were no such problems in India because firstly, only very few drugs were available, and secondly, the pregnant woman enjoyed greater emotional stability under the loving care of elders. In present society, the problem has become acute with the introduction of innumerable drugs and the woman's dual responsibility of working in and outside the home. She suffers from a lack of the much-needed physical and mental rest, and for every complaint, takes a pill or two to keep herself going.

Concern about the use of drugs during pregnancy started in 1961 in West Germany when an apparently innocent sedative, *thalidomide*, became popular among pregnant women. It caused congenital deformities of the long bones of the limbs (arms and legs) in thousands of babies and had to be withdrawn. This was the only logical solution to the *thalidomide* disaster.

Since most of the drugs taken by a pregnant woman reach the unborn baby through the circulating blood, and our knowledge is based primarily on animal studies, it is best to minimize the use of drugs during pregnancy. If symptoms like vomiting due to pregnancy, or due to an associated disease become unbearable, and it is a must to take medication in such cases at least the drugs listed at the end of this chapter should be avoided.

Adverse effects of drugs vary with the age of the unborn in the uterus. To know more about these, the nine months period of pregnancy can be divided into two phases:

### Early Pregnancy: Formation of Embryo

From the start of the first trimester the cells of the fertilized ovum multiply rapidly to form an embryo, which after a period of 3 months, is called a foetus. In the early part of this trimester (up to 17 days) the teratogenic drugs (malformation-causing drugs) may kill the embryo.

Beyond this period, up to 55 days (period of organs formation) is the most vulnerable time when the drugs may cause teratogenic effects (physical defects or malformations). It has been estimated that the incidence is 1 to 2%, but it is not known as to how many of these are due to drugs. It is possible that besides the drugs used in a particular disease, the disease itself may be producing such effects.

### Period of Growth and Development: 56 days onwards

During this period the teratogenic effects are unlikely to occur as the shape of the foetus is completely formed. Some drugs may inhibit the growth and functional development of its organs. For example, *streptomycin* may damage the developing ears; *tetracyclines* are deposited in the teeth and growing bones, and may affect the colour and shape of teeth and the growth of bones.

At full term, the liver of the foetus is not fully mature and can't synthesize vitamin K-dependent clotting factors. At this period anticoagulant drugs or large doses of *aspirin* may cause bleeding in the foetus, although the clotting time of the mother's blood may remain near normal.

In the foetus, many of the enzymes which metabolize the drugs are also not developed. For this reason drugs like *barbiturates, morphine, pethidine* or *anaesthetics,* given at the time of delivery, may cause long-lasting respiratory depression in the newborn baby.

The adverse effects caused by some important drugs during pregnancy are given below. The formulation of the preparation intended for a pregnant women need to be studied carefully. If it contains any of the following drugs, it would be safer to avoid it or take in consultation with the doctor. It is a useful tip to remember, 'No drug is safe in pregnancy'. Since the list is not by far an exhaustive list and safety of newer drugs remains to be ascertained, it is urged that for any drug prescribed the readers should ensure the safety from prescriber before it is used during pregnancy.

### Drugs to Be Avoided During Pregnancy

**Aspirin** (DISPRIN) : It is commonly used for headache, fever, and pain. Large doses, if taken during the first trimester, may cause physical defects in the developing foetus, while large doses, during the latter part of the pregnancy, may lead to a bleeding tendency in the newborn baby, prolong pregnancy and labour.

**ACE-inhibitors** (CAPTOPRIL, ENALAPRIL) : Use of these drugs may cause underdevelopment of lungs, kidneys and other organs.

**Bishydroxy-Coumarin** : This drug is an oral anticoagulant. If taken during the last three weeks of pregnancy, it may cause a bleeding tendency in the newborn child, which may prove fatal.

**Busulphan** : It causes physical defects in the developing foetus during early pregnancy.

**Carbimazole (& methimazole)** : This is used in a hyper-functioning thyroid. It is best to stop these drugs four weeks before the expected date of delivery as it may alter the activity of the thyroid in the newborn baby.

**Chloramphenicol** : It is used in typhoid. If taken during the last few weeks of pregnancy, the foetus may die due to circulatory collapse or bone marrow depression.

**Chloroquine** : It is used in malaria. It may be responsible for permanent deafness and defects in vision in the newborn baby.

**Clomiphene** : This drug is used in cases of sterility to induce ovulation. It may cause multiple pregnancies and foetal malformations.

**Cortisone (& Prednisolone)** : It is a corticosteroid. If taken during the later part of pregnancy, it may cause deficiency of adrenal hormone on withdrawl of the drug. It delays growth and promotes infection.

**Cyclizine** : Its effects are same as *chlorocyclizine.*

**Cyclophos-Phamide** : This has the same effects *busulphan.*

**Dexamethasone** : Its effects are the same as *cortisone.*

**Dexamphetamine** : This is used as a slimming drug. It may cause developmental defects of the heart in the foetus, if taken during pregnancy.

**Diazepam** : An anti-anxiety drug, if taken in a large quantity during late pregnancy, it may cause lowering of the body temperature and muscular weakness in the newborn baby.

**Diazoxide** : It may lead to abnormal distribution of foetal hair formation and hypoglycaemia in the new born baby.

**Discoumarol** : Its effects are the same as *bishydroxycoumarine.*

**Dihydrogesterone** : It is likely to produce male characteristics in female babies.

**Estrogens** : If taken during pregnancy, they may cause vaginal cancer in the female children at a later age and feminization of male offspring.

**Ethionamide** : This is an anti-tubercular drug. Its use during pregnancy may cause physical defects in the foetus.

**Ethisterone** : The effect of this drug are similar or *dihydrogesterone.*

**Furosemide** : A diuretic (increases urine output), it should not be used during pregnancy as it may cause the death of the foetus due to decreased circulation.

**Glibenclamide** : It may cause prolonged hypoglycaemia in neonates (newborn babies) if taken during late pregnancy.

**Hydralazine** : It increases the heart rate of newborn babies.

**Hydroxy-progesterone** : The effects are the same as those of *dihydrogesteron.*

**Indomethacin and other pain relievers (NSAIDS)** : This drug is sometimes used in rheumatoid arthritis. If used during the early part of the pregnancy, it may cause physical defect (premature closure of ductus) in the foetus.

**Iodides** : These are ingredients of many cough mixtures and also used in a hyerfunctioning thyroid. Their use during pregnancy may alter thyroid function in the newborn babies. It may also affect their mental functions.

**Lithium Carbonate** : This is an antidepressant drug. If taken during the first trimester it may cause physical defects in the foetus and poor suckling in the neonate.

**Meclizine** : Its effects are common to *chlorcyclizine*

**Melphalan** : This has the same effects as *busulphan.*

**Methyldopa** : Destruction of red blood cells (hemolytic anaemia) and decreased activity of the intestines occurs.

**Morphine** : A potent pain reliever, causing addiction. The newborn babies of addicted mothers may be premature and exhibit withdrawal symptoms. The chances of death among such babies are very high.

**Nitrofurantoin** : Commonly used in urinary tract infection its use should be avoided during the last few days of pregnancy as it may cause bursting of red blood cells, specially in individuals who are genetically deficient in certain enzymes.

**Norethisterone** : The same effects occur as in *dihydrogesterone.*

**Norethynodrel** : The same effects occur as in *dihydrogesterone.*

**Opium** : The same effects occur as in *morphine.*

**Oral contra-ceptives** : These are used by women for birth control but if by any chance pregnancy occurs, the doctor should be consulted because of the possibility of adverse effects on the foetus.

**Pethidine** : The same effects occur as with *morphine.*

**Phenobarbitone** : The effects are the same as with *barbiturates.*

**Phenytoin** : This is an anti-epileptic drug. If taken during the last few days of pregnancy, the newborn baby may suffer from bleeding disorders (hypoprothrombinaemia and haemorrhage). The use of anti-epileptic drugs may cause physical defects in the foetus.

**Prednisolone** : This produces the same effects as *cortisone.*

**Primaquine** : It is an anti-malaria drug. If taken during pregnancy, the newborn baby may suffer from haemolysis and jaundice.

**Primidone** : The effects are the same as with *phenhytoin.*

**Progesterone** : The same effects occur as with *dihydrogesterone*.

**Propranolol** : This is used in some heart disorders and high blood pressure. Its use should be avoided during pregnancy as it may cause slowing of the heart rate and decrease of blood sugar in neonates.

**Propylthiouracil** : The same effects occur as with *carbimazole.*

**Purgatives** : These are used in constipation. Strong purgatives may cause abortion.

**Pyrimethamine** : Sometimes used in malaria, its use may cause foetal malformation.

**Quinine** : Now *quinine* is used in *chloroquine-resistant* cases of malaria. Use in early pregnancy may cause abortion. It has been associated with deafness and vision defects in offspring, if taken during pregnancy.

**Salbutamol** : It increases the heart rate in newborn babies.

**Stilboesterol** : The same effects occur as with *estrogen*.

**Streptomycin** : This is an anti-tubercular drug. It may produce deafness and weakness of the muscles in the newborn baby if taken during pregnancy.

**Sulfonamides** : These drugs should be avoided during the last few days of pregnancy as they may cause jaundice in newborn babies. These drugs may also combine with the haemoglobin of red blood cells (methaemoglobenaemia) rendering it unable to carry oxygen.

**Tetracyclines** : These antibiotics, if taken during pregnancy, are deposited in developing bones and lead to discolouration of teeth of the foetus. They impair bone growth of the foetus.

**Tolbutamide** : The effects are the same as with *glibenclamide.* It may also cause a decrease in platelets, causing bleeding.

**Trimethoprim** : This drug is used in certain infections. It may increase blood bilirubin.

**Valproic acid** : This can cause defects of spinal cord.

**Vitamin A& Isotretinoin** : Large doses, If taken during pregnancy, may cause developmental defects of head and face in the foetus, specially in the urinary and genital system. (*Isotretinoin* never used).

**Vitamin D** : Very large doses should be avoided during pregnancy. It may cause mental retardation and defects in bones.

**Vitamin K** : Large doses during pregnancy may produce jaundice in the newborn baby.

**Warfarin** : The same effects occur as with *bishydroxycoumarin.*

**Note:** Exposure to X-ray radiation must be avoided during pregnancy especially in the first six months as it may cause malformation of the foetus.

## Use of Drugs during Breast-feeding

Many drugs enter into human milk in very low concentrations so that suckling child is not harmed. However, a few drugs may pass into breast milk in quantities sufficient to harm the suckling infant. If the mother has to take medicine, and the medicine is relatively safe, she should take it 30 to 60 minutes after breast feeding or 2 to 4 hours before next feed.

A number of antibiotics can be detected in breast milk. *Tetracyclines* are found in concentration of about 70% of the mother's blood level. So they may be avoided. Sedatives and sleepaids also can cause poor suckling and drowsiness in breast fed-infant. Other drugs with possible effects on breast feeding infant are shown in table. It is recommended that these drugs should be taken under medical advice.

| *Drugs* | *Effect on infant* |
|---|---|
| *Ampicillin* | Minimal- possible diarrhoea |
| *Alcohol* | In large quantities may affect infant |
| *Iodides* | Thyroid suppression possible |
| *Isoniazid* | Vitamin $B_6$ deficiency possible |
| *Propylthiouracil* | Can suppress thyroid function |
| *Theophylline* | Can cause restlessness and sleeplessness |
| *Radio active substance use* | Breast feeding is contraindicated for several weeks |
| *Anti cancer drugs* | Breast feeding is contraindicated for several weeks |

# 46

# Smoking and Effects of Drugs

It is well established by scientific studies that smoking is injurious to health in many ways. The tobacco contains nicotine which leads to addiction by raising brain dopamine levels. Studies show that even one cigarette a month may cause habit and young smokers become addicted within 2 days of regular smoking. Smoking is linked to mutation in p53 gene which is the causal factor in cancer.

The most common effect of tobacco smoke on a drug is the increase in the rate of its inactivation in the body. Nicotine, the main ingredient in a cigarette, causes nausea and vomiting in non-smokers but not in smokers. Smoking increases the activity of certain enzymes in the liver. Out of about 300 compounds found in cigarette smoke, a certain class of these known as polycyclic aromatic hydrocarbons are thought to be responsible for stimulating (inducing) liver enzymes. As a result, smokers as compared with non-smokers, may require larger or more frequent doses of drugs which are thus metabolized in the liver. Tolerance (decreased effect) to certain drugs after prolonged use can also be caused by additional enzyme induction that results from smoking. Another effect of smoking which may lead to altered drug action is that it increases the heart rate, blood pressure, oxygen demand of the heart tissues, and cardiac rhythm abnormality (arrhythmia). These factors greatly increase the unpredictability of drug therapy in smokers.

**Risks of smoking**

| Premature death | Smokers die 5-8 years earlier |
|---|---|
| Life threatening heart attacks | 2 times |
| Lung and other cancers | 10 times |
| Strokes and paralysis | 2-3 times |
| Stomach Ulcers | 4 times |
| Age related macular degeneration | 2 times |
| Cataract | 2 times |
| Blood cancer, prostate, colon, Alzheimer's disease, osteoporosis Low birth weight, genital cancers | Greater chances |

## Drug Interaction Due to Smoking

**Theophylline** (AMINOPHYLLINE, DERIPHYLLIN, THEOLONG, THEOMAC)
This is a frequently prescribed as a bronchodilator to relieve and prevent symptoms of asthma, chronic bronchitis, and emphysema. In smokers, the drug is more rapidly eliminated from the body than in non-smokers, and thus its level in the blood decreases faster, reducing the duration of action. Some heavy smokers may require as much as one and a half to two times the maintenance dose of *theophylline*. This effect is long lasting. It may take six months to three years to return to normal after smoking is stopped.

**Propranolol** (INDERAL, CORBETA), **Metoprolol** (METOLAR, BETALOC)
This is drug which belongs to the class of beta-blocking agents which are used to control high blood pressure, angina pectoris (severe chest pain), cardiac arrhythmias, migraine headaches, and to improve the chances of survival of the patient after a heart attack. In smokers the drug is cleared faster from the body than in non-smokers and thus, there is a reduced level of the drug in the blood, resulting into inadequate therapeutic effect.

**Pentazocine** (FORTWIN, PENTAWIN, SOSEGON)
*Pentazocine* is a pain reliever and is required in larger doses by smokers because of its increased rate of metabolism.

*Phenothiazines* like *chlorpromazine* (LARGACTIL), *trifluoperazine* (TRINICALM, LACALM), *thioridazine* (MELLERIL) are required in larger than usual doses in smokers as compared to non-smokers due to their increased rate of metabolism. The same is true for *tricyclic antidepressant* drugs like *imipramine* (DEPSONIL, ANTIDEP, TENCODEP), *desipramine* (NORPRAMINE), *amitriptyline* (SAROTENA), *trimipramine* (SURMONTIL), and *doxepin* (SPECTRA).

**Sedatives**
Sleep-producing and anxiety-relieving agents are affected by smoking. Heavy smokers are known to show markedly diminished effects of drugs such as *diazepam* (VALIUM, CALMPOSE), *chlordiazepoxide* (LIBRIUM), *lorazepam* (LARPOSE), and *oxazepam* (SEREPAX).

**Heparin** (BEPARINE)
This drug prevents the clotting of blood and is important in treating such conditions as thromboembolic disease, in which clotted blood fragments threaten to block blood vessels. In smokers the *heparin* level in the blood decreases 50% more rapidly than in non-smokers.

**Frusemide** (LASIX, SALINEX)
This is a drug used in hypertension and edema, and shows lesser effects amongst smokers.

**Vitamins**
Smoking has been shown to lower the blood level of the indispensable Vitamin $B_{12}$ (*methylcobalamin*) by causing increased urinary excretion. Smokers also metablise Vitamin C faster than non-smokers and thus require about 40% additional dose of the vitamin.

## Oral Contraceptives

Women who use oral contraceptives are strongly advised not to smoke. Cigarette smoking increases the risk of such serious cardiovascular side effects of oral contraceptives such as stroke, heart attack, and sudden blockage of blood vessels (thromboembolism). The risk increases with age and the number of cigarettes smoked per day, and is more marked in women above 35 years of age and those who smoke more than 25 cigarettes a day.

**Benefits of Cessation of Smoking**

- Reduced risk of ageing and early death
- Less heart and brain diseases
- Less breathlessness and lung disease
- Increased survival even in those who quit smoking at the age of 65 years
- *It is never too late to quit smoking!*

## Cessation of Smoking

The relative ineffectiveness of the drugs described above, must be understood in the right perspective. If you are a smoker and suffer from high blood pressure, heart disease, asthma, or any mental disorder, and taking any of the above drugs, make sure that the adjustment of dosages is done in a proper way.

Only when faced with serious health problems do smokers think seriously of quitting smoking. They are advised to make a serious effort to stop smoking before their problems get out of hand.

There are some drugs which can help smokers quit smoking. It should be remembered that these medicines do not help without motivation and education.

***Nicotine Replacement:*** In the form of chewing gum, sprays, inhalers and pills is helpful.

**Nicotine Patch (NICOTINELL-TTS** 10, 20, 30 $cm^2$ patch releases 7, 14, 21 mg nicotine in 24 hours respectively). One may start with a higher dose and then gradually reduce the doses.

**Nicotine gum** (GUTKA, NULIFE 1mg, 2mg, 4mg) is also available in India. It is useful in smokers who smoke over 20 cigarettes a day..

**Bupropion** (SMOQUIT-SR, NICOTEX) **Varencline** (CHAMPIX) are also used.

# 47

# Medicines: Their Safe and Correct Usage

••••••

Medicines should be used exactly as prescribed by the doctor. *Do not* change the amount of medicine to be taken or stop the medicine without consulting the doctor. Always read the label carefully before use. They may contain warnings and precautions pertaining to condition or prescription. In case of any doubt or clarification consult the doctor or the pharmacist. Check medications before use. If they are not of the same size or colour as the usual prescription, immediately check with the pharmacist.

**Safe Use of Medicines:** Always ensure that the doctor knows:

- about any other prescriptions or non-prescription drugs (such as laxative, pain relievers, vitamins cough and cold medicines) being taken simultaneously;
- about any allergies to food, pollen, or other drugs;
- about diet habits;
- about pregnancy or breast-feeding;
- about any major surgery of abdomen and bowels.

> Make sure that the medicine you are using is within the 'Expiry Date' as indicated on the label.

Most people experience few or no side effects from drugs. Most of the side effects often disappear during the course of the treatment. However, if the use of medicine is bothersome and causing unusual reactions, consult the doctor immediately. Similarly consult the doctor immediately if skin rash, hives, itching, swelling of the face, or difficulty in breathing develops. These are signs of a hypersensitive (allergic) reaction to the medicine. Many drugs have chemical structure, which may cause reactions akin to known medicine causing allergy. Keep a record of drugs, which have caused you allergy in the past.

**Safe Storage of Medicines:** Medicines should be stored in a cool and dry place. *Do not* store medicine in bathroom cabinets, kitchen cabinets, near a stove or area of excessive heat, or in the

---

* Chapter contributed by Dr N.K. Gurbani, Professor and Head of Department of Pharmacy, Public Health Training Centre, S.M.S. Hospital, Jaipur.

refrigerator. Only those medicines which are labelled 'Store in a cool place or refrigerate' should be refrigerated. Tablets and capsules can be kept at room temperature. Medicines like insulin should be kept in the lower compartment of refrigerator.

Medicines should always be kept out of the reach of children. If available, childproof containers are preferred. These are devised in a way that children cannot open them. *Never* share medicines with other family members or friends even if their symptoms seem to be similar.

*Do not* take or save old medicines; many may decompose after a period of time. They should be destroyed. Liquid lotions and suspensions, which are to be applied locally over skin, should be kept separate from those syrups and tonics to be taken by mouth. There have been instances when 'Liquid dettol' was mistakenly taken orally in place of 'Liquid antacid'.

### How to Administer Ear Drops

Wash hands thoroughly with soap and water just before starting. For accuracy and to avoid contamination, another person should insert the eardrops when possible. These days eye and eardrops are available in soft plastic containers with nozzle or with droppers fixed on top.

*Do not* insert the dropper or tip of the container in the ear. Avoid touching the dropper against the affected ear or any other surface.

Hold the container in the hand for a while to warm to near-body temperature. *Do not* heat in boiling water. If the drops are in a suspension form, shake well for ten seconds before use. Lie sideways or tilt the affected ear up for the ease of administration.

**Do not...**

- Insert dropper or tip of the container in the ear.
- Heat the container in boiling water.
- Allow water to get into the eardrops or wash the dropper.
- Refrigerate, unless instructed.

In order to allow the drops to run:

- In adults: hold the earlobe up and back.
- In children: hold the earlobe down and back.
- Instill the prescribed number of drops in the ear. Maintain the ear tilted for about 2 minutes, or insert a soft cotton plug, as recommended.

Consult the doctor if condition persists or becomes worse, or any itching or burning occurs in the ear for more than a few minutes after use. Keep container tightly closed when not in use.

*Do not* allow water to get into the eardrops or wash the dropper. *Do not* refrigerate, unless instructed by the doctor or the pharmacist.

### How to Administer Eye Drops

Single application formulations (applicaps) are preferred. However, eye drops and ointments are available in small containers and can be used repeatedly. Particular care should be observed to prevent contamination of contents. The person administering the drops should wash his/her hands thoroughly with soap and water before starting and after using the eye drops. Never rinse the dropper as it

**Do not...**

- Rinse the dropper. It may contaminate the drops.
- Touch the dropper to the eye, fingers, or any surface.
- Use eye drops that have changed colour or appear to have crystals or suspended particles in solution.
- Touch the tip of the ointment tube or cap to the eye, fingers or any surface.

may contaminate the drops. Contact lens wearers should remove the contact lenses before instilling the eye drops.

In order to allow the drops to run in:

- Gently pull lower eyelid of the affected eye downwards. Tilt head backwards, or if more convenient, lie down and look up at the ceiling. Hold the dropper above the affected eye (do not touch eye lashes or lids) and drop medicine inside lower lid while looking up, usually one drop is sufficient. *Do not* touch the dropper to the eye, fingers, or any surface.
- Release lower lid. Try to keep the affected eye closed [no squeezing] and *do not* blink for at least 30 seconds. Apply gentle pressure with fingers to the bridge of the nose (inside corner of the eye) for about one minute to prevent drainage of solution from the eye.
- If using more than one kind of eye drop at the same time, wait for at least 5 minutes before use of another eye drop.

If dropper is separate, hold it with the tip down. Replace it on the bottle and tighten the cap. Never use eye drops that have changed colour or appear to have crystals or suspended particles in the solution.

### How to Apply and Administer Eye Ointments

The person administering the ointment should wash his hands thoroughly with soap and water before and after using the eye ointment(s).

Contact lens wearers should remove their contact lenses before applying the eye ointment. To improve the flow of ointment, hold the tube (with the cap still on) in a hand for several minutes so that it may warm up before use.

**Application by Another Individual:** Lie down or tilt the head backwards and look at the ceiling. Gently pull the lower eyelid of the affected eye downwards. Squeeze a small amount of ointment (about 5 mm to 1 cm) inside the pocket of lower lid. *Do not* touch the tip of the tube or cap to the eye, fingers, or any surface.

**Self-Application:** Keep the head tilted backwards just slightly. Squeeze a small amount of ointment (about 5 mm to 1 cm) inside the lower lid. *Do not* touch the tube tip or cap to the eye, fingers, or any surface. Use a tissue paper or clean cloth or cotton to wipe off any excess ointment around the eye. Always clean the tip of the ointment tube with a tissue paper or cotton after use.

If using more than one kind of ointment at the same time, wait for about 10 minutes before using the other ointment. Blinking helps spread the ointment easily.

**Co-Administration of an Eye Drop and Eye Ointment:** Instill the eye drops first as explained. Wait for 5 minutes and instill the eye ointment as directed.

**Caution:** Some eye drops or ointments may cause blurring of vision for a short time after applying. Use preferably at bedtime. Be careful not to drive or operate dangerous machinery until vision has cleared.

**Do not...**

- Use drops and sprays for more than 5 days unless instructed.
- Touch the side of the dropper to the inside of the nose as it may cause sneeze and/or contaminate the dropper.
- Share the dropper with anyone to prevent spread of infection.
- Shake the plastic squeeze bottle of nose sprays.

Inform or consult the doctor immediately if condition becomes worse or if itching or burning occurs for more than a few minutes after use. Some eye ointments sting for a short time after use. Keep eye drop or ointment container tightly closed when not in use. *Do not* refrigerate unless instructed by the doctor or pharmacist or indicated on the label.

### How to Administer Nose Drops and Sprays

Wash hands thoroughly with soap and water just before starting. The patient should blow his nose gently just before using the nose drops or the spray. Inform or consult the doctor if the condition becomes worse or if any stinging, burning, or drying of the nasal mucosa occurs.

*Do not* use for more than three to five days unless instructed by the doctor.

**Nose Drops:** If a dropper is supplied separately, squeeze rubber bulb to fill the dropper with the proper amount of medication. Sit on a chair with the head tilted as far back as possible, or lie down on a bed with the head extending slightly over the edge of the bed, placing a pillow under the shoulders so that the head is tilted backwards. Insert the dropper into one nostril about 1 cm (approx.) or hold the dropper or plastic container just vertically above the nostril so that the drop falls directly into the nostril, and squeeze the prescribed number of drops into the nose. *Do not* change position for at least 2 minutes. Lean the head forward, inhaling and turning the head side to side. Refill the dropper by squeezing the bulb, and repeat the procedure for the other nostril. *Do not* touch the side of the dropper to the inside of the nose as it may cause sneeze and/or contaminate the dropper. Avoid use of the dropper by more than one person to prevent spread of infection.

**Do not...**

- Use more frequently or in quantities more than directed.
- Use for any other skin problem without consulting the doctor.
- Apply other creams, lotions, or cosmetics over medicine or mix products unless directed.
- Bandage unless directed.
- Spray into eyes, nose, or mouth.
- Use the spray near food. Some sprays contain alcohol.
- Smoke while using the spray or use spray near a fire, open flame, or heater. Alcohol may catch fire.
- Puncture, break, or burn the aerosol container even if empty.

After use, rinse the dropper with very hot water before putting it back into the container to prevent contamination. Keep the container tightly closed when not in use. *Do not* use solution that has discoloured or has suspended particles.

**Nose Sprays:** *Do not* shake the plastic squeeze bottle. Remove the cap. Hold the head upright to spray. Insert the nosepiece into the nostril, pointing it slightly backwards. To spray the prescribed amount, squeeze the bottle sharply and firmly while sniffing through the nose.

### How to Administer Oral Inhalers

There are two types of Inhalers:

1. Metered Dose Inhalers (MDI) and
2. Dry Powder Inhalers (DPI)

**MDI:** Read and follow the instructions exactly as supplied with the inhaler. Ensure that the canister is properly inserted into the inhaler unit. Remove the dust cap and shake the canister well before using. Hold the inhaler unit with the canister upwards. Breathe out fully and place mouthpiece well into the mouth, aimed at the back of the throat. Press the top of the canister firmly down inside the mouthpiece while simultaneously breathing in deeply. This releases one dose.

Release pressure on the canister and remove the unit from the mouth. Hold the breath in for 5 to 10 seconds; then breathe out slowly. The desired relief may not be immediate. Wait for the prescribed time before inhaling a second dose. Inform/consult the doctor if shortness of breath persists after the dose, or if the dose fails to provide the usual relief.

**DPI:** The capsule containing dry powder of active drug is inserted into the mouth of inhaling device. Its lower part is rotated while holding upper part. This breaks the capsule releasing drug into lower chamber. The open upper end of device is held firmly in mouth within lips after a full breath out. Now a deep breath is taken in so that powder is inhaled.

The dryness of mouth and sore throat, which occurs in some patients, can be cared for by rinsing the mouth with water or a mouthwash after the dose. Keep the mouthpiece clean. When not using the inhaler, store it with the dust cap on the mouthpiece (especially while in a pocket or purse) to prevent inanimate objects like paperclips, dust, or small coins from getting into the mouthpiece. Initially, there is some difficulty in proper use of these devices but repeated use allows a proper coordination to establish between placing or pressing the canister and deep breathing for inhalation.

## How to Apply Topical Skin Products (Creams, Ointments, Lotions, Aerosols, Sprays)

These products are for *External Use Only. Do not* place in the eyes, nose or mouth. Wash the hands thoroughly before applying the medicine. Clean the skin area each time before application, unless otherwise directed by the doctor. Gently pat dry the washed skin area with a clean towel. Wash hands immediately after applying the medicine. This avoids getting any medicine into the eyes, nose, or mouth accidentally.

*Do not* use more frequently or in quantities larger than directed. *Do not* use for any other skin problem without checking with the doctor. *Do not* apply other creams, lotions, or cosmetics over the already applied medicine or mix products unless directed by the doctor. Consult the doctor if the condition persists or becomes worse, or if a constant irritation, such as burning or itching (which was not there before) occurs.

**Creams and Ointments:** Apply a small amount of the medicine to the affected area and spread lightly. Only the medicine that is actually touching the skin will work. A thick layer is not more effective than a thin layer. *Do not* bandage the area unless directed by the doctor.

**Lotions:** Shake the liquid preparation well before using. Apply a small amount of the medicine to the affected part and spread lightly. Only the medicine that is actually touching the skin will work. A thick layer is not more effective than a thin layer. *Do not* bandage the area unless directed by the doctor. Lotions need not be rubbed rigorously.

**Aerosols/Sprays:** Shake the container well each time before using and even between sprays. Hold the container straight up and about 15 to 20 centimetres away from the affected skin. Spray the affected skin area for 2 to 3 seconds.

*Do not* spray into the eyes, nose, or mouth. *Do not* use the spray near food. Some sprays contain alcohol. Alcohol may catch fire. *Do not* smoke while using the spray or use the spray near a fire, open flame, or heater. *Do not* puncture, break, or burn the aerosol container even if empty. Store in cool place.

## How to Use and Apply Rectal Products (Creams, Ointments, Suppositories)?

These products are for *Rectal Use Only. Do not* place in or near the eyes, nose, or mouth. Wash hands before use. Wash and gently dry the rectal area before use. Wash hands immediately after use to prevent any medicine from getting into the eyes, nose or mouth.

Take a missed dose as soon as possible but if it is almost time for the next dose, skip the missed dose and continue the regular dosing schedule. *Do not* use twice the amount prescribed. Consult the doctor if the condition persists or becomes worse; or if a constant irritation such as burning or itching (which was not there before) occurs. *Do not* use leftover medicine for other rectal problems without first consulting the doctor.

**Outside the Rectal Area:** Apply a small amount of the cream or ointment to the rectal area and rub in gently. Tissue paper or cotton may be used to avoid using the medicine directly on the finger.

**Inside the Rectal Area:** Attach the plastic applicator tip onto the opened tube. Lubricate the applicator tip with a small amount of medicine to make the insertion easier. Lie down sideways and insert the applicator tip into the rectum and gently squeeze the tube. Remain sideways for a few minutes before getting up. After using this medicine, remove the applicator tip from the tube and wash the applicator tip with hot, soapy water. Replace the cap on the tube after each use.

**Rectal Suppositories:** Remove the wrapper and moisten the suppository with lukewarm water or hold it for a few seconds in the palms of the hands to soften it. If the suppository is too soft to insert, cool it in the refrigerator for about 15 minutes or run under cold water before removing the wrapper. Lie down sideways and use a finger to push the pointed end of the suppository well up into the rectum. A finger wrapped in plastic wrap (single finger glove or stall) may be used to avoid direct finger contact. Store the remaining suppositories in a cool, dry place to avoid melting.

## How to Apply Vaginal Creams and Pessaries

Wash hands with soap and water before and after every use. Use a sanitary napkin (rather than a tampon) to prevent staining of clothing and bed linen. Refrain from sexual intercourse, or have the partner use a condom to prevent reinfection. Inform your doctor immediately if the condition becomes worse or any vaginal discomfort, such as burning or irritation, from medication occurs. Use the medication as prescribed. Use continuously, even through the menstrual period.

**Vaginal Cream:** Remove the cap from the tube or medicine and screw the applicator to tube. Squeeze the tube and fill the applicator until the plunger is fully extended. Fill the applicator for the dosage prescribed. Unscrew the applicator from the tube. Lie on the back, raise knees and gently insert the applicator into the vagina as far as it goes comfortably. Press the plunger gently to release the cream. Keeping the plunger depressed, remove the applicator from the vaginal canal. Recap the tube. After each use remove the applicator and wash with soap and warm water to avoid reinfection.

**Pessaries (Vaginal Suppository):** Remove the wrapper from the suppository and place the suppository quickly into warm water just to moisten it. If an applicator is used, place the small end of the suppository into the applicator. Lie on the back, raise the knees and gently insert the applicator into the vagina as far as it goes comfortably. Press the plunger gently to release the suppository into the vagina. While the plunger is depressed, remove the applicator from the vaginal canal. After each use wash applicator and hands thoroughly with soap and water to avoid reinfection.

To summarise, proper use of medicines, provides the expected results and avoids harmful side effects. It is important to make sure that the medicine you are using is within the 'Expiry Date' as indicated on the label and to faithfully follow the directions of your doctor.

# 48

# Exercise and You

In the earlier times, calories stored as fat in the body was used in famines that were recurrent and prolonged. As such, the human use of food and nutrition in this time-period was more closely linked to survival and efficiency as opposed to a greater emphasis on fitness and enjoyment in today's world.

It is apparent that the human body has evolved to function under the circumstances related to scarcity of food. It is only in the last century that food has become plentiful and easily available and this change in availability has created multiple problems related to the excess ingestion of food.

## Nutrition Today

The food availability discussed above, combined with inactive lifestyles, has resulted in obesity, diabetes, and hypertension amongst other health problems in the USA and other western societies. With increasing wealth and industrialization in India as well, we are seeing similar patterns where obesity and related problems are reaching alarming proportions.

These patterns forecast an ominous future for health and lifestyle patterns of individuals. We need to address these consequences of inactive lifestyles without with great urgency, to prevent health problems in the future that are too far-reaching and complicated to reverse.

Research and proven data clearly indicate the importance of exercise and its benefits for both the young and the elderly. In spite of our Indian traditions of Yoga, morning walks and fasting, we Indians seem to have abandoned these very important lifestyle traditions. In fact, we have one of the highest rates of heart attacks and diabetes (*raj rog*), which cause a decrease in our life span and quality of life.

Fortunately, all these maladies can be controlled and reversed largely with life style modifications.

* Chapter contributed by Dr Rohit Dandiya, Chief of the Staff and Chairman of Board of Palm Beach Gardens Medical Center Heart Institute.

## How to Solve this Problem
## What you need to know about exercise but never asked:

It is never too late to begin exercising regularly. Studies have shown that even a group of elderly people gained more than twice their muscle strength (170% to be exact!) and increased their walking speed by 50%. And this was only after 8 weeks of regular exercise with weights! This is particularly impressive as the age group of elderly people ranged from 65 to 98!

### Longevity

Physical activity is clearly central to a healthy life, and results in comfortable and satisfying aging. After the age of 65, regular exercise can prolong life by 6 years. This requires regular sustained exercise as an integral part of one's lifestyle and not an occasional 'weekend warrior' approach.

### Diabetes

It is proven that exercise can not only delay, but also prevent the onset of diabetes. Once diabetes has developed, exercise can reverse and diminish its ill affects. This also requires concurrent change in diet and weight reduction. Scientifically speaking, exercise empowers the insulin secreted by the body to work more efficiently, thereby reducing insulin resistance, which is central to the onset of Type 2 Diabetes (adult onset) — the most common form of diabetes.

### Hypertension

This common malady can be reversed and better controlled with exercise and other modalities. This 'silent killer' needs to be addressed promptly and will require medications in addition to exercise. Remember, hypertension is the single most important cause of strokes.

### Heart Disease

It is a well-known fact that heart disease, heart attack, and angina (chest pain from reversible shortage of blood to the heart) are all positively affected with careful exercise under supervision. It is important to remember that regular exercise can also prevent coronary artery disease that results in heart attacks.

### Other Benefits

A healthy exercise regime can have far-reaching effects on your physical and mental life, providing improvement or reversal to a host of other maladies. In fact, depression can be reversed by the release of endorphins, a happy chemical released from the brain in response to exercise. Sleep disorders, balance, and dementia are also positively affected by a lifestyle with regular exercise. Overall, people who exercise have more self-confidence, which comes from feeling and being stronger.

## So, How Can This Be Done?

Quite simply, one needs to exercise at least 30 minutes but, preferably 40 to 50 minutes a day. Any exercise should always be for a sustained period of at least 10 to 15 minutes. The total daily exercise can be split into two or three sessions.

Exercise does not have to be intense where profuse sweating and windedness is the norm. Almost equal benefit can be achieved by pleasant brisk walking. Some say the benefits improve by walking fast enough to make speech difficult during walking.

There are three types of exercises with specific benefits:

### 1. Aerobic

Aerobic exercise includes brisk walking, running, dancing, and swimming. This has a beneficial effect on the heart, lungs, and cholesterol profile. The good cholesterol (HDL), which protects the heart increases and the bad cholesterol (LDL) decreases. Endurance, the ability to perform activities for prolonged periods, is also enhanced.

Simple tricks to add to daily exercise are to avoid lifts and escalators as well as walking, not driving, to the markets whenever possible. When waiting at railways stations and airports, walk around your surroundings instead of sitting and reading. Also, malls are a great place to walk in air-conditioned comfort in the middle of the summers. Perhaps you should leave your wallets behind as you could lose both your weight and money if you do not!

### Concept of Target Heart Rate:

To get the maximum benefit of aerobic exercise a target heart rate has to be reached which can be calculated individually.

The formula is as follows:

Heart Rate = (220 - Age) x 0.85

For example, for a 60-year-old man, the target heart rate would be:

(220-60) = 160… (160 x 0.85) = 136 beats of heart rate per minute.

### 2. Resistance exercise

Weight lifting and strength training is not just for young men. All other groups of people, including the elderly, both men and women, benefit from it.

As one ages, there is a 1% loss of muscle (also known as sarcopenia) per year. Therefore, at the age of 80 more than a quarter of muscle mass can be lost. Consequently, muscles 'hang' in older people, resulting in frailty, instability, falls and joint pains. Lack of self-confidence and self-esteem often results from these reactions also.

Thankfully, regular exercise will reverse these changes and increase the size and power of muscles. To do so, it is important to exercise regularly for about 20 minutes, three times week. At a practical level, join a local gym and if possible, get a personal trainer at least for a couple of months to learn safe and effective exercising habits. This is money well spent; skip a few dinners in a restaurant per month to conserve calorie intake, money and time.

*A note for women*: Resistance exercise will specially benefit postmenopausal women. It will especially reverse and delay the onset of osteoporosis, where bones become weak and porous and break easily.

### 3. Stretching

A few benefits from the stretching of muscles are suppleness, mobility and range of motion of joints. This form of exercise should be done carefully as there is a potential for injury if done incorrectly.

Yoga has been proven to benefit the body in many different ways much beyond simply stretching; it has been accepted in various Western societies and is commonly practiced in India as well. Fortunately, almost every neighborhood in India has its own Yoga centre and should be tried.

Pilates is another form of stretching which combines some modalities of weight resistance. Do not think of Pilates as something for women only, it is very strenuous and will get you gasping for breath, with tired and aching muscles!

### Final Thoughts

With the incorporation of these simple and highly effective practices into your daily life, one will find the quality of their physical and mental health substantially improved. Exercise and nutrition are crucial to healthy living and with the adaptation of the above suggestions into a regimen, one will enjoy a happier and healthier life.

# 49

# Preventive Check-ups for a Healthy Body*

••••••

This unique machine, the human body that carries our mind, makes us enjoy the beauty of this earth, enables us to act on our impulses and desires, takes us from place to place, eventually slows down. As time goes by it needs some maintenance and repair. No matter who, what and where we are, this is bound to happen though the extent may vary.

Routine check up visits are advised on an yearly basis to pre-empt, diagnose, correct any reversible illness and address lifestyle issues. The current recommendation is to do these exams after the age of 40. Individual variation in health and availability of resources will dictate the final frequency of these check ups. Depending on these factors above, the following tests and exams are included in a good yearly physical exam:

### 1. Vital Signs

Blood pressure (which should be below 120/80), height, weight, waist size, pulse.

### 2. Complete Physical Exam

This should include a full body check up as well as tests for hearing, glaucoma, vision. Details of this exam will depend on the individual needs and discretion of the examining doctor.

### 3. Laboratory Tests

*Blood*

- CBC — Tests mainly for anemia, clotting abilities of the blood, and leukemia
- Comprehensive Chemistry Exam — includes tests for diabetes, kidney and liver
- PSA test for men to judge the health of the prostate gland.
- Complete — Cholesterol Profile includes HDL, LDL, and Triglycerides

*Urinalysis*

To screen for diabetes, protein in the urine. Glycohemoglobin and urine for microalbumin for diabetics. These are useful tests for managing diabetes.

* Chapter contributed by Dr Rohit Dandiya, Chief of the Staff and Chairman of Board of Palm Beach Gardens Medical Center Heart Institute.

### 4. Other Tests

***Colonoscopy:*** The recommendation is to get a colonoscopy every 5 years; this test is done to look for colon cancer. This test is advised after the age of 50; those with a family history colon cancer should get this done at the age of 40 or sooner.

Procedure: *A fibro-optic* tube is inserted in the rectum by a trained colon specialist and the colon is visualized directly. This is an involved test and requires the colon to be completely cleaned by strong purgative prior to the test. The patient is advised to stay away from work on the day of the test. Most doctors use a mild anesthetic that makes this a painless ( but nevertheless a messy) procedure. Those patients whose lives have been saved by early diagnosis of colon cancer will attest to the usefulness of this test. Ronald Reagan, a past president of the USA was found to have pre-cancer of the colon and benefited by this procedure.

**Stress Test (AKA Treadmill Test):** This is a test done for the assessment of the condition of the heart. The goal of the test is to see how the heart performs under increasing workload. This is done by walking on a treadmill machine at increasing speeds and inclination. During this test the heart rate, rhythm and other parameters are constantly monitored.

This test is indicated for the following groups of people:

- Those with a strong family history of heart disease, and diabetes.
- Individuals embarking on a strenuous exercise program.
- Those with *'Atypical Chest Pains'* – a chest pain that does not fit the usual guidelines of heart pain.

**Note:** Patients with *typical chest pains* should probably not get a stress as this may precipitate a heart attack. Such patients would probably benefit from a diagnostic cardiac angiography and intervention as clinically indicated.

Most commonly performed stress tests are:

*Nuclear stress test* - a radioactive dye is injected at the peak of exercise and the heart is then scanned for deficiency of blood supply.

*Echo stress test*- essentially similar but, instead of injecting a dye, the heart is directly visualized for wall movement abnormalities that occur if there is a decrease in blood supply.

### In addition to the above tests, the following tests are advised for females

**Mammogram** a type of X-ray for the surveillance of breast cancer should be done yearly or every other year. A self-breast exam is advised as well. This test is advised after the age of 40. Those with a family history of breast cancer may need to start getting mammograms before the age of 40.

**Yearly Pap Smear is** advised for all sexually active women and involves taking a smear from the cervix to look for cancer.

**Bone Density** is recommended for all postmenopausal women. In this age group of women, bones start thinning causing osteoporosis, which can cause increased incidence of fracture of the bone. Once diagnosed osteoporosis can be arrested with many available medications

With these simple routines, exercise and lifestyle moderation, the human body will continue to work at its peak and avoid the genetic liabilities and misuse that it encounters during its lifetime.

Appendix 1

# Some Abbreviations Commonly Used in Prescriptions

| | |
|---|---|
| ac | before meals |
| ad lib | as much as wanted |
| ad | alternate day |
| Amp | Ampoule |
| bid or bd | twice a day |
| BE | both eyes |
| caps | Capsule |
| cms | take next morning |
| D&C | dilatation and curettage |
| day | 24 hours |
| garg | Gargle |
| gr | Grain |
| gtt (gatta) | a drop (0.6 ml) |
| haust | a single dose (draught) |
| hs | at bedtime |
| ic | in-between the meals |
| im | Intramuscular |
| Inj | Injection |
| iv | Intravenous |
| lin | Liniment |
| Liq | Liquid |
| mist | Mixture |
| nocte | at night |
| od | once a day |
| pc | after meal |
| qh | every hour |
| qid | four times a day |
| qs | as much as necessary |
| sc | subcutaneously |
| sos | whenever needed |
| ss | one half |
| stat | immediately |
| suppos | suppository |
| syr/syp | syrup |
| tab | tablet |
| tid or tds | three times a day |
| tr | tincture |
| tsf | teaspoonful (4 or 5 ml) |
| ung. (oint) | ointment |
| 1 x 2 or 1 x 3 | one dose to be taken twice or three times a day, respectively. |

Appendix 2

# Some Important Diagnostic Laboratory Tests and Their Normal Values

| **Laboratory Test** | **Normal Values/Range** |
|---|---|
| Alkaline phosphate | 4-13 K.A. units of blood |
| Bilirubin | Direct 0-0.4 mg/100 ml of serum<br>Indirect 0.2-1.0 mg/100 ml of serum<br>Total 0.2-1.0 mg/100 ml of serum |
| Bleeding Time (BT) | 1-5 minutes |
| Calcium | 9-11 mg/100 ml |
| Cholesterol | 150-230 mg % |
| Differential Leukocyte Count (DLC) | |
| Polymorph (P) | 60-70% |
| Eosinophil (E) | 1-4% |
| Basophil (B) | less than 1% |
| Monocytes (M) | 1-6% |
| Lymphocytes (L) | 20-35% |
| Erythrocyte Sedimentation Rate (ESR) | *Westergren* — men 3-5 mm in 1 hour<br>women 4-7 mm in 1 hour<br>*Wintrobe* — men -9 mm in 1 hour<br>women -20 mm in 1 hour |
| Glucose fasting (Auto 70-110 mg/100 ml of blood analyzer method) | |
| Haemoglobin (Hb) | Adult male 13 to 18 g/100 ml<br>Adult female 12 to 16 g/100 ml |
| Platelets | 1.5-3.5 lacs per cmm |
| Prothrombin Time | 11-14 sec. |
| Prostate Specific Antigen | 0-4 ng/ml |
| Red Blood Cells (RBC) | Adult male 4.5 to 5.5 million per cmm<br>Adult female 4.1 to 4.8 million per cmm |
| Urea | 10-40 mg/100 ml of blood |
| Uric Acid | 3-6 mg/100 ml of blood |
| White Blood Cells (WBC) | 4,000 to 10,000 per cmm |
| Carcino Embryonic Antigen(CEA) | 0-5 ng/ml |

| | |
|---|---|
| SGOT(AST) | 0-35 Units/Lit |
| SGPT(ALT) | 7-56 Units/Lit |
| CK-MB | <16 units/Lit |
| CK 32-267 Units/Lit | |
| Glycosylated Hb($HbA_{1c}$ | 4-7 mg% |
| Total cholesterol | <200 mg% |
| HDL-cholesterol | 30-70 mg% |
| LDL-Cholesterol | <130 mg% |
| Triglycerides | <165 mg% |
| $T_4$ 5-11 mcg/100ml | |
| T3 95-190 ng/100 ml | |
| TSH 0.4-6 mcUnits/ml | |
| Serum B12 | 140-820 pg/ml |
| CD4 Count | 350-1725 cells/mcL |
| Potassium | 3.5-5.0 mEq/Lit |
| Sodium | 135-145 mEq/Lit |
| Chloride | 101-112 mEq/Lit |
| Fetoprotein | 0-15 ng/ml |

## Local Pain Relieving Preparations

A number of drugs are now available as local gels, creams, ointments and liniments (need rubbing) for relief of sport injuries, sprains and joints paints. Some of these are :

| | |
|---|---|
| *Diclofenac* 1% gel | VOVERAN EMUGEL, RELAXYL gel, DICLORIL gel (contains *methyl salicylate* and *menthol* also) |
| *Ibuprofen* 10% gel | RIBUFEN gel |
| *Nimesulide* 10% gel | NIMULID gel |
| *Piroxicam* 0.5% gel | DOLONEX gel |
| *Naproxen* 10% gel | NAPROSYN gel |
| *Flurbiprofen* 5% gel | FROBEN gel |
| *Capsicum oleoresin* 5% | ALGIPAN (contains *Histamine, methyl nicotinate* and *glycol Salicylate* also) |
| *Methyl-Salicylate cream* 4-5% | MEFTAL FORTE gel, AXANE cream (contains *menthol* & camphor) ETHNORUB (contains *Mephensin* 5% & *Iodine* 0.5%) |
| *Alphalinoleic acid* 3% | XEROFLAM gel (contains *diclofenac, methyl-salicylate menthol*). |

It is believed that these preparations have local effects and lack significant effects on other body organs. It appears that tall claims are made for their effects by manufacturers. A simple oil of winter green (methyl salicylate), camphor in oil or warm/hot fomentation may also provide comparably equal relief. A slight massage done increases warmth and blood flow that also contributes relief. Nevertheless they are useful in common joint disorders such as osteoarthritis, sprains, backache and pains arising from soft tissues such as muscles and tendons. These should never be applied on broken skins, abrasions or tears.

# Index of Diseases


Abdominal pain 13-15
Acne 187-190
AIDS 179, 182-183, 217
Allergic conjuctivitis 76
Allergy 16-19
Alzheimer's disease 35
Amoebiasis 20-23
Angina, unstable 90-92
Angina pectoris 85-90
Anginal pain 85
Anxiety 24-27, 122
Arthritis 109-112, 217, 223
Asthma 36-41, 219-220, 224
Atherosclerosis 84

Bacterial Infection 75
Benign Prostatic Enlargement 178
Bronchitis, acute & chronic 36

Cancer 218
Cataract 76
Chest Pain 85
Chronic alcoholism 244-248
Congestive heart failure 93-96
Conjunctivitis 76
Constipation 42-47
Coronary Heart disease 93-96
Cough 48-53

Dandruff 191
Depression 122
Diabetes mellitus 54-64, 218
Diarrhoea 65-69
Dry eye 76
Dysmenorrhoea (Painful menstruation) 80

Epilepsy, petil mal, grand mal, psychomotor 70-74
Erectile dysfunction 173-175

Flatulence 13
Fungal infection 76, 190-191

Gastro-intestinal disorders 85
Gastroenteritis 204
Giardiasis 23
Glaucoma 77
Gonorrhoea 183-184
Gout, acute, chromic 112-113

Haemorrhage 144
Headache 127, 139
Heart failure 93-96
Heart attack 85
Hepatitis 249
High blood pressure 97-108
Hookworm 199
Hypertension 219

Impotence 173-175
Insomnia 170-172
Irritable bowel syndrome 69
Ischaemic Heart Disease 84-92

Lice Infestations 187
Liver Diseases 219

Malaria 114-117
Mania 118-126
Menopause 82
Menorrhagia (excessive menstriation) 81
Menstruation, scanty 82
Mental depression 118-126
Methyl alcohol poisoning 248
Migraine 127-131
Motion sickness 135
Myocardial infarction 90-92

Nausea 132-135
Neuralgia 248
Neurosis 122

Obesity 236-239
Obsessive compulsive disorder 27
Osteoarthritis 111
Osteoporosis 136-138

Palpitation 27
Paralysis 28
Parkinson's disease 149-152
Pediculosis *see* Lice Infestations
Pelvic Pain 80-81
Phobia 27
Pimples *see* Acne
Pinworm 199
Premature ejaculation 175-176
Premenstrual syndrome 81
Protozoal Infections 20-23
Psychosis 122

Ringworm 190
Reflux esophagitis 159
Rheumatoid Heart Disease 223
Rheumatoid arthritis 110
Roundworm 198-199

Scabies 185-186
Schizophrenia 122
Seborrhea 191
Shocks 224
Sleeplessness *see* Insomnia
Spondylitis 109
Syphilis 184

Trachoma 75
Trichomoniasis 23
Tuberculosis 192-197
Typhoid 249

Ulcers, duodenal, gastric, peptic 153-159
Urinary stress incontinence 82
Urticaria 26

Vaginal discharge 79
Viral Infection 76
Vitamin A Deficiency 77-78
Vomiting 132-135

Worm infestations 198-201

# Index of Medicines

This index lists Medicines both by their Generic and Brand names. Generic names are in italics and Brand names in capitals.


A-TOCOFEROL 215
AABLAQUIN 116
*Abacavir* 182
*Abatacept* 111
ABAVIR 182
ABSOLUT 68
*Acarbose* 57, 59
ACCUCHEK 55
*ACE-inhibitors* 95, 96, 105, 256
*Acebutolol* 100
*Aceclofenac* 110, 141, 144
*Acesulfame* 64
*Acetamenophen* 141, 142
*Acetazolamide* 253
ACETEN 104
*Acetone* 188
*Acetylcysteine* 51
ACHROMYCIN 251
ACIVIR 76
ACLENE 189
ACNEDERM 189
ACNESOL 189
*Activated methypoly siloxane* 14
ACTRAPID 62
*Acyclovir* 76, 180-181
*Adapalene* 189
ADAPEN 189
ADBETA 101
ADCEF 208
ADMENTA 35
*Adrenergic beta-blockers* 101-102
ADROYD 226
AEROCORT INHALER 38
AEROCORT ROTACAPS 38
*Agar-agar* 43
AGAROL 43, 44, 45
*Albendazole* 186, 199, 200, 250
ALBUCID 75, 204
ALBUTEROL 38
*Alcohol* 52, 188, 244-248, 259
ALDACTIDE 95
ALDACTONE 189
ALDINE-D 19
ALDOMET 103
*Alendronate* 137
ALERCET-DC 19
ALEX 49, 50, 52, 53
ALFUSIN 178
*Alfuzosin* 178
ALGESIN-O 144
*Alginic acid* 155
ALGIPAN 148
ALLEGRA 17
ALLERCROM 76
*Allopurinol* 113
ALMINTH 200-201
ALOHA 234
ALPHA CALCIDOL 137
*Alpha-adrenergic recepter blockers* 102-103
ALPHABON 137
ALPHAGAN 77
*Alphalinoleic acid* 148, 215
ALPRAX 25, 171
ALPRAX- PLUS 25, 26
ALPRAX-FORTE 26
ALPRAX-SR 25
ALPRAX-Z 26
*Alprazolam* 25-26, 154, 171, 254
ALPROSTADIL 175
ALTACEF 208
*Alteplase* 91
ALTHROCIN 206
ALUDROX 154
*Aluminium hydroxide* 154-155
*Aluminium oxide* 188
AMACE 106
AMALAKI CHURNAM 218
*Amantadine* 152
AMANTREL 152
AMARYL 57, 59
*Amavatha tailam* 217
AMBRODIL 49
AMBROLITE 49
*Ambroxol* 19, 49, 51, 206, 208
AMBULAX 26
AMBULAX-HD 26
AMBULAX-M 26
AMCOLD 49
AMENOVA 165
*Amidopyrine* 141
*Amikacin* 196, 207, 250, 254
*Amiloride* 95
*Amineptine* 121
*Aminoglycosides* 207, 254
AMINOPHYLLINE 261
*Aminophylline* 39
*Aminosalcyclic acid* 195
*Amitriptyline* 119, 121, 131, 261
AMLODAC 106
*Amlodipine* 88, 106, 107
AMLOKIND-L 106
AMLOPRESS-Z 106
AMLOVAS-AT 106
*Ammonium chloride* 49, 50, 52
*Amodiaquine* 114, 117
*Amoxapine* 119, 254
*Amoxycillin* 69, 159, 180-181, 205, 206, 208, 250
AMOXYVAN 205
*Amphetamine* 33, 118, 172, 242
*Ampicillin* 65, 68, 180-181, 205, 208, 250, 259
AMPICILLIN 68
*Amritkalash* 219
ANABOLEX 226
*Anaesthetics* 256
*Analgin* 142, 144
ANAMOL 141

ANATENSOL 123
ANCOLAN 133
ANDRACTIM 226
ANDRE 76
*Androgenic progestins* 187
*Androgens* 187, 190
ANDROZ 174
ANGIOPRIL 104
*Angiotensin receptor blockers* 103-105
ANGISED 85
ANGISPAN-TR 87
ANTABUSE 247
*Antacids* 154-156, 254
ANTEPAR 200
*Anti-serotonin drugs* 130
*Antibiotics* 254
*Anticoagulants* 253
ANTIDEP 261
*Antidepressants* 173, 176, 254
*Antiemetics* 250
*Antiglucoma drugs* 253
*Antipsychotic* 173, 254
ANTOXID 81, 216
ANTRENYL 14
ANXIPAR 26
ANXIT-FORTE 26
ANXIT-PLUS 26
ANXIZIDE 25
APIDIN 146
AQUAVIRON 177, 226
ARFLUR 143
ARICEP 35
ARIDUS 125
ARINAC 49
*Aripiprazole* 125, 126
ARJUNA 218
ARJUNA RISHTHA 218
ARKAMIN 103, 131
ARTAGEN 143
*Arteether* 116
*Artemether* 116, 117
ARTESTAR 116
*Artesunate* 116, 117
ARTIRAN 113
*Ascorbic acid* 215
ASCORIL-D 50
*Aspartame* 64
*Aspirin* 30, 31, 37, 50, 90, 91, 92, 104, 108, 113, 128, 139-146, 154, 158, 251, 256
ASPRITO 125
*Astemizole* 207, 212
ASTHAFEN 18, 41
ASTHALIN 38, 51
ATARAX 18, 26, 172
*Atenolol* 30, 87, 90, 101, 102, 105, 106, 108, 130, 254
ATIVA 19, 74
ATIVAN 25
ATORVA 30
*Atorvastatin* 30
*Atovaquone* 116
*Atropine* 13, 67, 92
AUGMENTIN 205
AURONOFFIN 111
AUROTHIAMALTE 111
AUTRIN 234
AVIL 17, 52
AVOMINE 132, 135
AXANE 148
AXIFER 234
AXURA 35
*Azathioprine* 111
*Azelaic acid* 189
*Azelastine* 17
AZEP 17
AZIDERM 189
AZIFAST 207
AZILECT 152
AZITHRAL 207
AZITHRAL-XP 80
*Azithromycin* 75, 80, 180-181, 197, 207, 250
AZIWOK 207
AZONA 125
AZOSTAT 80
AZUCON 57

B-LONG 81
BABYLAC 68
BACIROM 209
*Bacitracin* 207
BACTRIM 204
BAG 187
*Balsalazine* 69
BAMBUDIL 40
*Bambuterol* 40, 41
BARALGAN 144
*Barbiturates* 256, 258
BAYER'S TONIC 232
BCG 249
BECADEX 232
BECELAC 68
BECLATE 40
BECLATE INHALER 224
*Beclomethasone* 38
*Beclomethasone dipropionate* 40, 224
BECOSULES 235
BECOZINC 232
BECOZYM-C FORTE 235
*Belladonna* 135
BENADRYL 52, 172
Benazepril 106
BENDY-PLUS 186
BENECID 113
BENFAG 228
BENFAGE FORTE 216
*Benfotiamine* 228
*Benidipine* 87
*Benserazide* 151
BENSPAR 151
BENYLIN 50
BENZAC-CC 188
*Benzafibrate* 30
BENZALIP 30
*Benzathine penicillin* G 180-181, 205
*Benzodiazepine* 26, 171, 243
*Benzoic acid* 212
*Benzonatate* 53
*Benzoyl peroxide* 188, 189
*Benzyl benzoate* 186
BEPARINE 261
BEPLEX FORTE 235
BESTOZYME 232
*Beta blockers* 87
*Beta-adrenergic receptor blockers* 130
BETACAPS TR 101
BETACARD 101
BETACORTIL 251
BETADAY 40
BETADINE 80
BETAGAN 77
*Betahistine* 135
BETALOC 101, 261
*Betamethasone* 223, 224, 251
BETANASE 57
BETAPRESS 77
BETASPAN 101, 130
BETAVERT 135
*Betaxolol* 77
BETNELAN 223, 251
BETNESOL 223
BETNOVATE 190
*Bhallataka* 217
*Bhang* 122, 178, 242

BIDURET 95
*Bifidobacterium* 69
*Biguanides* 57, 58
BILOVAS 34
BIO VITAL 232
BIOCILLIN 205
BIOFER 234
BIOFFIN 45
BIOTAX 208
*Biphosphonates alendronate* 137
*Bisacodyl* 254
*Bisacodyl* 45
*Bishydroxycoumarin* 256, 257, 259
BISOLVON 49
*Bisoprolol* 96, 102
BLUCEF 208
BLUMOX-P 69
BONMAX 138
BRAN 238
*Bran* 254
BRENTO 221
BRICANYL 38, 39
BRICAREX 51
BRICAREX EXPECT 49, 51
BRIMOCOM 76
*Brimonidine eye drops* 77
*Bromhexine* 38, 49, 50, 51, 206
*Bromides* 187, 190
*Bromocriptine* 152
BRONCHO PLUS 38
BRONKOTAB 38
BRONOLAX 52
BROZEDEX 49
BRUFEN 142
*Buclizine* 17
BUDECORT 18
BUDESOL 38
*Budesonide* 18, 40, 224
BUFEX PLUS 141
*Bulaquin* 116
*Buprenorphine* 90, 139, 142
*Bupropion* 119, 121, 241, 262
BUSCALM 26
BUSCOPAN 14
BUSPIN 26
*Buspirone* 26
*Busulphan* 256, 257, 258
*Butenafen* 212
BUTOP 212
*Butylbromide* 14
*Butyprophenones* 124
*Caffeine* 32-33, 140, 154, 172, 210, 241
CALCIGARD RETARD 88
CALCIPLUS (OYSTER SHELL) 137
*Calcitonin* 138
*Calcium antagonists* 131
*Calcium carbonate* 137, 155
*Calcium channel blockers* 87-88, 106-107
*Calcium citrate* 137
*Calcium entry blockers* 102
*Calcium gluconate* 94
*Calcium hydroxy apatite complex* 137
*Calcium lactate* 137
*Calcium phosphate* 137
*Calcium Polycarbophil* 43
CALCIUM SANDOZ 137
CALMPOSE 25, 171, 261
CALPLUS 137
CALPOL 141, 144
CALPOVIT 137
CALSYNAR 138
CAMPICILLIN 68
CANCER GAJ KESRI 218
CANDESAR 96, 105
*Candesartan* 96, 105
CANDID Gel 80
CANDITRAL 191
CANESTEN 181
*Cannabis* 178, 242
CANTAR 105
CANTHARADIN 177
CAPOCIN 196
CAPOTEN 95
*Capreomycin* 196
*Capsicum oleoresin* 148
CAPTOPRIL 104, 256
*Captopril* 95, 96, 104
*Carbamazepine* 71-72, 120, 125, 126, 207
CARBATOL 71
*Carbenecillin* 205
*Carbenoxolone* 158
*Carbidopa* 151, 152
*Carbimazole* 256, 258
*Carbocysteine* 51, 206
CARBOTARD 60
*Carboxymethylcellulose* 76, 155
CARDACE-H 104
CARDILATE 87
CARDIVIT 216
CARDULES 106
CARITEC 87
CARLOC 102
CARTIGEN 112
CARTILLAMINE FORTE 112
CARTILLAMINE LUBRIJOINT 112
CARTIVIT 112
*Carvedilol* 87, 96, 102
*Castor oil* 254
CATASPA 14
CAVIT-PM 216
*Cefaclor* 208
*Cefadroxil* 208, 250
CEFAXONE 208
*Cefazolin* 208
*Cefdinir* 208, 209
*Cefepime* 209
*Cefetamet Pivoxil* 208, 209
*Cefixime* 181, 208, 209
CEFIZOX 208
CEFOGEN 208
*Cefoperazone* 208
*Cefotaxine* 208
*Cefpirome* 209
*Cefpodoxine* 208, 209
*Cefprozil* 208
CEFROM 209
*Ceftazidime* 208
*Ceftibuten* 208
*Ceftizoxine* 208
*Ceftriaxone* 80, 180-181, 184, 208, 254
CEFTUM 208
*Cefuroxime* 180-181, 208
*Celecoxib* 145
CELECT 145
CELIB 145
CELICA 121
*Celiprolol* 87
CELLUBRIL 43
*Centchroman* 166
*Cephalexin* 208, 250
*Cephaloridine* 209
*Cephalosporin* 68, 113, 207, 252
*Cephalosporins* 208, 209
CEPODEM 208
CERELOID 34
*Cervical caps* 163
CETADEP 121
*Cetirizine* 17, 18, 19, 49
CETRIZET-DC 19
CETZINE 19

CHAMPIX 262
*Charas* 122, 178, 242
*Chemoprophylaxis* 193
CHERANA 50
CHERICOF 50
*Chitraka* 216
*Chlophedianol* 50
*Chloramphenicol* 67, 75, 209, 251, 257
*Chlorcyclizine* 258
*Chlordiazepoxide* 25, 26, 171, 261
CHLORFORMIN 57
*Chlorocyclizine* 257
CHLOROMYCETIN 251
*Chloroproguanil* 116
*Chloroquine* 114, 115, 116, 117, 172, 250, 257
*Chlorphedianol* 53
*Chlorpheniramine* 17, 19, 49, 50, 52
*Chlorpramazine* 123, 124, 149, 254, 261
*Chlorpropamide* 57, 254
*Chlorthalidone* 100
*Cholestyramine* 31
*Chondroitin Sulphate* 112
*Chromium Picolinate* 60
CHROMOTOP 41
*Chyavanprasha* 219, 220
*Ciclasonide* 40, 224
CICLOHALE 224
*Ciclopirox olamine* 212
CIFRAN 209
*Cimetidine* 118, 156, 173, 254
CIMETIGET 156
CINARYL 49
*Cinnarizine* 133, 135
CINZAN 135
CIPLACTIN 130
CIPLAR 101
CIPLORIC 113
CIPLOX 209
CIPRIL-H 104
*Ciprofloxacin* 172, 181, 184, 197, 209-210
*Cisapride* 46, 69, 134, 207, 210-212
*Cisplatin* 134
*Citicoline* 152
CITINOVA 152
*Citolapram* 121
CIZA 134
CLAFORAN 208
CLARIBID 207
CLARIMAC 207
*Clarithromycin* 159, 197, 207
*Clavulanic acid* 205
*Clemastine* 17
CLEXANE 91
*Clidinium* 14
*Clidinium Br* 14
*Clindamycin* 189, 210
CLINDY 189
CLINICAL 137
CLISTIN-DMR 52, 53
*Clobazam* 74
*Clobetasone* 186
CLOFRANIL 27, 119
CLOMIN 14
*Clomiphene* 257
*Clomipramine* 27, 119
CLONAFIT 27
*Clonazepam* 27, 74, 126
*Clonidine* 103, 108, 131
CLONORIL 27, 74
CLOPAZ 124
CLOPEVAS 91
*Clopidogrel* 90-92, 140
*Clotrimazole* 80, 181, 190, 191, 212
CLOX 205
*Cloxacillin* 205, 206
*Clozapine* 124, 125
CNN 206
*Co-levodopa* 152
*Co-timoxazole* 203, 204
COBADEX FORTE 232, 235
*Cocaine* 178, 242
CODEINAE CO 50, 53
*Codeine* 50, 52, 67, 139, 142, 144, 145, 146, 147, 242
*Codeine phosphate* 146
CODINE LINCTUS 53
CODOMOLINDON 146
COF-Q LOZENGE 53
COFURA 52
*Colchicine* 112
COLIMEX 14
COLINOL 14
*Colistin sulfate* 68
COLIVAN-D 14
COLOREX 69
COLOSPA 14, 15
COLOX 43, 44
COMBIFLAM 251
COMBITHER 116
COMBIVIR 182
COMBUTOL 195
*Condoms* 162-163, 183
CONFIDO 176
CONTIFLO 178
CONTRAMAL 147
CONVIRON 234
*Copper T* 163
CORAL-F 26
CORBETA 261
CORBIS 102
COREX 50, 53
COREX-DX 50
*Corticosteroids* 118, 154, 187, 190, 195, 222-226
*Cortisone* 257, 258
COSCOPIN LINCTUS 53
COSOME 52
*Cotrimoxazole* 58, 180-181, 250
COVERSYL 104
CREMAFFIN 43, 44, 45
CREMALAX 43, 44
CROCIN 141, 144
*Cromolyn* 18, 41
CROMOLYN 41
*Cromolyn sodium* 18
*Crotamiton* 186
CROTORAX 186
CURCUMIN 215
CVP GYNAE 81
CYCLIZINE 133
*Cyclizine* 17, 133, 134, 135, 257
CYCLOPAM 14
*Cyclophosphamide* 257
CYCLORINE 196
*Cycloserine* 196
*Cyclosporine* 30
CYCLOZOBID 14
CYNOMYCIN 206
CYP-L LIQUID 232
*Cyproheptadine* 17, 130
CYSTAPEN-V 205
CYSTICIDE 200-201
CYSTRAN 15
CYTOGARD 89
CYTOLOG 158
CZCOLD 19

*D-penicillamine* 111
*D-propoxyphene* 14, 142, 254
DAKTARIN 190
DALCIN 210

*Danazol* 80, 81
DANCURE 191
DANDRID 191
DANOZEN 80
DAONIL 57, 59
*Dapsone* 195
DARKTARIN 212
DASLIN 52
DAZOLIC 21
DBI 57, 58
DBI-TD 57, 58
DDRETRO 182
DEBUNASE 91
DECADRON 223, 251
DECADURABOLIN 226
*Deflazacort* 223
DEFZA 223
*Dehydroemetine* 22
DELETUS-D 50, 53
DELTACORTIL 223
*Demeclocycline* 206
DEMOLOX 119
DENFOS 137
DENOL 158
*Deoxycorticosterone* 226
DEPAKOTE 73
DEPIDOL 124
DEPNON 121
DEPSONIL 119, 261
DERIPHYLLIN 39, 261
*Deriphylline* 39
DERIVA-C 189
*Desferrioxamine* 229
*Desipramine* 254, 261
DESLOR 17
*Desloratidine* 17, 19
DESOGESTRAL 165
*Desogestrel* 165
*Desoxycorticosterone acetate* 223
DETIGON LINCTUS 50
DETRUSITOL 15
DEWORMIS 200-201
*Dexamethasone* 134, 223, 224, 251, 257
*Dexamphetamine* 257
*Dexchlorpheniramine* 52
DEXEDRINE 33
DEXONA 223, 251
DEXORANGE 234
*Dextromethorphan* 19, 49, 50, 51, 52, 53
*Dextropropoxyphene hydrochloride* 146
*Dextropropoxyphene* 139, 140, 141, 144, 146, 147
*Dhanawantara taila* 221
DHE 129
DIABINESE 57
DIABOSE 59
*Diacerein* 112
DIADEMIL 100
DIAMICRON 57
DIAMIG 57
DIANUTRIN 232
*Diaphragm* 163
DIAT-AIM 60
*Diazepam* 18, 25-27, 69, 92, 120, 154, 157, 171, 243, 247, 250, 253, 254, 257, 261
*Diazoxide* 257
DIBIZIDE-M 59
*Diclofenac sodium/potassium* 14, 110, 143, 144, 148
DICLORIL 148
DICLOSPAS 14
*Dicyclomine* 14, 143, 145
*Dicyclomine HCL* 14
*Didanosine* 182
*Diethyl carbamazine* 200-201
DIETMANN 60
DIGENE 155
*Digitalis* 60
*Digoxin* 31, 89, 94, 95, 195, 254
DIHYDERGOT 129
*Dihydralazine* 106
*Dihydroergotamine mesylate* 129
*Dihydrogesterone* 257, 258
*Diiodohydroxyquin* 22
*Diiodoquin* 22
DILANTIN SODIUM 71
DILANTIN-P 71
DILIGAN 133, 134
DILOSYN 52
*Diloxanide furoate* 21-22
*Diltiazem* 87, 88, 89, 106
DILZEM 87, 88, 89
DILZEM-SR 88
DIMAG POUSHTAK RASAYANA 221
DIMAGHEEN SYRUP 221
*Dimenhydrinate* 17, 133
*Dimethicone* 155
*Dimethindine* 17
*Dioctyl sodium sulfoccinate* 43, 44
*Diphenhydramine* 17, 49, 50, 52, 172, 242
*Diphenoxylate* 67, 69
*Diphenylhydantoin* 71
*Diphyenoxylate* 251
DIPROEX 131
*Dipyrone* 142
*Discoumarol* 257
DISIPAL 151
*Disopyramide* 195
DISPRIN 140, 144, 251, 256
*Disulfiram* 247
*Diuretics* 95, 100, 101, 254
DIVALPROEX 73
*Divalproex sodium* 131
DOCA 223
DOCABOLIN 226
*Docusate* 43
DOLONEX-DT 148
DOMADOL 147
*Domperidone* 133, 157, 159, 259
DOMSTAL 133
DOMSTAL-O 133, 159
DONECEPT 35
*Donepezil* 35
DONOLEX 143
*Dopamine* 92, 132, 149, 150
DOSLAX 43
DOXACARD 102, 178
*Doxazosin* 102, 178
*Doxepin* 119, 254, 261
DOXINATE 133, 134
DOXOBID 39
*Doxophylline* 39
*Doxycycline* 111, 116, 117, 180-180, 189, 206, 254
*Doxylamine* 133, 134
DPT 249
DRAMAMINE 17, 133
DRISTAN 19
*Dronabinol* 134
*Drospirenone* 165
*Drotavarine* 14
DROTIN 14
DROTINPLUS 14
DROXYL 208
DULCOLAX 45
DULOJOY 121
*Duloxetine* 121
DUMASULES-Z 234
DUOLIN 38

DUOLUTON-L 165
DUOTROL 51
DUOVA 40
DUPHALAC 45
DUPROST 178
DURABOLIN 226
DURAGESIC 148
*Dutasteride* 178
DYCERIN 112
DYMIC 141
DYNASPIRIN 140, 144
DYSMEN 14
DYTOR 95

E-PREG 134
EBAST 17
*Ebastine* 17
EBIZA-L 215, 216
ECODERM 212
*Econazole* 212
ECONORM STIB 68
ECOSPRIN 251
EFAVIR 182
*Efavirenz* 182
EFCORLIN 223
EMALMATHER 116
EMBRIL 111
EMESET 134
EMETIL 124
*Emetine* 22
EMSCAB 186, 187
EMYCIN 206
ENACE 95, 104
*Enalapril* 48, 92, 95, 104, 105, 256
ENAM 104
ENCELAX 45
ENCEPHABOL 34
ENCORATE 73
ENDOPACE 133
ENDRINE 19
ENEMA 69
*Enoxaparin* 91
ENSELIN 57
*Entacapone* 152
ENTEROQUINOL 22
ENTOFORM 69
ENVAS 104
EPHEDREX 50
*Ephedrine* 19, 52, 108, 150, 172
EPIDOSIN 14, 15
EPILEX 73
EPITIC 72
EPITOP 73
EPSOM SALT 44
EPTOIN 71
EQUAL 64
EQUILIBRIUM 25
ERGOPHEN 128
ERGOTAMINE 128
*Ergotamine tartrate* 128-129
ERIX 174
EROTID 175
*Erythrityl tetranitrate* 87
ERYTHROCIN 189
*Erythromycin* 30, 174, 180-181, 189, 206-207
ERYTOP 189
ESAM 106
ESDEP 121
ESIFLO 40
ESKAZINE 123
ESLO 106
ESOFAG 157
*Esomeprazole* 157
ESOZ 157
*Estrogen* 257, 258
*Etanercept* 111
ETERNEX 171
*Ethacrynic acid* 207
*Ethambutol* 193, 195-197
ETHAMSYL 81
*Ethamsylate* 81
*Ethinylestradiol* 165
*Ethinylestradiol* 166
*Ethionamide* 196, 257
*Ethisterone* 257
ETHNORUB 148
*Ethoheptazine* 146
*Ethosuximide* 73
*Ethyl alcohol* 241
*Ethylmorphine* 14
ETO-SABETOL 38
*Etoricoxib* 110, 112, 144, 145, 204
ETROBAX 145
EUDENA 188
EUREPA 57, 59
EVACUOL 45
EXELON 35
EXIFINE 191
EXIPLON 53
EXPENT 200-201
*Ezetimide* 31
EZETIP 31
FALCIGO 116
FALCIRID 116
FALSICARE 116
FALSIQUIN 116
*Famotidine* 156, 159, 204
FAMTAC 156
*Famyclovir* 181
FEBREX PLUS 49
FEELGOOD 134
FEFOL SPANSULE 234
*Felodipine* 88, 106
FEMILON 165
*Fenofibrate* 30
FENOLIP 30
*Fenoverine* 14, 15
*Fentanyl* 139, 142, 148
FERISAN 234
FEROMALT 234
FEROX 234
FERRIUM 234
FERROCHELATE 234
FESOVIT-SPANSULE 234
*Feverfew* 131
FEXO 17
*Fexofenadine* 17, 19
FIBOGYL 43
FIBOTAB 43
FIBROPIL 43
FIFA 234
FINAST 178
*Finasteride* 178
FINCAR 178
FINTAL 18
*Fintal* 41
FINTOP 212
FLAGYL 21
FLAVEDON 89
*Flavoxate* 15
FLEXILOR 144
FLEXON 141, 251
FLEXPEN 62
FLOCHEK 14, 15
FLOHALE 40
FLOHALE INHALER 224
FLOMON 76
*Fluconazole* 76, 80, 81, 190, 191, 211
FLUDAC 27, 80, 121, 176
FLUDECAN 124
*Fludrocortisone* 223
FLUNARIL 131
*Flunarizine* 131
FLUNIL 121

*Flunisolide* 18, 40
*Fluoromethlone* 76
*Fluoroquinolone* 68, 209-210, 254
*Fluoxamine* 119
*Fluoxetine* 27, 119, 120, 121, 172, 176, 254
*Fluphenazine* 123-124
*Fluphenazine deconate* 124-125
*Flurbiprofen* 142, 148
FLURICORT 223
FLUTICASONE 224
*Fluticasone* 40
*Fluticasone propionate* 40
*Fluvastatin* 30
FLUVOXIN 121
FML 76
FORACET 141
FORATEC 40, 147
FORISTAL 17
*Formoterol* 40
FORTAGESIC 147
FORTUIS 30
FORTUM 208
FORTWIN 147, 261
*Fosphenytoin* 71
*Framycetin* 207
FRISIUM 74
FROBEN 148
FRUSELAR-C 95
*Frusemide* 101, 261
FUNGICIDE 191, 212
FUNGIZOLE 191
FURADANTIN 211
FURAMIDE 21
*Furazolidone* 67
*Furosemide* 95, 207, 257
FUROXONE 67
FURSEMENE 95
*Fusidic* acid 211
FUSIDIN 211

GAB 186
*Gabapentin* 27, 73, 172
*Galantamine* 35
GAMASCAB 181
*Gamma benzene hexachloride* 186, 187
GAMMADERM 186, 187
GANATON-TOTAL 159
*Ganja* 122, 178, 242
GARLIC PEARLS 219
GASTRILCER 158
GATE 75
*Gatefloxacin* 75, 210
GATIFAX 75
GELUSIL 155
GEMBAX 210
GEMEF 210
*Gemeprost* 169
*Gemfibrozil* 30
*Gemifloxacin* 210
GEMPAR 30
*Gentamicin* 207, 254
GI KIT 159
GINKOCER 34
*Ginkocer* 34
GIRFUNGIN-P 190
GLAXENNA 45
*Glibenclamide* 57, 59, 254, 257, 259
GLIBURIDE 57
*Gliclazide* 57, 59
*Glimepiride* 57, 59
GLIMER 57
GLINATE 57, 59
GLIPIMET 59
*Glipizide* 57-59
*Glitazone* 57, 58
GLOBAC-XT 234
GLUCOBAY 57, 59
*Glucocorticoids* 113, 225, 226
*Glucomannan* 60
*Glucometer* 55
GLUCONORM-P 59
GLUCORED 59
*Glucosamine* 112
*Glutamic acid* 35
GLUTANEURAL 36
GLUTIM 77
GLYAHA LOTION 189
*Glyburide* 57
*Glyceryl trinitrate* 85-86
GLYCHEK M 59
GLYCINORM-M 59
GLYCIPHAGE 57, 58, 59, 239
*Glycolic acid* 189
GLYCOMET 57, 58
GLYNASE 57
GLYNASE-MF 59
GRAMONEG 210
*Granesetron* 134
GRANICIP 134
GRANISET 134
GRILINCTUS 50, 52
*Griseofulvin* 190, 191, 211
GRISOVIN-FP 190, 211
*Guaiacols* 49
*Guaiaphenesin* 49, 50, 51, 52
*Guaicolate* 19
*Guargum* 60
*Guddoochi* 217
*Guggul* 218
*Guggulipid* 31, 217, 218
*Guggulsterones* 218
GUGLIP 31
GULDIBIT 218
GUM TONE 221
GUTKA 262
GYNACEA 216
GYNISTA 138
GYNODAKTARIN 80, 212

HAEM UP 234
*Halofantrine* 116
*Haloperidol* 123, 124, 125, 126, 149
*Hamycin* 212
HCQs 111
HELIBACT 159
HELIGO 159
HELIKIT 159
HEMATRINE 234
HEMFER 234
HEMGLOB 234
HEMMSYNERAL 234
*Heparin* 90, 91, 92, 261
HEPASULFOL-AA 19
*Hepatitis-B* 182, 249
HERBOLINE 220
*Heroin* 242
HIMCOLIN GEL 175
HIPRIL 106HISTAC 156
HP KIT 159
HUMAN INSULATARD 62
HUMAN MIXTARD 62
HUMAN MONOTARD 62
HUMAN RAPIMIX 62
HUMAN ZINULIN 62
HUMINSULIN 62
HUMOLOG 62
*Hyaluronan* 112
HYDERGINE 34
*Hydralazine* 105, 257
HYDRAZIDE 100
*Hydrochlorothiazide* 30, 96, 100, 101, 102, 103, 106
*Hydrocortisone* 40, 69, 223
*Hydrocortisone acetate* 223

*Hydroflumethiazide* 95, 100
*Hydromorphone* 142
*Hydroxy choroquine* 111
*Hydroxyprogesterone* 257
*Hydroxyzine* 17, 18, 26, 172
HYLAX 113, 121
*Hyoscine* 135
HYOSCINE 135
*Hyoscine-N* 14
HYPERICIN 121
HYPNOTEX 171
HYPONID 218
HYTHALTON 100

I TOTOR-OD 46
I-PILL 166
I-VIT 216
*Ibandronate* 138
*Ibuprofen* 33, 49, 108, 110, 139-146, 148, 250
IBUPROXYVON 146
IFIRAL 18
IGOL 43
ILDAMEN 90
ILETIN-L 62
ILETIN-NPH 62
IMFERON 229
*Imidapril* 104
*Imipramine* 119, 254, 261
IMMODIUM 67
IMMUNOSE 216
IMPRIMA 212
INCIDAL 17
*Indapamide* 100, 104
INDERAL 130, 261
*Indinavir* 182
INDIVIR 182
INDOCAP 143
*Indomethacin* 37, 104, 108, 110, 112, 113, 114, 143, 154, 257
INSLATARD 62
*Insulin* 60-64, 225
INSUMAN 62
INTAZIDE 69
*Iodides* 187, 190, 257, 259
*Ipratropium* 38, 40
IPRAVENT 40
*Irbesartan* 105
IRET 189
IREX 234
IROVEL 105
*Isabgol* 46, 67, 69, 254
ISOFLAV-CR 215
ISOGEL 43
ISONEX 194
*Isoniazid* 190, 193-197, 259
*Isopropamide* 14
ISOPTIN 87
ISORDIL 86, 96
*Isosorbide dinitrate* 86, 87, 96
*Isosorbide mononitrate* 87
*Isotretinoin* 189, 259
ISOTROIN 189
ISOVAC 43
ITASPOR 191, 211
ITOKINE 134
ITOKINE-T 46
ITONORM 46, 134
*Itraconazole* 76, 191, 211
ITRAL 76
*Itropride* 46, 134, 159
IUD 163
*Ivermectin* 186, 187, 200
IVERMECTOL 180, 181, 186, 200

JECTOFER 229
JOINACE 112
JOINCERIN 112
*Joshanda* 219, 220
JOSHINA 220
JULAX 45

K-CARB 59
K-CARE 57
*Kanamycin* 196, 207
*Karpastatyade taila* 221
KARPIN 212
KEFLOR 208
KEFLOXIN 208
KEMADRIN 151
KENACORT 186, 223
KENALFIN 145
KERUTIN-C 81
KETASMA 41
*Ketoconazole* 30, 80, 174, 190, 191, 195, 207, 211, 212
*Ketoprofen* 110, 143, 148
KETOROL 145
*Ketorolac* 145
KETOTIF 18
*Ketotifen* 18, 41
KETOVATE 191, 212
KETOVATE CREAM 80
KETOVENT 18
KETOZOLE 190, 191
KEYNET 191
KHAMIRA ABRESHAM ARSHADWALA 219
KILPANE 144

L-COT KIT 159
L-DEPRENYL 152
*L-norgestel* 166
LACALM 261
*Lacidipine* 88, 106
*Lactitol* 45
*Lactobacilli* 68, 206
*Lactulose* 45
LADOGAL 80
LAMIDUS 72
LAMITOR 72
LAMIVIR 182
*Lamivudine* 182
*Lamotrogine* 72
LANOXIN 94
*Lansoprazole* 157, 159
LANTAS 62
LANZAP 157
LANZOL 157
*Larcanidipine* 106
LARGACTIL 123, 124, 261
LARIAGO 114
LARODOPA 150
LARPOSE 25, 74, 171, 261
LASILACTONE 95
LASIX 261
*Latanoprost eye drop* 77
LATOCOM 77
LAXICON 43
LAZINE-D 19
LEDERCORT 223
LEDERMYCIN 206
*Leflunomide* 110
LEFRA 110
LEFUMIDE 110
LENTARD 62
*Lercanidipine* 88, 199
LEREX 88
LERKA 106
LESURIDE 134
LEVAMISOLE 200
*Levetiracetam* 73
*Levobunolol* 77
LEVOCET 17, 19
*Levocetirizine* 17, 19, 41
LEVODAY 210
*Levodopa* 125, 150, 151, 152, 172
*Levodropropizine* 53
*Levofloxacin* 59, 184, 197, 210

LEVOLIN 39
LEVOMAX 210
*Levonorgestrel* 165, 169
*Levorphanol* 142
*Levosalbutamol* 39
*Levosulpiride* 134
LEVROX 73
LIBRAX 14
LIBRIUM 25, 171, 261
*Lignocaine* 176
LIMICAL BISCUITS 238
*Lincomycin* 189
*Lindane* 181
*Linezolid* 209
LINOX 209
LIPEZET 31
LIPIGARD 30
LIPOPHAGE 239
LIPRIL 104
*Liquid paraffin* 44, 254
LIQUORICE 211
LISICARD 104
*Lisinopril* 48, 95, 104, 106
LISTRIL 95, 104, 106
*Lithium carbonate* 126, 258
*Liv-52* 219
LIVO-LUK 45
LIVOMYN 219
LIVOTRIT 219
LIZOLID 209
LOBATE 186
LOCULA 75, 204
*Lodochlorhydroxyquinoline* 22
LOKIT 157
LOMAC 157
LOMORIN 91
LOMOTIL 67, 251
LONGIFENE 17
LONOXI 144
LOPAMIDE 67
*Loperamide* 67, 68, 69, 251
*Lopinavir* 182
*Loratidine* 17, 19, 50
*Lorazepam* 25, 27, 74, 126, 171, 261
LOREXANE 186, 187
LORFAST 17, 19
*Lornoxicam* 110, 144
LOSACOR 105
LOSAR 96
LOSARTA 106
*Losartan* 96, 105, 106
LOTEL 76
LOTEPRED 76
*Lotoprednol* 76
*Lovastatin* 30
LOXAPAC 125
*Loxapine* 125
LOXOF 210
LOZAP 125
LOZAPINE 124
*Lumefantine* 116, 117
LUMINAL 72
*Lumiraxocib* 145
LUMIRAXOCIB 145
LUPUS 223
*Lvermectin* 180-181
LYCOGOLD 216
LYCORED 82
LYCOVIT 216
LYDOXYL 208
LYNX GEL 189
LYZOLIN 208

M-CAM 143
*Mafenamic acid* 82
MAGADOL 141
MAGNAMYCIN 208
*Magnesium hydroxide* 44, 155
*Magnesium sulfate* 44, 254
*Magnesium trisilicate* 155
MAGSULF 44
MAHAGABA 228
*Mahamasha taila* 221
*Mahanarayava taila* 221
MAJORAL 140
MALAPRIM 116
MALARID 116
MALARWIN 116
*Malathion* 187
MALOCIDE 116
MAMOFEN 138
MANDRAX 240
MANOHEXY 151
MAREZINE 17, 133
*Marijuana* 242
MAXICEF 209
MAZETOL 71
MCBM 228
*Mebendazole* 199, 200, 201
MEBENDAZOLE 200-201
*Mebeverine* 14, 15
MEBEX 200-201
*Mebhydroline* 17
*Mebrophenhydramine* 17
MEBRYL 17
*Meclizine* 17, 133, 135, 258
MECOLIFE 228
MECONEURON 228
MEDILICE 187
MEDISLIM 239
*Medroxy progesterone acetate* 166
*Mefenamic acid* 14
MEFLIAM 116
*Mefloquine* 115, 117
MEFLOTAS 115
MEFTAL 143, 148
MEFTAL-SPAS 14
*Megaldrate* 155
*Meglitinides* 59
*Melatonin* 26, 171
MELIDENS 141, 144
MELLERIL 123, 124, 261
MELO 143
MELOPRESS 171
*Meloxicam* 143
*Melphalan* 258
*Memantine* 35
MENOEASE 216
*Menthol* 49, 50, 52
MEOLAR 101
*Meperidine* 242, 254
*Mephenamic acid* 143
*Mephenytoin* 71
*Meprobamate* 120
MERIZYME 232
MESACOL 69
*Mesalazine* 69
MESANTOIN 71
METACIN 141, 144
METAKELFIN 116
*Metamizol* 142
*Metformin* 57, 58, 59, 239, 254
*Methadone* 142, 146, 242, 243
*Methaqualone* 242
*Methdilazine* 17, 52
*Methimazole* 256
*Methotrexate* 110
*Methycobalamin* 261
*Methyl cellulose* 43, 238
METHYL CELLULOSE GRANULES 238
*Methyl polysiloxane* 155
*Methyl prednisolone* 113, 223
*Methyl salicyclate* 148
METHYLCOBAL 228
*Methyldopa* 103, 118, 258
METHYNEURON 228

*Metoclopramide* 133, 134, 251, 254
METOLAR 261
*Metoprolol* 87, 92, 96, 101, 102, 130, 261
METRODERM 189
METROGYL 21
*Metronidazole* 21-23, 67, 80, 82, 172, 180-181, 189, 200-201
*Mezlocillin* 205
MEZOL 76
*Miconazole* 80, 190, 191, 212
MICRODOX 80, 189, 206
MIFEGEST 169
*Mifepristone* 166, 169
*Miglitol* 57, 59
MIGRATAN 129
MIGTOL 57
MILICAL 137
MILK OF MAGNESIA 44
*Minaserin* 121
*Mineralocorticoids* 226
MINIPRESS 102
*Minocycline* 111, 189, 206
*Minoxidil* 105
MINTOP 105
MIRAPREX 152
MIRT 121
MIRTAZ 121
*Mirtazapine* 121
MISOPROST 158, 169
*Misoprostol* 158, 166, 169
MITS LINCTUS 50
MIXTARD 62
MMR 249
*Modafinil* 34
MOISOL 76
*Monoamine Oxidase inhibitors* 119, 121
MONOCEF 208
MONOTRATE 87
MONTAIR 41
MONTELAST 41
*Montelukast* 41
*Morphine* 90, 124, 139, 142, 145, 146, 240, 242, 256, 258
*Mosapride* 46, 69, 134, 159
MOSID 46, 134
MOX 205
MOX-P 68
MOXICIP 210
MOXIF 210
*Moxifloxacin* 75, 197, 210
MOXIKIND 68
MOZEP 124
MT PILL 166, 169
MUCAINE 155
MUCOGUARD 157
MUCOLITE 49
MUCOSOL 51
MULTILOAD-250 163
MULTIZAC 216
*Mupirocin* 211
*Musk* 178
MYAMBUTOL 195
MYCIN 70
MYCOCID 190
MYCONIP 80
MYCOSTATIN 212
MYOBID 196
MYOSTAL 218
MYOVIN OINTMENT 87
MYSOLINE 72

*Nabumetone* 144
NADIBACT 189, 210
*Nadifloxacin* 189, 210
NAF 138
*Nalidixic acid* 210, 250
NALTIMA 243
*Naltrexone* 243
NAPROSYN 143, 148
*Naproxan* 144
*Naproxen* 110, 112, 143, 144, 148
NASIVION 19
NATAMET 76
*Natamycin* 76
NATCAL 137
*Nateglinide* 57, 59
NATELIDE 59
NATRILIX 100
NATURE CARE 43
NATUROLAX 43
NAVOLET 62
NEBASULF 207
NEBICARD 102
*Nebivalol* 102, 106
NEBRACIN 75
*Neem* 117
NEEM 220
NEFOMAX 145
*Nefopam* 145
NELFIN 182
*Nelfinavir* 182
NEMOCID 200
NEOCALM 124, 132
NEOGADINE 232
NEOLORIDINE-D 19
*Neomycin* 68, 192
NEOTOMIC 45
NEOTREXATE 110
NEPHRIL 100
NEPHROGESIC 15
NERVE-UP 228
NERVITONE 232
*Netilmicin* 207
NEUKIND ORTHO 112
NEURABOL 226
NEUROBION FORTE 232
NEUROCETAM 34
NEUROKIND 228
NEURONTIN 73, 172
NEVIMUNE 187
*Nevirapine* 182
NEXPRO 157
*Niacin* 31, 113
*Nialamide* 119
NIALIP 31
NIASPRIN 31
NIBUFLAM 144
NICARDIA 87-88
NICARDIA-CD 87, 106
*Nicergoline* 35
NICORAN 89
*Nicorandil* 89
NICOTEX 262
*Nicotinamide* 31
*Nicotine* 241
*Nicotine patch* 262
NICOTINELL-TTS 262
*Nicotinic acid* 31
*Nifedipine* 87-88, 89, 106, 107, 156, 254
NIM-SPAS 14
NIMEGESIC 145
*Nimesulide* 14, 110, 144, 145, 148, 204
NIMODIP 35, 106
*Nimodipine* 35, 106
NIMSAID 145
NIMULID 148
NIMUPAIN 145
NISE 145
NISHA 218
NISHA AMLIKI 218
*Nitazoxanide* 21, 23
NITCOL 21
*Nitrates* 87, 89, 96
*Nitrazepam* 171

*Nitrendipine* 88, 106
NITREPEN 106
NITRODERM TTS SKIN PATCH 87
*Nitrofurantoin* 15, 258
*Nitroglycerine* 85-86, 87, 90
NIZRAL 190
NOBELSPAS 14, 145
NOCTURIN 15
NOMIGRAIN 131
*Nonoxynol* 167
NOOTROPIL 34
*Norethisterane* 82, 165, 258
*Norethynodrel* 258
NORFLOX 68, 210, 251
NORFLOX-TZ 251
*Norfloxacin* 68, 210
NORGEST 165
*Norgestimate* 165
*Norgestrel* 165
NORLEVE 166
NORMABRAIN 34
NORMAGUT 46
NORMALIP 30
NORMAXIN 14
NORMOSPAS 14
NORPRAMINE 261
*Nortriplyline* 254
NOSCAPAX 53
*Noscapine* 53
NOVALGIN 142
NOVAMIX-30 FLEX 62
NOVAPIME 209
NOVELON 165
NOVOLET 62
NOVOPEN 62
NOWORM 200
NSAIDS 154, 257
NUCOPE 19
NUFORCE 80
NULIFE 262
NUMLO-L 106
NUTRASWEET 64
NUTRISAN 232, 235
NYOX 144
*Nystatin* 212

OBESTAT 239
OBRA 75
OCCUMOX 75
OCUGOLD 216
ODOXIL 208
OFLOMAC 210
*Ofloxacin* 181, 197, 210
OLAMIN 212
*Olanzapine* 125, 126
*Olapatidne* 76
OLAPIN 125
*Olestra* 239
OLIZA 125
OLOPAT 76
*Omalizumab* 41
*Omeprazole* 133, 157, 159, 204, 254
OMEZ 157
OMEZAC 157
OMEZOL 157
OMIDOM 159
OMILCAL 137
OMNACORTIL 251
OMNATAX 208
*Ondansetron* 134, 250
ONE TOUCH HORIZON 55
*Opium* 258
OPTIPRESS 77
OPTISOL 75
*Oral contraceptives* 118, 164, 165, 166, 195, 258, 262
ORAP 124
ORINASE 57
ORLICA 239
*Orlistat* 239
*Ormeloxifene* 138
ORNIDA 21
*Ornidazole* 21, 23, 82
*Orphenadrine* 151
ORPHIPAL 151
ORS 66
ORTHOBID 145
*Osartan* 106
OSONIDE 40
OSTEOCALCIUM 137
OSTEOPHOS 137
OSTOFEN 143
OSTOGARD 112
OTRIVIN 19
OVRAL 128, 165, 166
OVRAL-G 165
OVRAL-L 165
*Oxacillin* 205
*Oxazepam* 25, 254, 261
Oxcarbazine 72
OXECARB 72
*Oxeladin* 53
*Oxethazine* 155
OXETOL 72
OXICON 212
*Oxiconazole* 212
*Oxprenolol* 101
OXYACE 216
OXYBUTYNIN 15
*Oxycodone* 142
*Oxyfedrine* 90
*Oxymetazoline* 19
*Oxymorphone* 142
*Oxyphenonuim Br* 14
*Oxypurinol* 113
*Oxytetracyline* 206
OXYVIT 216

*P-piperdinoethoxy* 14
PACITANE 123, 151
*Palonaratron* 134
PALTHER 116
PALUTHER 116
PALZEN 134
*Pamidronate* 138
PANTA DOM 159
PANTODAC 157
*Pantoprazole* 159
*Papaverine* 175
*Para-aminosalicyclate* 196
*Paracetamol* 14, 19, 49, 50, 112, 128, 139-147, 250, 254
PARACIN 144
PARAXIN 251
*Parecoxib* 145
PARKIN 151
PARKITOP 152
*Paromomycin* 22
PAROTIN 121
*Paroxetin* 26, 121
PAROXIB 145
PARVON 14
PEDIA-3 49
PEDICLORYL 171
PEFLOX 210
*Pefloxacin* 181, 210, 254
PEFLOYSN 210
PENEGRA 174
*Penicillin G* 180-181, 184
*Penicillins* 37, 113, 184, 204-209, 223, 254
PENIDURE-LA 205
PENIVORAL 205
*Pentaerythrityl tetranitrate* 87
PENTAWIN 147, 261

*Pentazocine* 139, 141, 142, 144, 146, 147, 261
*Pentobarbitone* 171
PENTOCID 157
*Pentoprazole* 157
PEPSIGARD GEL 158
PERIACTIN 17
PERIGARD-D 104
*Perindopril* 104
PERINORM 133, 251
PERITOL 130
PERITRATE 87
PERITRATE SA 87
PERLIFE 185
*Permethrin* 180-181, 185, 187
PERMITE 185
PERMITE CREAM RINSE 180-181
PERNOX GEL 188
PERSOL FORTE 186, 188
*Pethidine* 67, 124, 139, 146, 242, 254, 256, 258
*Phenazopyridine* 15
PHENERGAN 17, 132, 172
*Phenformin* 57, 58
*Pheniramine* 17
*Pheniramine maleate* 52
*Phenobarbital* 72, 120, 190, 258
*Phenobarbitone* 71, 112
*Phenolphthalein* 45
*Phenothiazides* 119, 123, 261
*Phenothiazines* 120, 124, 132, 133
*Phenoxymethyl penicillin* 205
PHENSEDYL 50
*Phentolamine* 175
*Phenylephrine* 19, 49
*Phenylpropanolamine* 18, 19, 49, 50, 52, 108
*Phenytoin* 71, 72, 156, 157, 190, 211, 212, 258
*Pholcodine* 51, 53
PHYTORAL 190
PIFLASYN 191
*Pimozide* 124, 254
*Pinda tailum* 217
PIOGLIT 57, 58
*Pioglitazone* 57, 58, 59
PIOZONE 57, 58
*Pipazethate* 53
PIPEN 14
*Pipenzolate* 14
*Piperacillin* 205
*Piperazine* 199
*Piperazine citrate* 200-201
PIPRACIL 205
PIPRAPEN 205
*Piracetam* 34
*Pirenzepine* 156
*Piribedil* 35, 152
PIRITON 52
PIROX 143
*Piroxicam* 110, 143, 144, 148
PLAGERIL 91
PLENDIL 106
PNV 134
PODOCEF 208
POLARAMINE 52
POLYCAP 30
POLYCOBAL 31
*Polycosanol* 31
POLYCROL FORTE GEL 155
*Polyethylene* 45, 188
POLYFER 234
*Polymyxin* 207
POLYRON 234
*Polythiazide* 100
POLYZEE 232, 235
*Potassium channel openers* 89
*Potassium iodide* 49
PRACTOCLYSS 45
*Pramipexole* 152, 172
PRAMIPREX 152
*Pramlintide* 60
*Praziquentel* 200
PRAZOPRESS 102, 178
*Prazosin* 102, 107, 176, 178, 254
*Prednisolone* 40, 69, 111, 113, 223, 224, 225, 251, 258
PREGABALIN 228
PREGAD 228
PREGNIDOXIN 134
*Prenoxdiazine* 50
PRENOXID 50
PRIMACIP 116
*Primaquine* 116, 258
*Primidone* 72, 258
PRIMOLUT-N 82
PRIMOSA 82
PRIMOVLAR 130
*Primrose oil* 82
*Probenecid* 113, 181
PROBOFEX 234
PROCADAX 208
*Procain penicillin* 205
*Procaine* 205
*Procaine penicillin G* 180-181
*Prochlorperazine* 132-133, 254
PROCTINAL 152
*Procyclidine* 151
*Progesterone* 190, 257
*Promethazine* 17, 50, 132-133, 135, 172
*Promethazine theoclate* 132,135
*Propoxyphene* 146-147
*Propranolol* 27, 37, 87, 93, 101, 102, 105, 107, 108, 118, 120, 130, 131, 156, 254, 257, 261
*Propylthiouracil* 258, 259
*Prostaglandin* 175
PROTOLOC 157
PROVAKE 34
*Proxicam* 112
PROXYTAB 141
PROXYVON 141, 146
PRUGO 18
PSEUDAFED 18
*Pseudoephedrine* 19, 49, 50, 52
*Psyllium* 43
PULMICORT 40
*Purgative* 65, 258
PYLOBACT KIT 159
PYLOKIT 159
PYLOMAX KIT 159
PYOPEN 205
PYRALDINA 195
*Pyrantel pamoate* 200
*Pyrazinamide* 113, 193, 195, 197
*Pyrentel* 199
PYRIDIUM 15
*Pyridoxine ($B_6$)* 82, 134, 194
*Pyrimethamine* 116, 117, 258
*Pyritinol* 34
PYZINA 195
PZA 195

QUEL 125
*Quetiapine* 125
QUINARSOL 115
*Quinidine* 156, 195
Quinine 115, 116, 250, 257
*Quinolones* 210
QUINTOR 209

R-COMPOUND 218
*Rabeprazole* 133, 134, 157, 159
RABETO PLUS 157
RACE LOC 67

*Racecadotril* 67, 68
RALISTA 138
*Raloxifene* 138
RALZAL 17
RAMACE 95, 104
*Ramipril* 48, 92, 95, 104, 105, 106
*Ranitidine* 156, 157, 159
RANITIN 156
RANTAC 156
RAPIMIX 62
RAPITUS 53
RARICAP 234
*Rasagiline* 152
RASTINON 57
RAXIT 121
REAL ONE 125
RECHARGE 216
RECIPER-D 157
REDOTRIL 67
REFLIN 208
REGISTRONE 82
REGLAN 133, 251
REGURNIL SYRUP 134
REJOINT 112
REKAST-L 41
RELAXYL 148
RELENT 49
*Repaglinide* 57, 59
*Reserpine* 100, 106, 118, 149
RESOCHIN 114
*Resorcinol* 188
*Resperidone* 124, 125, 126
RESPIDON 124
RESPREN 19
RESTYL 25
*Resveratrol* 31
RESVITA 31
*Reteplase* 91
RETHERMA-C 19
RETOVIR 182
REVITAL 215, 232
REVODOL 147
RHOFENID 148
RIDAURA 111
RIDOL 67, 251
RIFA 194
*Rifabutin* 197
*Rifampicin* 26, 113, 174, 193-197, 212
RIFAMPIN 194
RIMACTANE 194
*Rimonoband* 239
RIMOSLIM 239
RINOSTAT 19
RIOMONT 239
*Risedonate* 137
RISOPHOS 137
RISOWEEK 137
*Ritonavir* 182
RIVADEM 35
*Rivastigmine* 35
RIZACT 129
*Rizatriptan* 129
*Rofecoxib* 204
ROLES 157
ROLES-D 133
ROLETRA 19
ROMELAST 67
*Ropinirole* 152, 172
ROPITOR 152
ROSCILIN 205
ROSICON 57, 58
*Rosiglitazone* 57, 58, 59
ROSINORM 58
*Rosuvastatin* 30
ROTANE 156
ROVACOR 30
ROVAMYCIN 207
*Roxatidine* 156
ROXID 207
ROXITHRO 207
*Roxithromycin* 207
ROZIDOL 124
RULIF 17
RUMALAYA 218
RUMAYOG 218
RUMAYOG-GOLD 218
RUPAL 17
*Rupatadine* 17
RUPIZ 17
*Rutin* 82

*S-amlodipine* 88, 106
*S-citalopram* 121
SAAFI 221
*Saccharin* 64
SAHELI 166
SALAZOPYRIN 69, 111
*Salbactum* 205
*Salbutamol* 38, 40, 49, 51, 258
*Salicylic acid* 188
SALINEX 261
SALLAKI 218
SALMETER 40
*Salmeterol* 40
SALZA 111
SANTEVINI PLUS 232
SAQUIN 182
SAROTENA 119, 131, 261
*Sarpgandha* 100, 219
SARTACE-H 106
SAT ISABGOL 67
*Satenolol* 101
*Satranidazole* 21, 23
SATROGYL 21
SCABALCID LOTION 186
SCABEX 186, 187
SCABICARE 186
SCABINDON OINTMENT 186
SCABITIN 186
SCABNIL 185
SCALPE NUFORCE 191
SCARAB 186, 187
*Scopolamine* 135
*Secnidazole* 21, 23, 80
SECTRAL 101
*Sedatives* 176, 261
SEDOSOLVIN 49
SELDAN 191
SELDRUFF 191
*Selegiline* 152
*Selenium* 191
SELGIN 152
SELSUN 191
*Senna* 45
SENNOSIDE 45, 46
SEPTRAN 204
*Sequinqvir* 182
SERENACE 124-126
SERENATA 121
SEREPAX 261
SERETIDE 40
SERLIFT 121
SERMION 35
SEROBID 40
SEROFLO ROTACAPS 40
SEROQUIN 125
SERPASIL 100, 106
*Sertraline* 25, 27, 121
SEVISTA 138
SHANKHPUSHPI 221
*Sibutramine* 239
SIBUTREX 239
*Sildenafil* 174, 175
SILVEREX 204
SILVERSHEILD 204
*Silversulphadiazine* 204
SIMCARD 30

*Simethicone* 155
SIMROSE 82
*Simvastatin* 30-31
SINAREST PAED 49
SINOPIN 88
SINOPRIL 106
SIQUIL 132
*Sitagliptin* 60
SIZAPEN 124
SMOQUIT SR 262
*Sodium citrate* 49, 52
*Sodium cromoglycate* 41
*Sodium fluoride* 138
*Sodium tetraborate* 188
*Sodium thiosulfate* 212
*Sodium valproate* 73
SOFRA-TULLE 207
SOFRAMYCIN 207
SOFSENNA 45
SOFT DROPS 76
SOLUMEDROL 223
SOMAZINA 152
*Sorbitol* 45, 64
SORBITRATE 85, 86, 87
SOSEGON 147, 261
SOVE 171
*Spanish fly* 177
SPARFLOX 210
*Sparfloxacin* 197, 210
SPASMINDON 14
SPASMO-PROXYVON 14
SPASMOPRIL 14
SPECIAL CHYAVANPRASHA 220
SPECTRA 119, 261
*Spermicides* 167
*Spiramycin* 207
SPIROMIDE 95
*Spironolactone* 95, 96, 189
SPORIDEX 208
SPORLAC 68
*St. John's wort* 121
STABLON 121
STALEVO 152
STAMLO 106
*Statin* 30, 31
STAVIR 182
*Stavudine* 182
STELABID 14
STEMETIL 132
*Stilboesterol* 258
*Streptokinase* 91, 92
*Streptomycin* 193, 196, 207, 256, 259
STRESSNIL 171
STUGERON 135
SUBDU 146
*Sucralfate* 157-158
SUCRALITE 64
*Sucralose* 64
SUDIN 19, 50
SUDIN KID 49
SULABH 45
SULBACIN 205
*Sulbactum* 205
*Sulfacetamide* 75, 204
*Sulfadiazine* 67
*Sulfadoxine* 116, 117
*Sulfamethoxazole* 116, 181, 204
*Sulfamethoxypyrazine* 116
*Sulfasalazine* 69, 111
*Sulfonamides* 67, 203-204, 259
*Sulfonylureas* 57, 58, 59
*Sulfupyrazone* 113
*Sulphur* 188
*Sulphur ointment* 186
SULQUIN 115
SUMATRIPTAN 129
SUMENTA 219, 221
SUMITREX 129
SUMOFLAM 145
SUPACEF 208
SUPRADYN 232, 235
SUPRESSA 50
SUPRIMOX 206
SURAKTA 221
SURFAZ 212
SURMONTIL 119, 261
SURVECTOR 121
SUSTANON 226
SWEETEX 64
SWEETFREE 64
SWEETONE 64
SYLATE 82
SYMBAL 121
SYNTARIS 18, 40, 224
SYSCAN 190, 211
SYSPRIDE 134

*Tacrine* 35
*Tadalafil* 175
*Tamoxifen* 138
*Tamsulosin* 178
TANCODEP 261
TARAKESHWARA RASA 218
*Tazobactum* 205
TAZOBID 205
TEARNATURAL 76
TEFROLI 219
*Tegaserod* 46, 69
TEGIBS 46, 69
TEGRETOL 71
*Telezenpine* 156
TELIMED 105
TELMA 105
*Telmisartan* 105
TELSAR-H 105
*Tenecteplase* 91
TENOLOL 101
TENORIC-50 101
*Tenoxicam* 143
TENSIMIN 101
TENTEX ROYAL 175
TERAPRESS 102
*Terazosin* 102-103
TERBEST 191
TERBIDERM 212
*Terbinafine* 191
*Terbinafine* 212
*Terbutaline* 38, 49, 51
TERFED 17
*Terfenadine* 17, 207, 212
*Teriparatide* 138
TERRAMYCIN 206, 251
TESTANON 177
*Testosterone* 177, 226
*Tetracyclines* 22, 65, 67, 68, 75, 111, 180-181, 189, 206, 251, 254, 255, 259
TETRADEP 121
*Tetramisole* 200-201
*Thalidomide* 134, 255
THEMIBUTOL 195
THEO ASTHALIN 38
THEOBRIC 39
THEOLONG 261
THEOMAC 261
*Theophyiline* 38-39, 121, 154, 156, 207-210, 259, 261
*Thiacetazone* 196
*Thiazide diuretics* 100-101
*Thiazides* 95, 100, 101, 105, 138, 173, 254
*Thiocolchicoside* 145
THIOGESIC 145
*Thioridazine* 123-124, 261
THIORIL 124
*Tiagabine* 73

TIATE 40
*Ticarcillin* 205
*Ticlophos* 171
TIDOMET FORTE 151
TIDOMET PLUS 151
TIDOMET-LS 151
TIMO-5 77
TIMOLD 77, 253
*Timolol maleate* 77, 130
TINADERM 212
TINAGYL 21
TINEAFAX 212
*Tinepline* 121
TINI 21
TINIBA 21
*Tinidazole* 21-23, 80-81, 159, 180-181
TIOMATE 40
*Tiotropium* 40
TIOVA 40
TITOMAX 182
TOBITIL 143
*Tobramycin* 75
TODAY 167
*Tolbutamide* 57, 254, 259
*Tolcapone* 152
TOLDIN 143
TOLNADERM 212
*Tolnaftate* 212
TOLTER 14
*Tolterodine* 14, 15
*Tolu* 49
TONATE 46, 134
TONOFERON 234
TOPAMATE 73
TOPCEF 208
TOPCID 156
TOPDIN 121
TOPIRAIN 73, 131
*Topiramate* 73, 126, 131
TOPIVAL 73, 131
TORLEVA73
TORMOXIN 206
TOVEGYL 17
TOZAAR-H 105
TOZAART 105
*Tramadol* 139, 147
TRAMAZAC 147
*Tranexamic acid* 82
TRAPE 81
TRASICOR 101
*Trazodone* 119, 121
TRAZONIL 121
*Trazonil* 254
*Tretinion* 188-189
*Triamcinolone* 186, 189
*Triamterene* 95
TRIBET 59
TRICAINE 155
TRICLORYL 171
TRIDAZOLE 21
*Trifluoperazine* 123, 124, 132, 133, 261
*Trifluperidol* 124
*Triflupromazine* 132-133
TRIGLYCOMET 59
*Trihexyphenidyl* 151
TRIKA 25
*Trimetazidine* 89
*Trimethoprim* 203, 204, 259
*Trimipramine* 119, 261
TRINICALM 261
TRIPERIDOL 124
*Tripolidine* 50
*Triptans* 129
TRIQUILAR 165
*Trithioparamethoxy phenylpropene* 19
TRIVASTAL 35
TRIVASTAL-LA 152
TROMUNE 182
TROPAN 15
*Tropesetron* 134
TRPHYLLIN 39
TRYMO 158
TRYPTOMER 131
TURMIX 215
TUSQ-X 51
TUXYLIX 50
TUXYNE 50
TX 81

U-KARE 163
ULCEKON 157
ULCERFATE 157
ULCIBAN 156
ULGEL 155
UN-WANTED 166
UN-WANTED-72 166
*Undecylenic acid* 212
UNIENZYME 232
UNIENZYME MPS 232
UNIMEZOL 21
UNIPRIDE 134
URIKIND 15
URIMAX 178
URISPAS 15
UROFLOX 68, 210
*Urokinase* 91, 92

VALANCE 131
*Valdecoxib* 204
VALENT 96, 105
VALERON 145
*Valethomate* 14, 15
VALIUM 25, 261
VALPARIN 73
*Valproate* 207
*Valproic acid* 259
VALPROL 73
VALSAFE 145
*Valsartan* 96, 105
*Vancomycin* 210
*Varencline* 262
*Vasaka* 49
VASOGRAIN 128
VASOTOP 35
VASOTRATE 87
VELOZ 157, 159
*Venlafaxine* 26, 119, 121
VENLAR 121
VENLIFT 121
VENTORLIN 38, 51
*Verapamil* 87, 88, 89, 93, 106, 126
*Verdenafil* 175
VERMIN-A 186
VERTIGON 135
VERTIN 135
VERTSAR 135
VESPARAX 26
VFEND 211
VIDYARTHI AMRIT 221
VIGA MOX 75
VIMLIV 219
VIROVIR 181
*Vishamusti tailam* 217, 221
VITAZYME 232
VITOXID-OD 216
*Voglibose* 57, 59
VOLIBO 57
VOMINATE 134
VOMISET 134
*Voriconazole* 191, 211
VOVERAN 143
VOVERAN EMUGEL 148

WALAMYCIN 68

WALAPHAGE 58, 59
WALAVIN-FP 190
WALFORMIN 59
*Warfain* 31, 92, 121, 156, 157, 195, 210-212, 259
WESTEL 132
WINOFIT 216
WORMIN 200-201
WYCORT 223
WYGESIC 146
WYSOLONE 69, 223, 251

XALATAN 77
XEELO 216
XEROFLAM 148
XIPAMID 100
XOLAIR 41
*Xylitol* 64
XYLOCAINE 176
*Xylometazoline* 19

Z&B 232
*Zafirlukast* 41
ZAHA 75
*Zaleplon* 171
ZANLOP 171
ZANOCIN 210
ZAPLON 171
ZARONTIN 73
ZASO 171
ZEDEX 50
ZEDOTT 68
ZEET 17
ZENTEL 200-201
ZEPRO 26
ZEPROM 26
ZEROCID 159
ZEROFAT 239
ZICOID 163
*Zidovudine* 182
*Zinc Pyrithione* 191
ZINETAC 156
*Ziprasidone* 125
ZIPRIL-H 104
ZIPSYDON 125
ZISPER 124
ZOCON 76, 211
ZOLDEM 171
ZOLDRO 138
ZOLEDRON 138
*Zolendronate* 138
ZOLINOX 171
*Zolpidem* 171, 254
ZONAP 171
*Zopiclone* 171, 254
ZOPICON 171
ZORPEX 156
ZOVANTA KIT 159
ZOXANIDE 21
ZUVAIR 41
ZYLOAD 163
ZYLORIC 113
ZYME-Q 10 215, 216
*Zytonin* 171

## Authors' Postscript

We hope you have found this book useful and informative. The ever expanding and newer research efforts continue to yield a lot of information, and newer discoveries in the field of medicine. Our endeavour is to sift through this plethora of information and to present the relavent facts in an easy-to-understand format and to answers many of the questions an ordinary individual may have. To achieve a better understanding of what our readers expect from us, we invite you to share your views, ideas, and thoughts which you feel would make the book better and more comprehensive.

We invite you to write to us at the following address:

Dr P.C. Dandiya/Dr J.S. Bapna
C/o Orient Paperbacks
5A/8 Ansari Road
Darya Ganj
New Delhi-110 002